PACS

PACS
Picture Archiving and Communication Systems in Biomedical Imaging

H.K. Huang, D.Sc., FRCR (Hon.)

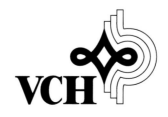

H.K. Huang
Professor and Vice Chairman
Director, Laboratory for Radiological Informatics
Department of Radiology
University of California, San Francisco
530 Parnassus Avenue, Rm CL-158
San Francisco, CA 94143-0628
and
Faculty, Bioengineering Graduate Program
UCSF/UC Berkeley

This book is printed on acid-free paper. ∞

Library of Congress Cataloging-in-Publication Data
Huang, H.K., 1939–
    PACS : Picture Archiving and Communication Systems in biomedical imaging / H.K. Huang.
        p.   cm.
    Includes bibliographical references and index.
    ISBN 1-56081-685-6 (alk. paper)
    1. Picture archiving and communication systems in medicine.   2. Diagnostic
imaging.   I. Title.
    R857.P52H83   1996
    616.07′54—dc20   95-38928
                                                                                          CIP

© 1996 VCH Publishers, Inc.

Printed in the United States of America

ISBN 1-56081-685-6 VCH Publishers, Inc.

Printing History:
10 9 8 7 6 5 4 3 2 1

Published jointly by

VCH Publishers, Inc.	VCH Verlagsgesellschaft mbH	VCH Publishers (UK) Ltd.
333 7th Avenue	P.O. Box 10 11 61	8 Wellington Court
New York, New York 10001	69451 Weinheim, Germany	Cambridge CB1 1HZ
		United Kingdom

To my wife, Fong,
for her endurance,
and to my daughter, Cammy,
for always teaching me the ways of a young mind.

Foreword

1. PACS and Technological Advances in the Diagnostic Image Industry

William M. Angus, M.D., Ph.D.
Senior Vice President
Philips Medical Systems, Inc.
Shelton, Connecticut

Born nearly a century ago in a physicist's laboratory, the art and science of diagnostic imaging developed as the direct result of a major technological discovery. This discipline has achieved its present level of clinical and technological sophistication as a result of a highly interactive process involving medical practice, the research community, and industry. Since the earliest days, clinicians have defined medical need while scientists explored and extended technological boundaries. Industry played an equally vital role in converting concepts to actual products, engineered and manufactured to facilitate the practice of imaging and to provide safe, reliable performance in the clinical setting. Although a hundred years have past, the fact remains that no other field of medicine is so closely allied with, and dependent upon, technological advancement.

This century has witnessed the refinement of the X-ray tube, a vast proliferation of patient positioning devices, and the introduction of automatic X-ray exposure devices, automatic film processors, the electron optical image intensifier, the computed tomograph, and the magnetic resonance imager, as well as nuclear and ultrasound imaging technology.

It would be wrong to underestimate the tremendous technological and industrial resources devoted to the development of these technologies, yet one might expect that the research community and industry would either possess such resources or have the wherewithal to acquire them. A far more vexing problem, especially to industry—toolmaker to the imaging practice—is that of executing technology in a way that makes its operation both safe and nearly transparent to the user. Regular and intense interaction between applications and engineering personnel in industry and those engaged in various aspects of practice—including more than a little "trial and error" and "back to the drawing board" activity—have traditionally provided the basis for safe and user-friendly designs. After so many years of close cooperation the know-how involved in proper execution of imaging technology has become nearly intuitive.

With these problems under control if not completely solved, imaging practice now confronts a new problem, that of managing the integration, presentation, communication, and archiving of the huge volume of data produced by modern imaging modalities. Solving this problem, which is aggravated by growth and aging of the population, becomes even more urgent in the face of increasing demands for greater efficiency and economy in the provision of health care.

More than a dozen years ago, a method for addressing this problem was proposed, the picture archiving and communication system, known by the acronym, PACS. The PACS was to handle all diagnostic image information in the form of digital electronic signals. It was an unfortunate obstacle to the timely development of the PACS concept that conventional radiography, which accounted for more than 75% of image information to be digitized, did not exist in digital format.

In the early 1980s, the introduction of a remarkable new technology, computed radiography, provided a means to decouple the traditional method of simultaneous acquisition, recording, and display of radiographic information. This technology allows the wide dynamic range of data detected by fluorescent screens to be scaled, processed, and appropriately displayed on media having a relatively narrow dynamic range. As a by-product of its intended purpose, the computed radiographic system provided conventional radiographic data in the form of digital electronic signals; thus, the missing link in the PACS concept had been found.

Development of PAC systems has been fraught with technological difficulties, especially in a field in which technology changes so rapidly that its state-of-the-art status is often valid for less than a year. One of the greatest technological challenges is, in fact, the development of platforms that do not become obsolete with the arrival of new technologies but, rather, accept and benefit from them. Past and present performance indicates that industry has and will continue to solve these problems. As always, the greater problem is the safe and user-friendly execution of the technology. In the area of PACS development, this problem has assumed monstrous proportions.

PACS invades every phase of imaging practice—the primary diagnostic, the consultative, the communicative; furthermore, it invades the entire environment in which diagnostic imaging practice functions. Although the imaging industry, albeit only recently computer literate, possesses a century of knowledge, insight, and intuition about imaging practice, this is not enough to cope with a problem as large and diverse as PACS development. The trial-and-error approach is prohibitively expensive in development of software-based systems. The computer and communication industries have a better handle on the technologies but know virtually nothing about the requirements of medical practice. If PAC systems are to improve the quality, efficiency, and economics of imaging practice, a new breed of experts must be sired, a breed of engineers, physicists, computer scientists who, on the one hand grow up and live with the practice and, on the other hand, can set proper examples and develop meaningful communication with the industry.

Dr. H.K. Huang is a pioneer in developing this new breed and has created the proper environment for its growth and eventual maturation. In the past 15 years, Bernie has trained three dozen doctoral and postdoctoral candidates; he has organized, developed, and assembled two full-function PAC systems; he and his colleagues have been engaged in numerous applied research programs and have authored literally hundreds of presentations and papers in the field of diagnostic image management and communication. All the results of his activities are carefully collated and generously distributed to everyone (including industry) who desires to learn from them. He stands ready and willing to consult with those who seek his very special brand of practical advice and is a gracious host to visitors who desire to study his laboratory and functioning PAC systems. His activities have sparked the development of similar programs at other academic institutions, thus providing a pool from which both industry and medical institutions can draw highly qualified young people to assist in the planning and execution of properly adapted and user-friendly medical information management systems.

It is the opinion of this author that the medical imaging practice and the industry owe Dr. Huang a great debt of gratitude for all that he has done in our behalf, as well for the gift of this wonderful book, which lays a foundation for the future training of imaging scientists. It is entirely appropriate that this volume is published during the year in which we celebrate the 150th birthday of Wilhelm Conrad Röntgen, another great teacher whose remarkable discovery just 100 years ago marked the beginning of our practice and the industry that serves it.

2. PACS-Related Research in Medical Imaging
Professor Heinz U. Lemke, Ph.D.
Technical University of Berlin
Berlin

Since the first meeting on PACS at the beginning of the 1980s, we have experienced a speedy development of enabling technologies for the generation, management, and communication of digital medical images. Initially, however, there was a delay in the widespread acceptance and actual use of these technologies in clinical environments. Doubts about cost-effectiveness, but also the lack of standards and clearly defined system implementation strategies, can be held responsible for this delay.

The hesitation to install PACS is gradually giving way to a more enthusiastic approach, with many institutions reevaluating the role of PACS for their clinical settings. This is also due to the untiring PACS research and development effort of Bernie Huang, formerly at UCLA and now at UCSF. Digital radiology and PACS are now with us, and their development promotes the achievement of cost-effective and user-friendly systems. An increasing number of papers presented on successful PACS installations in scientific/medical meetings, such as the Computer-Assisted Radiology (CAR) conference series, demonstrate that PACS developments have reached sufficient maturity to warrant their widespread acceptance. A comprehensive book on PACS and related topics is urgently needed for teaching of students and as a reference to practitioners.

After reviewing the breadth of issues covered, and knowing that they have been authored by one of the world's experts on PACS and his team, I feel confident in using this book in my own teaching at the Technical University in Berlin. This book not only provides an understanding of the fundamentals of digital radiology and PACS, but also gives valuable references to current technological developments. I am convinced that all those who face difficult decisions with regard to the allocation of limited resources in the health care sector will profit from the accumulated wisdom in this book.

The more general reader who is concerned about health care is likely to acknowledge the widespread changes now under way, induced by technology and other driving forces. Together with these developments, PACS will lead to a breakdown of traditional boundaries within and between primary, secondary, and tertiary care. New infrastructures in health care will therefore evolve. We may partially blame or thank PACS for this and of course those, like Bernie Huang, who champion the work on PACS and so effectively spread the news about its developments.

3. PACS and the Practice of Medical Imaging
Edward V. Staab, M.D., Professor and Chairman
Department of Radiology
University of Florida
Gainesville, Florida

Health care delivery systems are progressively converting to digital formats for better and more cost-effective communications. This trend has been accelerated by changes in the health care socioeconomic environment in the United States. The movement from a hospital-based system to widely integrated, multiple-provider networks, which work largely in a distributed outpatient setting, has put constraints on the current processes. Better communications can help to alleviate these stresses. Over the past few years there has been a change in the orientation of medical and administrative leaders from watchful waiting to a focused demand for more robust information systems. This includes a need for better communication of images.

Digital communication in radiology is very demanding because of the large databases created by the information in images. Progressive improvement in the components of a digital image system is taking place. Today, useful complete systems can be assembled. The technology is still maturing at a rapid rate, but the fundamental knowledge to put together these systems is reasonably well defined.

Dr. Huang and his colleagues, during the formative years of this field, have gathered the necessary ingredients of talented people, adequate resources, administrative support, and vision to make PACS work. Dr. Huang successfully obtained peer review support for these efforts. He has provided the vision and direction in a field where research findings must be taken into the workplace and developed to achieve useful systems. I do not believe there is a better group to collate the information about the infrastructure that is needed to understand PACS and digital radiology.

Much needs to be done to make these systems faster, more reliable, and less expensive. But beyond that we should be looking to improve the diagnostic process. Dr. Huang's insight into what the future holds is greatly appreciated.

This book should serve as a text for many and an excellent reference for most of us as we develop our PACS.

Preface

Picture archiving and communication systems (PACS) is a concept perceived in the early 1980s by the radiology community as a future method of practicing radiology. PACS consists of image acquisition devices, storage archiving units, display stations, computer processors, and database management systems. These components are integrated by a communications network system. During the past 10 years, technologies related to these components became mature, and their applications have gone beyond radiology to the entire health care delivery system. As a result, PACS for special clinical applications as well as large-scale, hospital-wide PACS are being installed throughout the United States and the world.

A literature search related to PACS reveals that there are about two thousand publications, several edited books, several special issues in journals, and three chapters in my earlier book, *Elements in Digital Radiology*. Although these publications provide, chronologically, documentation on research and development advancement of PACS during the past decade or so, they lack coherence in the subject matter. This book is an attempt to introduce this topic systematically, based on the most recent research and development results. Although originating in the radiology community, the PACS concept can be applied to any scientific field that requires the handling of voluminous pictures and textual data. We anticipate that this field will continue to grow in the next 5 years. This book will serve as a foundation for the future training of people entering this area of work.

I owe a debt of gratitude to Dr. Edmund Anthony Franken, Jr., past chairman of the Department of Radiology, University of Iowa, for getting me interested in this field in 1981. Later, Dr. Gabriel Wilson, then the chairman of the Department of Radiological Sciences at UCLA, offered me an opportunity to launch a PACS project in the department. He provided the initial financial support to establish the Image Processing Laboratory, which later became the Medical Imaging Division. In the ensuing years, Drs. Zoran Barbaric, Robert Leslie Bernett, acting chairmen, and Dr. Hooshang Kangarloo, past chairman of the department, all provided generous support to the project. We also received from the National Institutes of Health (NIH) three large long-term grants in PACS, and we established collaboration from private industry including (in chronological order) Technicare Corporation; Gould/DeAnza Graphic System Division; Light Signatures, Inc.; Konica; IBM Corporation; ADAC Laboratories; Philips Medical Systems, Inc.; Mitsubishi Electronic Corporation; 3M; and Kodak. As a result of these efforts, a large-scale PACS was released for clinical use in early 1992. This UCLA PACS was developed with the Department of Radiology in mind and lacks the expanded, open architecture design that is necessary for a hospital-integrated PACS.

In October 1992, Dr. Ronald Arenson, chairman of the Department of Radiology, UCSF, offered me an opportunity to build a second PACS. Kathy Andriole (computed radiography), Todd Bazzill (network), Andrew Lou (acquisition and display), and Albert Wong (PACS controller), who were part of the core team that built the first PACS, also joined UCSF. In addition, Yuki Ishimitsu and Jun Wang came from UCLA to UCSF to finish their Ph.D. dissertations. At UCSF we recruited several staff members, some postdoctoral fellows, and our assistant, Laura Snarr. Together, we established the Laboratory for Radiological Informatics.

Meanwhile, the NIH has continued supporting our laboratory. We also received new support from IBM Almaden Research Center; the CalREN (California Research and Education Network) Program by Pacific Bell; HPCC (High Performance Computing and Communication) Program sponsored by the NLM (National Library of Medicine); Abe Sekkei, Japan; Lumisys; and Sun Microsystems.

It took us about 18 months to complete the second-generation PACS infrastructure including the interface to the hospital and radiology information systems and to the departmental Macintosh users. We released image workstations one by one for clinical use beginning early in 1994. The next step in our PACS growth is to obtain hospital commitment for deployment of many image workstations to the radiology department as well as in the hospital. In the research area, we are moving toward image content base information retrieval, online PACS three-dimensional rendering, and distributed computing in a PACS environment.

From our experience during the past 12 years, we can identify some major contributions in advancing PACS development. Technically, the first laser film digitizers, developed for clinical use by Konica and Lumisys, the development of computed radiography (CR) by Fuji and its introduction from Japan to the United States by Dr. William Angus of Philips Medical Systems, and the large-capacity optical disk storage by Kodak all are critical. Also highly significant are parallel transfer disk technology, 2000-line and 72 Hz display monitors, the system integration methods developed by Siemens Gammasonics and Loral for large-scale PACS, the DICOM committee's effort in standardization, and the asynchronous transfer mode (ATM) technology for merging local area network and wide area network communications.

In terms of events, the annual SPIE PACS and Medical Imaging meeting and EuroPACS are the continuous driving force for PACS. In addition, every two years the Computer-Assisted Radiology (CAR) meeting, organized by Prof. Heinz Lemke, and the Image Management and Communication (IMAC) Conference organized by Dr. Seong K. Mun, provide a forum for international PACS discussion. The InfoRAD Section at the Radiological Society of North America (RSNA) organized in 1933 by Dr. Laurens V. Ackerman with the live demonstration of DICOM interface, sets the tone for industrial PACS open architecture. The annual RSNA refresher courses in PACS organized first by Dr. C. Douglas Maynard and then by Dr. Edward V. Staab, provide continuing education in PACS to the radiology community.

In 1992 *Second Generation PACS,* Michel Osteaux's edited book, gave me confidence that PACS is moving toward a hospital-integrated approach. When Dr. Roger A. Bauman became editor-in-chief of the then new *Journal of Digital Imaging* in 1988, the consolidation of PACS research and development publications became possible. Colonel Fred Goeringer instrumented the Army's project in medical diagnostic imaging support (MDIS) systems, resulting in several large-scale PACS installations that provide major stimulus and funding for the PACS industry.

All these contributions have profoundly influenced my thoughts on the direction of PACS research and development as well as the contents of this book. This book summarizes our experiences in developing the concept of digital radiology and PACS during the past 10 years. Selected portions of the book have been used as lecture materials in graduate courses on medical imaging and advanced instrumentation at The University of California at Los Angeles, San Francisco, and Berkeley. We hope that this book will inspire more researchers to become interested in this field. Together we can move one step closer to the reality of a digital-based health care environment.

H.K. (Bernie) Huang
San Francisco and Agoura Hills, CA

Acknowledgments

Many people provided assistance during the preparation of this book—in particular, some of my graduate students, postdoctoral fellows, and colleagues from whom I have learned most. Chapters 2, 3, 4, and 5 are revisions from my book *Elements of Digital Radiology,* published in 1987. Some of the materials were originally contributed by K.S. Chuang, Ricky Taira, Brent Stewart, and Paul Cho. Many new materials were also added in these chapters. Chapter 6, on image compression, was completely rewritten, and some of the figures are extracted from Ben Lo's Ph.D. dissertation. Chapters 7, 8, 9, 10, and 11 are all new materials based on our research and development during the past several years.

Specifically, I am thankful for the contributions from Yuki Ishimitsu (Sections 3.2.4, 3.4), Jun Wang (Sections 3.3.2.2, 6.6), Kathy Andriole (Section 4.1), Stephen Wong (Sections 6.8, 11.2.1, 11.2.2, 11.2.7), Andrew Lou (Sections 7.5, 8.4.3, 9.3.3, 10.3.2), Todd Bazzill (Section 8.2 and 8.3), Albert Wong (Sections 8.5, 9.5, 9.6, 10.3.1, 11.1.3), Mike Moskowitz (Section 9.1.4.5), Xiaoming Zhu (Section 11.2.5), Mohan Ramaswamy and Joseph Lee (Section 9.6), Lloyd Yin (Section 7.4.1), and Paul Cho (Sections 9.1 and 9.2), and Ron Arenson for initiating the concept of the folder manager.

I also thank Prof. Gary Fullerton, University of Texas Health Sciences Center, San Antonio, who reviewed the original proposal and has provided continuous encouragement. Thanks also to the late Dr. Rita G. Lerner, consulting editor of VCH, for providing me the opportunity to write this book. Lastly, a special thank you to my assistant, Laura Snarr, B.S., for preparing the entire manuscript.

This book was written with the assistance of the following faculty and staff members of the Laboratory for Radiological Informatics at UCSF:

Katherine P. Andriole, Ph.D.
Assistant Professor

Todd Bazzill, B.S.E.E.
PACS Engineering

Andrew Lou, Ph.D.
Assistant Professor

Michael Moskowitz, Ph.D.
Postdoctoral Fellow

Jun Wang, M.S.
Ph.D. Candidate

Albert W.K. Wong, B.S.
PACS Manager

Stephen Wong, Ph.D.
Assistant Professor

Xiaoming Zhu, Ph.D.
Postdoctoral Fellow

and

Laura Snarr, B.S.
Administrative Assistant

Contents

List of Acronyms

1-D	one-dimensional
2-D	two-dimensional
3-D	three-dimensional
4-D	four-dimensional
ABF	air-blown fiber
ACR-NEMA	American College of Radiology–National Electrical Manufacturers' Association
A/D	analog-to-digital converter
ADT	admission, discharge, transfer
AL	aluminum
AMP	amplifier
AP, A-P	anterior–posterior
ATM	asynchronous transfer mode
Az	area under the ROC curve
BERKOM	Berlin Communication Project
BDF	building distribution center
BNC	a type of connector for 10 Base2 cables
CAD/CAM	computer-aided design/computer-aided manufacturing
CalREN	California Research and Education Network
CAR	Computer-Assisted Radiology (meeting series)
CCD	charge-coupled device
CCU	coronary care unit

CDDI	copper distributed data interface
CFR	contrast frequency response
CIE	Commission Internationale de L'Éclairage (International Lighting Commission)
CNA	campus network authority
CPU	central processing unit
CR	computed radiography
CRF	central retransmission facililty—head end
CRT	cathode ray tube
CSMA/CD	carrier sense multiple access with collision detection
CSU/DSU	channel service unit/data service unit
CT	computed tomography
CTN	central test node
D/A	digital-to-analog converter
DASM	data acquisition system manager
dB	a unit to measure signal loss
DC	the first coefficient of a mathematical transform
DCT	discrete cosine transform
DEC	Digital Equipment Corporation
DECRAD	DEC radiology information system
DF	digital fluorography
DICOM	Digital Imaging and Communication in Medicine
DIFS	distributed image file server
DIN/PACS	Digital Imaging Network/PACS (U.S. Army–MITRE Corp. project)
DOD	(U.S.) Department of Defense
DOM	distributed object manager
DRll-W	a parallel interface protocol
DS	digital service
DSA	digital subtraction angiography
	digital subtraction arteriography
DSC	digital scan converter
DSP	digital signal processing chip
eV	electronic volt
EuroPACS	Picture Archiving and Communication Systems in Europe
ECT	emission computed tomography
EIA	Electronic Industries Association
ESDI	enhanced small device interface
ESF	edge spread function
FCR	Fuji CR
FDA	(U.S.) Food and Drug Administration
FDDI	fiber-distributed data interface
FFBA	full-frame bit allocation algorithm

FFD	focus-to-film distance
FFT	fast Fourier transform
FID	free induction decay
FM	folder manager
FP	false-positive
FRS	fast reconstruction system
FT	Fourier transform
FTE	full-time equivalent
FTP	file transfer protocol
FWHM	full width at half-maximum
GEMS	General Electric Medical System
H and D curve	Hurter–Driffield characteristic curve
HI-PACS	hospital-integrated PACS
HIS	hospital information system
HL7	Health Level 7
HP	Hewlett-Packard
HPCC	high performance computing and communications
Hz	Hertz (cycles/second)
ICU	intensive care unit
ID	identification
IDEA	international data encrytion algorithm
IDF	intermediate distribution frame
IDNET	a GEMS imaging modality network
IFT	inverse Fourier transform
Im	imaginary part of a complex function
IMAC	image management and communication
InfoRAD	radiology information exhibit
I/O	input/output
IP	imaging plate Internet protocol
ISDN	integrated service digital network
ISO	International Standards Organization
JAMIT	Japan Association of Medical Imaging Technology
JND	just noticeable differences
JPEG	Joint Photographic Experts Group
k	1000
K	1024
kV(p)	kilovolt potential difference
LAN	local area network
lp	line pair
LRI	Laboratory for Radiological Informatics (UCSF)

LSF	line spread function
LUT	lookup table
mA	milliampere
MAN	metropolitan area network
Mbyte	megabyte ($= 10^6$ bytes)
MDIS	medical diagnostic imaging support systems
MIDS	medical image database server
MIMP	Mediware Information Message Processor—a computer software language for HIS used by the IBM computer
Modem	modulator/demodulator
MP	multiprocessors
mR	milliroentgen
MRI	magnetic resonance imaging
ms	millisecond
MTF	modulation transfer function
MUMPS	Massachusetts General Hospital Utility Multiprogramming System—a computer software language
MUX	multiplexer
NATO ASI	North Atlantic Treaty Organization, Advanced Science Institutes
NDC	network distribution center
NEC	Nippon Electronic Corporation
NFS	network file system
NIE	network interface equipment
NIH	(U.S.) National Institutes of Health
NINT	nearest integer function
NLM	(U.S.) National Library of Medicine
NM	nuclear medicine
NMSE	normalized mean square error
NTSC	National Television System Committee
OC	optical carrier
OD	optical density
OSI	open system interconnection
PA	posterior–anterior
PACS	picture archiving and communication system
PC	personal computer
PET	positron emission tomography
PGP	pretty good privacy
PICT	Macintosh picture format
PIP	Philips interface processor
PL	plastic

PMT	photomultiplier tube
PPI	parallel peripheral interface
ppm	parts per million
PSF	point spread function
PSL	photostimulable luminescence
PSNR	peak signal-to-noise ratio
PTD	parallel transfer disk
PVM	parallel virtual machine system
RAM	random access memory
RETMA	Radio-Electronics-Television Manufacturers Association [now EIA]
RAID	redundant array of inexpensive disks
Re	real part of a complex function
RF	radio frequence
RIS	radiology information system
ROC	receiver operating characteristic
ROI	region of interest
RGB	Red, green, and blue
S-bus	a computer bus used by SPARC
SCSI	Small computer systems interface
SMPTE	Society of Motion Picture and Television Engineers
SMZO	Social and Medical Center East (in Vienna, Austria)
SNR	signal-to-noise ratio
SPARC	a computer system manufactured by Sun Microsystems
SPECT	single-photon emission computed tomography
SPIE	International Society for Optical Engineering
SQL	Structured Query Language
ST	a special connector for optical fibers
T1	DS-1 private line
TCP/IP	transmission control protocol/Internet protocol
TDS	tube distribution system for optical fibers
TGC	time gain compensation
TIFF	tagged image file format
TP	true-positive
UCLA	University of California at Los Angeles
UCSF	University of California at San Francisco
UNIX	a computer operating system used by Sun and other computers
UPS	uninterruptible power supply
US	ultrasound
UTP	unshielded twisted pair
VAX	a computer system manufactured by Digital Equipment Corporation

VM	a computer operating system software used by IBM computers
VME	a computer bus used by older Sun and other computers
VMS	a computer operating system software used by DEC computers
VRAM	video RAM
WAN	wide area network
WORM	write once, read many
WS	workstation
WSU	working storage unit
XCT	X-ray transmission computed tomography
YIQ	Luminance, in-phase, and quadrature chrominance color coordinates
YCbCr	Luminance, and two chrominance coordinates used in color digital imaging

1

Introduction

1.1 Introduction

There are many advantages of introducing digital and communication technologies to the conventional film-based operation in radiology and medicine. For example, through the computer, it is possible to manipulate a digital image for value-added diagnosis, and through imaging plate technology and other imaging modalities it is possible to improve the diagnostic value while at the same time reducing the radiation exposure to the patient. Also, insofar as they promote a more efficient operating environment, digital and communication technologies can also reduce operating costs in health care delivery.

With all these benefits, the digital and communication technologies are gradually changing the method of acquiring, storing, viewing, and communicating diagnostic images and related information. One natural development along this line is the emergence of a digital radiology department and a digital hospital environment. A digital radiology department has two components: a radiology information management system (RIS) and a digital imaging system. The radiology information system is a subset of the hospital information system (HIS), which entails data management with respect to the patient (as opposed to images). The digital imaging system, sometimes referred to as the picture archiving and communication system (PACS), involves image acquisition, archiving, communication, retrieval, display, and processing. A digital hospital environment consists of the hospital information system, PACS, and other digital clinical systems. The combination of HIS and PACS is referred to as hospital-integrated PACS (HI-PACS). Up-to-date information on these topics can be obtained from the multidisciplinary literature, research laboratories of university hospitals, and medical imaging manufacturers, but not in a coordinated way. Therefore, it is difficult for a radiologist, hospital administrator, medical imaging researcher, radiological technician, or trainee in diagnostic radiology to collect and assimilate this information.

The purpose of this book is to consolidate PACS related topics into one self-contained text. Here the emphasis is on basic principles, augmented with current technological developments and examples on each topic.

1.2 Organization of This Book

PACS: Picture Archiving and Communication Systems in Biomedical Imaging consists of eleven chapters. Chapter 1 describes the history of PACS and PACS activities and related research in various countries. Figure 1.1, which charts the organization of this book, also gives an overview of digital radiology and PACS.

Chapter 2 describes the fundamentals of digital radiologic imaging. It is assumed that the reader already has some basic knowledge in conventional radiographic physics. This chapter introduces the basic terminology used in digital radiologic imaging and gives some examples. Familiarizing oneself this terminology will facilitate the reading of later chapters.

Chapters 3, 4, and 5 discuss radiologic image acquisition systems. Chapter 3 deals with the principles and procedures of conventional projection radiographic acquisition systems with films as output. Since conventional projection radiography is still responsible for 70% of current radiological examinations in a typical radiology department, we have to consider methods of converting these films to digital images. For this reason, the chapter includes a detailed discussion on various types of film digitizer, including the vidicon camera, the drum scanner, the photodiode detector, the charge-couple device camera, and the laser scanner.

Chapter 4 discusses some projection radiographic acquisition systems with direct digital images as output. These include laser-stimulated luminescence phosphor plate technologies and digital fluorography. All these acquisition systems are digital-based and utilize electro-optical technologies. Digital-based radiography allows digital subtraction; the temporal and dual-energy subtraction methods are discussed in-depth.

Chapter 5 discusses sectional imaging. Section 5.1 introduces the concept of image reconstruction from projections. Sections 5.2, 5.3, and 5.5 provide basic knowledge in transmission and emission computed tomography (CT), and magnetic resonance imaging. Section 5.4 discusses nuclear medicine and ultrasound imaging.

Note that Chapters 3, 4, and 5 are not a comprehensive treatise on sectional imaging. Instead, they provide basic knowledge in sectional images of the various types encountered in diagnostic radiology and microscopic imaging, emphasizing the digital aspect, instead of the physics of these systems. The reader should grasp the digital aspect of these imaging modalities, which form the imaging basis of a digital-based operation in a hospital environment. This digital imaging basis is essential for a thorough understanding of interfacing these imaging modalities to a PACS.

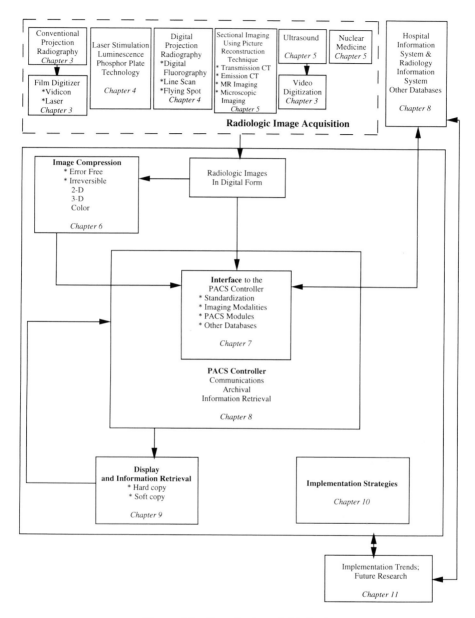

Figure 1.1   Organization of this book.

Chapter 6 covers image compression. After an image has been captured in digital form from an acquisition device, it is transmitted to a storage device for long-term archiving. In general, a digital image file provides a large storage capacity. For example, an average computed tomography study or two-view computed radiography comprises about 20 Mbytes. Therefore, it is necessary to consider how to compress an image file into a compact form before storage or transmission. The concept of reversible (lossless) and irreversible (lossy) compression are discussed in detail in Sections 6.3 and 6.4. Section 6.5 describes methods of measuring the quality of the reconstructed image from compressed data. Three-dimensional image data sets occur very often now in sectional imaging, and color images become important in Doppler ultrasound imaging. For these reasons, two current research topics on three-dimensional and color image compression are given in Sections 6.6 and 6.7, respectively. Finally, image compression raises certain legal and regulatory issues, which are discussed in Section 6.8.

Chapters 7, 8, 9, 10, and 11 cover topics in picture archiving and communication systems. The five major components of PACS—image acquisition, communications, databases, display, and information retrieval—are covered in Chapters 7, 8, and 9. In Chapter 7, we introduce the basic concept of PACS. Two industrial interface standards on data are discussed: Health Level 7, and the image format and communication protocols of ACR-NEMA (American College of Radiology–National Electrical Manufacturers Association) and the DICOM (Digital Imaging and Communication in Medicine), which have been adopted by the PACS community. Systematic methods of interfacing image acquisition devices with these standards are given. Many image preprocessing functions used during the interface are described in Section 7.6.

Chapter 8 discusses two topics: communication and databases. In image communication, both digital and analog methods are given. The latest technology in digital communication using asynchronous transfer mode (ATM) is described. In Section 8.5, the design of the PACS central node or the PACS controller is discussed in detail. Sections 8.6 and 8.7 describe the PACS interface with the hospital information system (HIS), and the radiology information system (RIS), and other medical databases. The two sections form the cornerstones of extending the PACS to a hospital-integrated PACS.

Chapter 9 discusses display (both soft copy and hard copy output) and information retrieval. Image processing and display functions are necessary to optimize the usefulness of the soft copy display methods (Section 9.3). Effective and efficient information retrieval is the ultimate test of acceptance of the PACS by users, and the methodology is given in Section 9.5. Finally, a section on physician's desktop information retrieval is provided as an example to highlight the usefulness of a hospital-integrated PACS in health care delivery.

Chapter 10 describes the system integration of PACS components into a daily clinical operational system. Methods of PACS system evaluation on subsystem throughput, system efficiency, and image quality are given in Section 10.3. This chapter is valuable for planning a digital-based operation environment.

Chapter 11 describes current trends in PACS development and future research directions. The three major development areas are large-scale PACS, teleradiology, and intensive care unit modules. The future research directions include medical image database management with image content indexing, online computation and three-dimensional rendering, and distributed computing in a PACS environment.

References are given at the back of the book. Some of them are referred to in the text for clarification and sources.

1.3 History of Picture Archiving and Communication Systems (PACS)

The term "digital radiology" was introduced by Dr. Paul Capp in the early 1970s. Lack of technological development to support the requirements of digital radiologists, however, prevented the concept from becoming popular until the early 1980s.

The First International Conference and Workshop on Picture Archiving and Communication Systems (PACS) was held in Newport Beach, California, in January 1982, sponsored by SPIE (the International Society for Optical Engineering). Thereafter, the PACS conference has been combined with the Medical Imaging Conference. The joint meeting has become an annual event, always held February in southern California.

In Japan, the First International Symposium on PACS and PHD (personal health data) was held in July 1982, sponsored by the Japan Association of Medical Imaging Technology (JAMIT). This conference, combined with the Medical Imaging Technology meeting, also became an annual event. EuroPACS (Picture Archiving and Communication Systems in Europe) has held annual meetings since 1984 and is a driving force for European PACS information exchange.

One of the earliest research projects related to PACS in the United States was the teleradiology project sponsored by the U.S. Army in 1983. A follow-up project was the Installation Site for Digital Imaging Network and Picture Archiving and Communication System (DIN/PACS) funded by the U.S. Army and administered by the MITRE Corporation in 1985. Two university sites were selected for implementation, the University of Washington at Seattle, with participation of Philips Medical Systems, and Georgetown University/George Washington University Consortium in Washington, D.C. with AT&T collaboration. The National Cancer Institute in the United States funded one of its first PACS-related research projects in 1985, under the title Multiple Viewing Stations for Diagnostic Radiology.

A meeting concentrating on dedicated PACS sponsored by NATO ASI (Advanced Study Institute) was PACS in Medicine, held in Evian, from October 12–24, 1990. Approximately 100 scientists from over seventeen countries participated. The ASI proceedings summarized international efforts in PACS research and development at that time. This meeting stimulated the medical diagnostic imaging support (MDIS) systems project sponsored by the U.S. Army Medical Command, which has been responsible for large-scale military PACS installations in the United States (see also Section 10.1.4.3)

1.4 PACS and Related Research in Various Countries

In this section, we summarize the PACS and related research and development in 15 countries based on recent literature (as of June 1995). The countries are Austria, Belgium, Denmark, France, Germany, Greece, Japan, Italy, South Korea, the Netherlands, Spain, Sweden, Switzerland, Turkey, and the United Kingdom.

Austria has installed a large-scale PACS project at the Social and Medical Center

East, known by its German acronym: SMZO. Details of this system are presented in Section 10.1.4. Another Austrian project is in the departments of Radiology, and Medical Informatics, Statistics, and Documentation, at the University of Graz using the SIENET (Siemens, Erlangen, Germany).

In Belgium, three institutes are active in PACS research: the University of Leuven (KUL), the University Hospital of Brussels (ULB), and the Pluridisciplinary Research Institute for Medical Imaging Science (PRIMIS) at the University of Brussels. At the KUL the PACS project's main application is to support research activities in acquisition techniques and image processing methods. The ULB, together with the PRIMIS group, started a multivendor installation PACS project. In addition, the ULB is working on an evaluation project in teleradiology. In Denmark, the Viborg Sygehus, a general hospital of 400 beds, installed a PACS (SIENET, Siemens) in 1989. And in 1992, the department was almost filmless except for mammography. In France, there are seven PACS projects, in Grenoble, Lille, Montpellier, Nantes, Rennes, and Villejuif. In Grenoble and in Rennes, PAC systems are in the university hospital with a special connection to neurosurgery. The University Hospital of Rennes recently assumed the major responsibility for the EuroPACS MIMOSA project, which aims at providing a generic framework for an information system dealing with the management of medical images within a medical institute. In Lille and Villejuif, PAC systems are designed into the university hospital infrastructure under the framework of a hospital information system project. In Montpellier, the PACS is designed for the university hospital instead of the radiology department. In Nantes, the PACS is confined to the nuclear medicine area. A recent project in the Hospital of Paris is the MIRIAM, a long-term integrated RIS–PACS project.

In Germany, there are three PACS-related projects, one each from the University of Hamburg, the University of Berlin, and the Rudolf Virchow University Hospital. The Hamburg project is related to the use of computed radiography (CR). The Berlin Communication Project (BERKOM), initiated in 1986, served as a test bed for future developments of broadband communication services, terminal devices, and applications. The project was shared by a spectrum of partners comprising 40 scientific institutions, 17 industrial companies, and 5 users. The BERKOM project has recently been replaced by an ATM research group DeTeBerkom. The third project is the recent BERMED project, a joint effort among the Rudolf Virchow University Hospital, the German Heart Institute, and the Technical University in Berlin, the design of the project is based on the Hewlett-Packard archive system (Palo Alto, CA).

In Greece, a new project, TelePACS 2.0, is being launched in Crete to support the health care network on the island.

In Italy, nine hospitals installed the turnkey CommView PACS system from AT&T and Philips. These hospitals are Mater Dei Clinic, Bari; Maggiore Hospital, Bologna; Castelfranco Hospital, Castelfranco; Sant'Anna Hospital, Ferrara; Messina Hospital, Messina; S. Gerardo Hospital, Monza; Cattinare Hospital and Maggiore Hospital, Trieste; and S. Paolo Hospital, Milan. The Collemaggio Hospital, L'Aquila, on the other hand, is developing its own PACS. Research activities in Italy include economic evaluation, metropolitan PACS, operational analysis, RIS–PACS integration, and teleradiology.

In Seoul, South Korea, a large-scale PACS has been installed in the Samsung Medical Center (see Section 10.1.5). The ASAN Medical Center is in the process of installing a large-scale system, designed and implemented by Hyundai Electronic, Ltd. (see Section 10.1.3.2).

PACS and related research in the Netherlands is concentrated in radiology and hospital information systems, the analysis of receiver operating characteristics (ROC), image quality evaluation, and modeling. A first-phase study was completed by a consortium, a cooperative effort between Utrecht University Hospital (AZU), BAZIS (a hospital information system organization), and Philips of Netherlands.

With more than 2000 CR systems in clinical use, Japan is very active in computed radiography. As for PACS, about 100 hospitals have already installed systems of various complexity. In Section 10.1.4, we describe a very-large-scale PACS project at Hokkaido University. Other major PACS installations are at Nagoya University, Osaka University, and Toshiba Hospital.

In the Vall d'Hebron Children's Hospital, Barcelona, Spain, a PACS project with the Philips CommView system was started in 1991, and the hospital continues to use the system.

Large-scale PACS installations do not exist in Sweden; however, at present there are two hospitals, Karolinska in Stockholm and Lasarettet in Lund, which have experience in limited PACS activities. Also, about 12 teleradiology systems are in use in Sweden or in these hospitals.

In Switzerland, a hospital-wide PACS project integrated within a hospital information system is in progress at the University Hospital of Geneva. In Turkey, a PACS project is being designed with the cooperation of two universities in Ankara. The system will be designed and implemented by Bilkent University and deployed at the Department of Radiology, Hacettepe University.

In the United Kingdom, there are two PACS projects, one in Hammersmith Hospital and the other in Conquest Hospital, Hastings, East Sussex. The Hammersmith Hospital project, the details of which are presented in Section 10.1.4.4, is supported by the British government.

Other countries also have PACS research and development efforts at various stages of design and implementation; thus the preceding list, by no means exhaustive, will increase as time progresses.

2

Digital Radiologic Imaging Fundamentals

2.1 Terminology

This chapter discusses some fundamental concepts and tools in digital radiologic imaging that are used throughout this text. These concepts are derived from conventional radiographic imaging and digital image processing. For an extensive treatment of these subjects, see the following materials, which are listed in the References at the end of the book:

Barrett and Swindell (1981)
Bertram (March 1970)
Bracewell (1965)
Brigham (1974)
Castleman (1979)
Cochran et al. (June 1967)
Dainty and Shaw (1984)
Gonzalez and Cointz (1982)
Rosenfeld and Kak (1976)
Rossman (1969)

Digital image. A digital image is a two-dimensional array of nonnegative integers $f(x,y)$, where $1 \leq x \leq M$ and $1 \leq y \leq N$ in which M and N are positive integers representing number of rows and columns. For any given x and y, the small square in the image represented by the coordinates (x,y) is called a picture element, or a pixel, and $f(x,y)$ is its corresponding functional value.

Digitization. Digitization is a process that quantizes or samples analog signals into a range of digital values. Digitizing a picture means converting the gray scales in the picture into a digital image.

About 70% of all radiologic examinations, including skull, chest, breast, abdomen, and bone, are acquired and stored on X-ray films. This process, which compresses a three-dimensional object into a two-dimensional image, is called projection radiography. An X-ray film can be converted to digital numbers with a film digitizer. The laser scanning digitizer is the gold standard among digitizers, because it can best preserve the resolutions of the original analog image. A laser film scanner can digitize a standard X-ray film (14 in. × 17 in.) to 2000 × 2500 pixels with 12 bits per pixel. Another method of acquiring digital projection radiography is computed radiography (CR), a technology that uses a laser-stimulated luminescence phosphor imaging plate as an X-ray detector. A laser beam is used to scan the imaging plate, which contains the latent X-ray image. The latent image is excited and emits light photons, which are detected and converted to electronic signals. The electronic signals are converted to digital signals to form a digital X-ray image.

The other 30% of radiology examinations, which include computed tomography (CT), nuclear medicine (NM), ultrasonography (US), magnetic resonance imaging (MRI), and digital subtraction angiography (DSA), are already in digital format.

Digital radiologic image. A digital radiologic image $f(x,y)$ is the digital representation of an image obtained by using radiologic procedures: conventional projection radiography, ultrasonography, computed tomography, or nuclear magnetic resonance. The coordinates of anatomical structures in the image are x and y.

Gray level value. The functional value $f(x,y)$ of a pixel (x,y) is called the gray level value (or gray level), a nonnegative integer. Depending on the digitization procedure or the radiologic procedure used, gray level values lie in the following ranges: 0 to 255 (8-bit), 0 to 511 (9-bit), 0 to 1023 (10-bit), 0 to 2047 (11-bit), and 0 to 4095 (12-bit). These gray levels represent physical or chemical properties of the structures in the object. For example, in an image obtained by digitizing an X-ray film, the gray level value of a pixel represents the optical density of the square area of the film. In the case of X-ray computed tomography (XCT), the gray level value represents the relative linear attenuation coefficient of the tissue; in magnetic resonance imaging (MRI), it corresponds to the magnetic resonance signal response of the tissue.

Image size. The dimensions of an image are the ordered pair (M, N), and the size of the image is the product $M \times N \times k$ bits, where 2^k is the gray level range. The following lists sizes of some common medical images:

CT	$512 \times 512 \times 12$
US	$512 \times 512 \times 8$
MRI	$256 \times 256 \times 12$
DSA	$512 \times 512 \times 8$, or $1024 \times 1024 \times 8$
NM	$128 \times 128 \times 16$
Microscopic image	$512 \times 512 \times 8$
Digitized X-ray film (14 inches by 14 inches)	$2048 \times 2048 \times 12$
CR	$2048 \times 2048 \times 10$ or other sizes dependent on the size of the plate

For most digital radiologic images, $M = N$ is chosen for convenience of operation; in this case, one speaks of a 12-bit 512 image, a 10-bit 1024 image, and so on. Figure 2.1 shows the relationship between a radiologic image, the image size, the pixel unit, and the gray level value.

Histogram. The histogram of an image is a plot of the gray level value (abscissa) against the frequency of occurrence of pixels of the gray level value in the entire image (ordinate). For an image with 256 possible gray levels, the abscissa of the histogram ranges from 0 to 255. The total pixel count under the histogram is $M \times N$. This histogram represent gray level distribution, an important characteristic of an image.

Video display. In visualizing a digital image, either of two methods may be used: print the digital image to film for a hard copy, or display it on a video monitor as a soft copy (volatile). To display a digital radiologic image on a video monitor, the gray level values are converted to analog signals compatible with conventional video signals used in the television industry. This procedure is called digital-to-analog (D/A) conversion. Video display monitors can be used to display a 512, 1024, or 2048 size image.

2.2 Density Resolution, Spatial Resolution, and Signal-to-Noise Ratio

Once an object of interest has been recorded as a digital image, we would like to know the image quality. The image quality is characterized by three parameters: spatial resolution, density resolution, and signal-to-noise ratio. The spatial resolution is a measure of the number of pixels used to represent the objects. The density resolution is the total number of discrete gray level values in the digital image. It is clear that N and k are related to spatial resolution and density resolution, respectively. A high signal-to-noise ratio means the image is very pleasing to the eyes, hence is a better quality image.

Figure 2.2 demonstrates the concepts of spatial resolution and density resolution of a digital image using a lymphocyte as an example. The left-hand column in Figure 2.2 shows digitized images of the lymphocyte with a fixed spatial resolution (21×15) and variable density resolutions (from top to bottom: 16, 4, and 2 gray levels). The right-hand column depicts the digital representation of the same analog image with a fixed density resolution (16) and variable spatial resolutions (from top to bottom: high, medium, low). Clearly, the digital image in the right upper corner is the best representation of the original analog image, having the highest spatial and density resolutions. The image in the lower left-hand corner, which has the lowest spatial and density resolutions, is a binary image. Spatial resolution, density resolution, and signal-to-noise ratio of the image are adjusted during image acquisition to accommodate the diagnostic requirement. A high resolution image requires a larger memory capacity for storage and longer time for image transmission and processing.

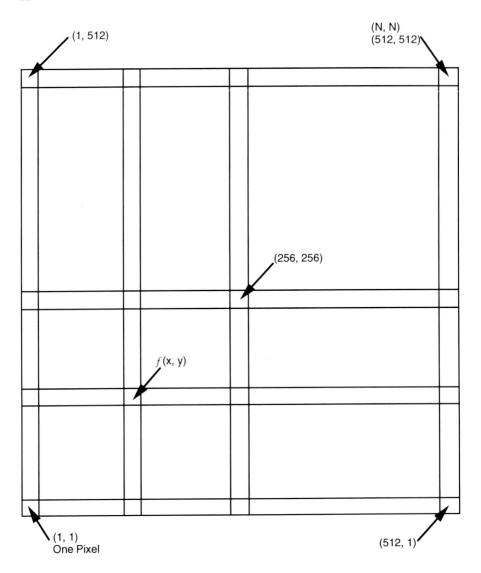

Figure 2.1 Terminology used in a radiologic image to indicate image size, a pixel, and its gray level value.

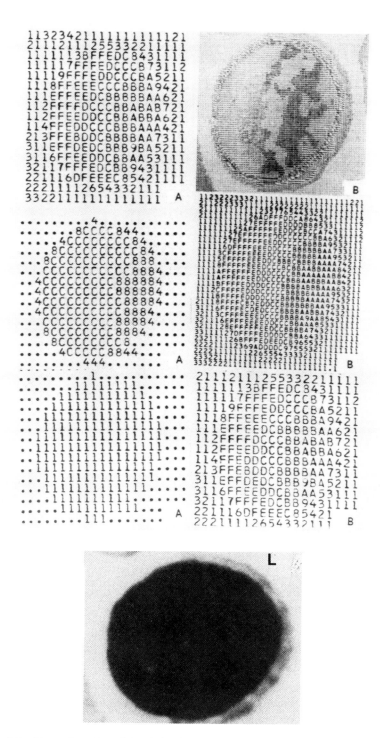

Figure 2.2 Illustration of spatial and density resolutions using a lymphocyte image (L) as an example. The 16 levels are represented by ·, 1, 2, 3, 4, 5, 6, 7, 8, 9, A, B, C, D, E, and F. (A) Fixed spatial resolution, variable density resolutions: 16, 4, and 2 gray levels. (B) Fixed density resolution (16 levels), variable spatial resolutions.

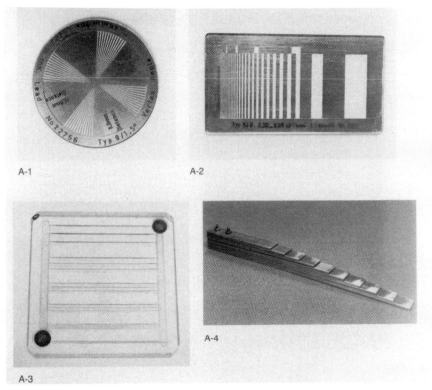

Figure 2.3 Some commonly used physical test objects and digitally generated test patterns. (A) Physical: 1, star-shaped pattern embedded in water contained in a circular cylinder; 2, high contrast line pair; 3, low contrast line pair; 4, step wedge. (B) Corresponding X-ray images. (C) Digitally generated 512 image: 1, high contrast (gray level = 0, 140; width of each line pair in pixel = 2, 4, 6, 8, 10, 12, 14, 16, 32, 64, and 128 pixels); 2, low contrast line pair: (gray level = 0, 40; width of each line pair in pixel = 2, 4, 8, 16, 20, and 28 pixels).

2.3 Test Objects and Patterns

Test objects or patterns (sometimes called phantoms), used to measure the density and spatial resolutions of radiologic imaging equipment, can be either physical phantoms or digitally generated patterns.

A physical phantom is used to measure a digital radiologic device performance. It is usually constructed with different materials shaped in various geometrical configurations that are then embedded in a uniform background material (e.g., water or plastic). The most commonly used geometrical configurations are circular cylinder, sphere, line pairs (alternating pattern of rectangular bar with background of the same width), step wedge, and star shape. Materials used to construct these configurations are lead, various plastics, air, and iodine solutions of various concentrations. The circular cylinder, sphere, and step wedge configurations are commonly used to measure spatial and density resolutions. Thus, the statement that an X-ray device

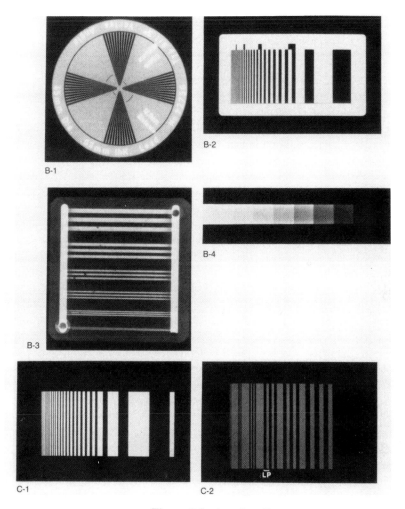

Figure 2.3 (*continued*)

can detect a 1 mm cylindrical object with 0.5% density difference from the background means that this particular radiologic imaging device can produce an image of the cylindrical object made from material that has an X-ray attenuation difference from the background of 0.5%; thus the difference between the average gray level of the object and the average gray level of the background is measurable or detectable.

A digitally generated pattern, on the other hand, is used to measure the display component performance of a digital radiologic device. In this case, the various geometrical configurations are generated digitally. The gray level values of these configurations are inputted to the display component according to certain specifications. A digital phantom is an ideal digital image. Any distortion of such images observed from the display component is a measure of the imperfections of the display component. Figure 2.3 shows some commonly used physical phantoms and digitally generated patterns, as well as the X-ray images of the physical phantoms.

2.4 Spatial Domain and Frequency Domain

If a digital radiologic image $f(x,y)$ is the gray level representation of anatomical structures in space, one can say that it is defined in the spatial domain. The image, $f(x,y)$, can also be represented as its spatial frequency components u,v through a mathematical transform (see Section 2.4.1). In this case, we use the symbol $F(u,v)$ to represent the transform of $f(x,y)$ and say that $F(u,v)$ is defined in the frequency domain. $F(u,v)$ is again a digital image, but it bears no visual resemblance to $f(x,y)$ (see Fig. 2.4). With proper training, however, one can use information displayed in the frequency domain to detect some inherent characteristics of each type of radiologic image.

The concept of using frequency components to represent anatomical structures might seem strange at first, and one might wonder why we even have to bother with this representation. To understand better, consider that a radiologic image is composed of many two-dimensional sinusoidal waves, each with individual amplitude and frequency. For example, a digitally generated "uniform image" has no frequency components, only a constant (dc) term. An X-ray image of the hand is composed of many high frequency components (edges of bones) and few low frequency components, while an image of a gall bladder plus contrast material is composed of many low frequency components (the contrast medium inside the gall bladder) but very few high frequency components. Therefore, the frequency representation of a radiologic image gives a different perspective on the characteristics of the image under consideration.

Based on this frequency information in the image, we can selectively change the frequency components to enhance the image. To obtain a smoother appearing image, therefore, we can increase the amplitude of low frequency components, whereas to enhance the edges of bones in the hand X-ray image, we can magnify the amplitude of the high frequency components.

Manipulating an image in the frequency domain also yields many other advantages. If, for example, we use the frequency representation of an image to measure its quality, we are led to the concepts of point spread function (PSF), line spread function (LSF), and the modulation transfer function (MTF), to be discussed in Sections 2.5.1.1, 2.5.1.2, and 2.5.1.4, respectively. In addition, radiologic images obtained from image reconstruction principles are based on the frequency component representation. Utilization of frequency representation also facilitates the explanation of how an MRI image is formed. (This is discussed in Chapter 5.)

2.4.1 The Fourier Transform (FT)

As discussed earlier, a radiologic image defined in the spatial domain (x,y) can be transformed to the frequency domain (u,v). The Fourier transform is one method for doing this. The Fourier transform of a two-dimensional function $f(x,y)$, denoted by $\mathscr{F}\{f(x,y)\}$, is given by:

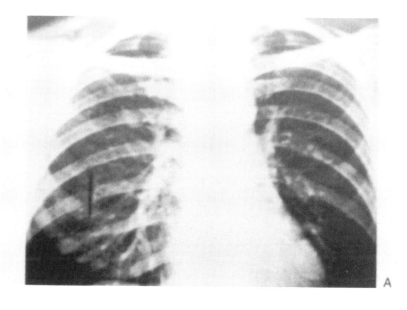

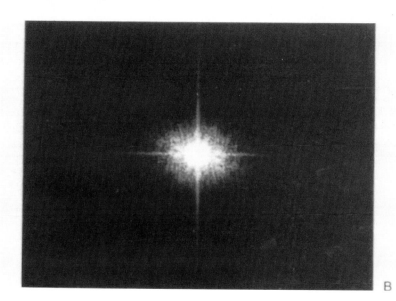

Figure 2.4 (A) A digital chest X-ray image represented in spatial domain. (B) The same digital chest X-ray image represented in frequency domain. The low frequency components are in the center and the high frequency components are in the periphery.

$$\mathscr{F}\{f(x,y)\} = F(u,v) = \int_{-\infty}^{\infty} \int f(x,y)\exp[-i2\pi(ux + vy)]dx\, dy \tag{2.1}$$

$$= \mathrm{Re}(u,v) + i\, \mathrm{Im}(u,v)$$

where $i = \sqrt{-1}$, and $\mathrm{Re}(u,v)$ and $\mathrm{Im}(u,v)$ are the real and imaginary components, respectively, of $F(u,v)$.

The magnitude function

$$|F(u,v)| = [R^2(u,v) + I^2(u,v)]^{1/2} \tag{2.2}$$

is called the Fourier spectrum of $f(x,y)$, and $|F(u,v)|^2$ the energy spectrum of $f(x,y)$, respectively. The function

$$\Phi(u,v) = \tan^{-1}\frac{\mathrm{Im}(u,v)}{\mathrm{Re}(u,v)} \tag{2.3}$$

is called phase angle.

Given $F(u,v)$, $f(x,y)$ can be obtained by using the inverse Fourier transform

$$\mathscr{F}^{-1}[F(u,v)] = f(x,y) \tag{2.4}$$

$$= \int_{-\infty}^{\infty} \int F(u,v)\exp[i2\pi(ux + vy)]du\, dv$$

The two functions $f(x,y)$ and $F(u,v)$ are called the Fourier transform pair. The Fourier transform enables us to transform a two-dimensional image from the spatial domain to the frequency domain and vice versa.

2.4.2 The Discrete Fourier Transform

The discrete Fourier transform is an approximation of the Fourier transform used to perform the transform on a digital image. For a square digital radiologic image, the integrals in the Fourier transform pair can be approximated by summations as follows:

$$F(u,v) = \frac{1}{N} \sum_{x=0}^{N-1} \sum_{y=0}^{N-1} f(x,y)\exp\left[\frac{-i2\pi(ux + vy)}{N}\right] \tag{2.5}$$

for $u,v = 0, 1, 2, \ldots, N - 1$, and

$$f(x,y) = \frac{1}{N} \sum_{u=0}^{N-1} \sum_{v=0}^{N-1} F(u,v)\exp\left[\frac{i2\pi(ux + vy)}{N}\right] \tag{2.6}$$

for $x, y = 0, 1, 2, \ldots, N - 1$.

The $f(x,y)$ and $F(u,v)$ shown in Eqs. (2.5) and (2.6) are called the discrete Fourier transform pair. It is apparent from these two equations that when the digital radiologic image $f(x,y)$ is known, its discrete Fourier transform can be computed with simple multiplications and additions, and vice versa.

2.4.3 The Fast Fourier Transform (FFT)

Although the procedure for computing the discrete Fourier transform of $f(x,y)$ is mathematically straightforward, in practice, Eq. (2.5) is seldom used to perform the transform because it involves too many multiplication and addition operations. Instead, the transform is performed line by line on the image with a one-dimensional (1-D) discrete Fourier transform defined by

$$F(u,Y) = \frac{1}{N} \sum_{x=0}^{N-1} f(x,Y)\exp\left[\frac{-i2\pi\ ux}{N}\right] \qquad (2.7)$$

for $u = 0, 1, 2, \ldots, N - 1$, where Y is constant representing a line of the image. Similarly, we use

$$f(x,V) = \sum_{u=0}^{N-1} F(u,V)\ \exp\left[\frac{i2\pi\ ux}{N}\right] \qquad (2.8)$$

for $x = 0, 1, 2, \ldots, N - 1$, where V is a constant representing a line of the 1-D Fourier transform of the image, to perform the inverse transform. The details of the procedure are described in Section 2.4.4.

Approximately N^2 operations are needed to transform one line of the image, where N is the number of pixels in the line. A technique for reducing the number of operations and computational time by properly grouping terms and operations is called a fast Fourier transform algorithm, or simply, FFT. A good FFT algorithm can reduce the number of operations from N^2 to $N\ log_2\ (N)$.

Table 2.1, which compares the number of operations required to perform one line of information for a conventional discrete Fourier transform and for the FFT, shows tremendous difference in number of operations required for the two transformations. The FFT method of performing the transform on one line of the image is called 1-D FFT.

Table 2.1 Comparison of the Number of Operations Required for Performing One Line of the Image Between the Conventional Discrete Fourier Transform and FFT (Unit: Number of Operations)

Image Size N	Type of Imaging*	Conventional FT N^2	FFT $N\ log_2\ N$
256	MRI	65,536	2,048
512	CT	262,144	4,608
1024	DF	1,048,576	10,240
2048	CR	4,194,304	22,528

* 256, image size 256 × 256; DF, digital fluorography; CR, computed radiography.

2.4.4 Performing a Two-Dimensional FFT
on a Radiologic Image

We are going to describe a method for performing a 2-D FFT using the 1-D FFT on an image at the programming level, since this topic has generally been ignored in textbooks.

Consider, for example, a 1024 radiologic image, each pixel consisting of 16-bit information (or less). To perform the 2-D FFT, a line buffer of 1024×64 bits is first set up in the computer memory. A line from the image that consists of 1024 pixels is then transferred into this line buffer (see A in Fig. 2.5). A 1-D FFT is performed on this line of information in the line buffer using Eq. (2.7) (Fig. 2.5, B). Note that the first, second, . . . , 1024th pixel value is the function value $f(0,Y)$, $f(1,Y)$, . . . , and $f(1023,Y)$ in Eq. (2.7). This convention will be used throughout this book.

The 1-D FFT of this line is 1024 complex numbers, each of which has a 32-bit real part and a 32-bit imaginary part. Only half (512×64) of this line buffer needs to be stored in a scratch image memory for further processing (Fig. 2.5, C). This is because $f(x,y)$ is a real-valued function, and the 1-D FFT of a real-valued function possesses some symmetric characteristics, as shown in the 8×8 numerical example given in Table 2.2. A second line from the original image is loaded into the line buffer, and a 1-D FFT is performed. The resulting 1-D FFT is stored in the second line of the scratch image memory. This procedure is repeated until the last line of the image has been transformed.

As an example, the 1-D FFT of the first line can be broken down as follows:

First line of the original image:

12.0	14.0	13.0	15.0	18.0	34.0	23.0	50.0

Real part of the 1-D FFT:

22.4	0.6	−0.8	−2.1	−5.9	−2.1	−0.8	0.6

Imaginary part of the 1-D FFT:

0.0	6.1	2.1	3.6	0.0	−3.6	−2.1	−6.1

Observe the symmetric property in the real part and the imaginary part; see also Figure 2.4, B).

At this point, the 1024×512 scratch image memory is filled up with the 1-D FFT information. A transpose operation is then performed on this 1024×512 array, which results in a 512×1024 array (Fig. 2.5, D). A 1024-pixel line from the transpose image is then loaded into the line buffer (Fig. 2.5, E). A 1-D FFT is performed on this line of information in the line buffer (Fig. 2.5, F), and the result is transferred to a line of the $512 \times 1024 \times 64$ bit image memory (Fig. 2.5, G).

This procedure is repeated until the 1-D FFT has been performed on all the 512

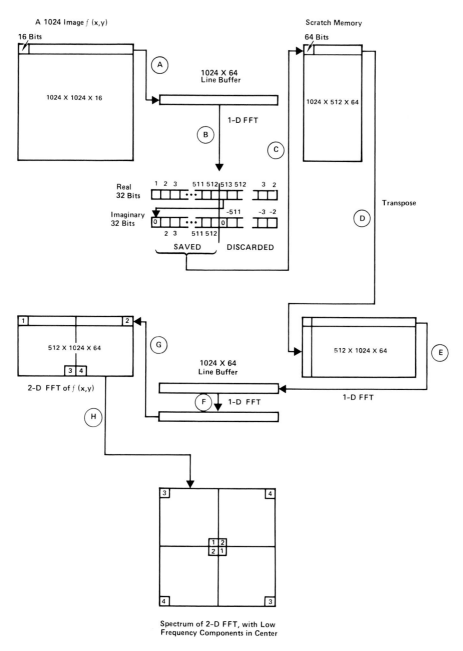

Figure 2.5 (A)–(H)   Step-by-step procedure for calculating the 2-D FFT using the 1-D FFT; see text and Table 2.2.

Table 2.2 An 8 × 8 Numerical Example Showing the Result of the 2-D FFT

The Original 8 × 8 Image

12.0	14.0	13.0	15.0	18.0	34.0	23.0	50.0
13.0	15.0	23.0	22.0	19.0	32.0	27.0	30.0
23.0	25.0	34.0	24.0	29.0	31.0	25.0	20.0
18.0	24.0	32.0	27.0	20.0	21.0	28.0	23.0
27.0	28.0	35.0	27.0	26.0	31.0	33.0	30.0
13.0	27.0	39.0	28.0	27.0	33.0	33.0	40.0
25.0	27.0	24.0	34.0	19.0	11.0	15.0	24.0
13.0	19.0	17.0	24.0	26.0	21.0	24.0	27.0

FFT (Real Part)

24.86	−1.80	0.41	−0.01	0.33	−0.01	0.41	−1.80
−0.54	0.18	0.55	−0.17	0.62	0.55	−0.29	−0.34
−1.52	−0.08	−0.34	0.17	0.80	−0.64	−0.25	1.12
−0.71	0.07	0.29	−0.68	0.31	−0.01	−0.86	−0.49
−1.33	−0.98	−0.63	−0.65	−0.05	−0.65	−0.63	−0.98
−0.71	−0.49	−0.86	−0.01	0.31	−0.68	0.29	0.07
−1.52	1.12	−0.25	−0.64	0.80	0.17	−0.34	−0.08
−0.54	−0.34	−0.29	0.55	0.62	−0.17	0.55	0.18

FFT (Imaginary Part)

0.00	−0.09	−0.89	0.91	0.00	−0.91	0.89	0.09
0.72	1.40	1.46	−0.09	−0.22	0.79	1.23	0.82
0.81	0.58	0.52	0.14	−0.09	0.38	−0.30	0.08
1.00	−0.06	0.58	0.08	0.13	0.79	0.49	0.60
0.00	−0.52	0.39	0.23	0.00	−0.23	−0.39	0.52
−1.00	−0.60	−0.49	−0.79	−0.13	−0.08	−0.58	0.06
−0.81	−0.08	0.30	−0.38	0.09	−0.14	−0.52	−0.58
−0.72	−0.82	−1.23	−0.79	0.22	0.09	−1.46	−1.40

lines in the transpose array, and the results are stored in the 512 × 1024 image memory. The outcome is then a 2-D FFT of the original image. This 512 × 1024 × 64 image memory contains the complete 2-D FFT information, because the 2-D FFT of a radiologic image $f(x,y)$, which is real, possesses some symmetric characteristics, as shown in part H of Figure 2.5.

Table 2.3 The Amplitude of the the FFT

0.05	0.69	0.74	1.11	1.33	1.11	0.74	0.69
0.34	0.69	0.65	0.10	1.23	0.78	0.99	0.79
0.80	0.22	0.62	0.59	1.72	1.12	0.39	0.74
0.66	0.19	1.56	1.41	0.90	0.89	1.27	0.96
0.33	0.91	0.98	1.80	24.86	1.80	0.98	0.91
0.66	0.96	1.27	0.89	0.90	1.41	1.56	0.19
0.80	0.74	0.39	1.12	1.72	0.59	0.62	0.22
0.34	0.79	0.99	0.78	1.23	0.10	0.65	0.69

The 1-D FFT algorithm is well established. We can select a suitable one from the literature and follow the procedure described here to obtain the 2-D FFT. The procedure described in Figure 2.5 can also be used to obtain $f(x,y)$ from its 2-D FFT by reversing the steps starting at G with the 512×1024 2-D FFT. The only differences are as follows: (1) before step B can be performed, the 512×64 bit line buffer must be extended to 1024×64 bits, as shown in Figure 2.5, B; and (2) Eq. (2.8) is used instead of Eq. (2.7) for the 1-D FFT. The result after step A is the original image.

To visualize the 2-D FFT, it is customary to display its spectrum. To do this, we perform a transformation on the pixels of the 512×1024 FFT, as shown in part H of Figure 2.5. The Fourier spectrum is computed for each pixel, as given in Eq. (2.2). The displayed Fourier spectrum has the low frequency components in the center and high frequency components at the periphery as in Figure 2.4, B. Traditionally, we use a logarithm scale to display the Fourier spectrum because of its large dynamic range.

The technique described here to perform the 2-D Fourier transform and to display the Fourier spectrum is not the only method; there are other algorithms available to achieve the same purpose. However, this method is probably the easiest to understand and to emulate. Typically, the results during and after a 2-D FFT are arrayed as in Table 2.2. Before displaying the amplitude values (Table 2.3), however, it is necessary to do some rearrangement of the low frequency components in the center and the high frequency components in the periphery.

2.4.5 Cosine Transformation Using the FFT

Another transform, the discrete cosine transform, can be expressed as the real part of the product of the $2N$-point discrete Fourier transform of $f(x)$, shown in Eq. (2.7), and a complex function.

Mathematically, this transform has the following form:

$$F(u) = \left(\frac{2C(u)}{N}\right) \mathrm{Re}\left[\exp\left(\frac{-iu\pi}{2N}\right) \sum_{x=0}^{2N-1} f(x)\exp\left(\frac{-iux\pi}{N}\right) \right] \qquad (2.9)$$

for $u = 0, 1, \ldots, N - 1, \ldots, 2N - 1$, where $f(x) = 0$, for $x = N, N + 1, \ldots, 2N - 1$, and $C(u) = (\frac{1}{2})^{1/2}$ for $u = 0$ but $= 1$ otherwise.

This transform can be used to perform image compression, reconstruction, and filtering. The principle of image compression and image reconstruction is covered in Chapter 6. The procedure of performing the discrete cosine transform is quite similar to that of the 2-D discrete FT, and is discussed here.

Consider again a 1024 image with 16-bit information in each pixel. The objective is to perform a 2-D discrete cosine transform of this image using the discrete FFT method. Figure 2.6 describes the procedure. One line of the image is first transferred to a 1024×64 bit line buffer (Fig. 2.6, step A). This 1024-line buffer is extended to a 2048×64 line buffer with pixels 1025–2048 filled with zeros (Fig. 2.6, B). For each $u, u = 0, \ldots, 1023$, a discrete FT with all 2048 pixels is performed (refer to

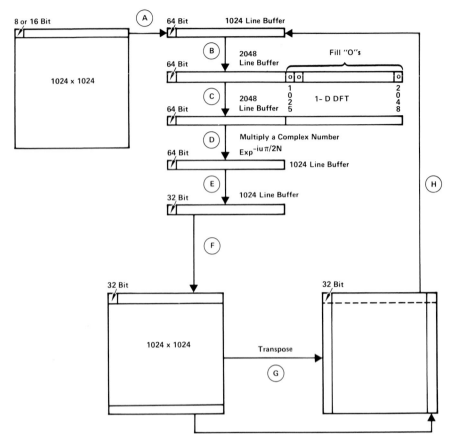

Figure 2.6 Step-by-step procedure on a programming level for computing the two-dimensional cosine transform using the discrete Fourier transform.

Eq. 2.9 and Fig. 2.6, C). Each transformed value is multiplied by a corresponding value $\exp(-\mathbf{i}u\pi/2048)$ (Fig. 2.6, D). The cosine transform $F(u)$ is the real part of this product multiplied by the constant $2C(u)/N$ (Fig. 2.6, E). The result is stored in a 1024×32 bit line buffer, which is used for carrying out the next step. Values in this line buffer are transferred to the first line of a $1024 \times 1024 \times 32$ bit scratch image memory (Fig. 2.6, F).

This procedure continues until the 1-D discrete cosine transform has been performed on all 1024 lines in the original image. At this point, the 1024×1024 scratch memory is entirely filled with the 1-D discrete cosine transform coefficients. A transpose operation is performed on this 1024×1024 image memory. The result is a transposed 1-D discrete cosine transform of the original image (Fig. 2.6, G).

One line in the transposed image is transferred to the 1024×64 bit line buffer (Fig. 2.6, H). A 1-D discrete cosine transform is again performed on this line of information following the same procedures as shown in Figure 2.6, (B–F). This procedure is repeated until the last line of information in the transposed matrix is completed. The result is a 2-D discrete cosine transform of the original image with coefficients in the scratch image memory, obtained using the discrete Fourier transform technique. In the scratch memory, the low frequency information is in the upper left corner and the high frequency information is in the lower right corner. Since the original image is real, the cosine transform contains only the 32-bit real part. No further rearrangement is required to display the spectrum of the cosine transform using the discrete Fourier transform technique, since the low frequency information is in the upper left corner and the high frequency in the lower right corner.

The method of using the discrete Fourier transform to perform cosine transform described here is not the only technique; other faster algorithms do exist. The technique described here, however, takes advantage of the 1-D discrete Fourier transform that is readily available in most laboratories. The theory of the cosine transform is dealt with in more detail in Chapter 6.

2.5 Measurement of Image Quality

Image quality is a measure of the performance of an imaging system used for a specific radiologic examination. Although the process of making diagnoses from a radiologic image is often subjective, higher quality images provide better diagnostic information. We will describe some physical parameters for measuring image quality based on the concepts of density and spatial resolutions and signal-to-noise level, introduced earlier.

In general, measurements of image quality can be divided into two categories: measurement of image unsharpness is inherent in the design of the instrumentation, while image noise, which arises from photon fluctuations from the energy source, and electronic noise accumulated through the imaging chain. Even if there were no noise in the imaging system (a hypothetical case), the inherent optical properties of the imaging system used might well prevent the image of a line pair phantom from giving sharp edges between black and white areas. By the same token, if a perfect imaging system could be designed, the nature of random photon fluctuation would introduce noise into the image.

Sections 2.5.1 and 2.5.2 discuss the measurement of sharpness and noise. This treatment is based on the established theory of measuring image quality in diagnostic radiologic devices. Certain modifications are included to permit adjustment for digital terminology.

2.5.1 Measurement of Sharpness
2.5.1.1 Point Spread Function (PSF)

Consider the following experiment. A small circular hole is drilled in the center of a lead plate, which is placed between an X-ray tube and an image receptor. An image of this plate is then obtained, which can be recorded by a film or by digital means

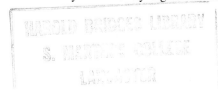

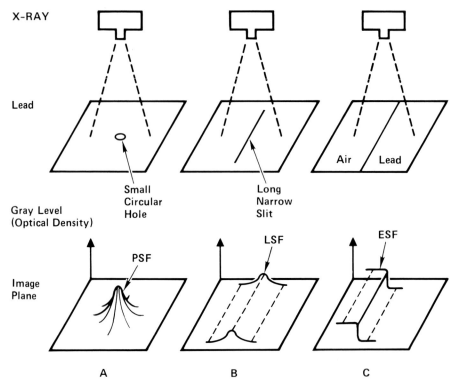

Figure 2.7 Experimental setup for defining (A) The point spread function (PSF), (B) the line spread function (LSF), and (C) the edge spread function (ESF).

and then displayed on a TV monitor (Fig. 2.7A). Upon measuring the gray level distribution of this image, we will see that the gray level (corresponding to the optical density) is comparatively high in the center of the image where the hole is located and decreases radially outward, becoming zero at a certain distance away from the center. Ideally, if the circular hole is small enough and the imaging system is a perfect system, we would expect to see a perfectly circular hole in the image, with gray level the same everywhere within the hole and zero everywhere outside. The size of the circle in the image would be equal to the size of the circular hole in the plate if no magnification was introduced during the experiment. However, in practice, such an ideal image never exists. Instead, a distribution of the gray level, as described earlier, will be observed.

This experiment demonstrates that the image of a circular hole in a lead plate never has a well-defined edge but has, instead, a certain *unsharpness*. If the circular hole is small enough, the shape of this gray level distribution is called the point spread function (PSF) of the imaging system (consisting of the X-ray source and the image receptor). The point spread function of the imaging system can be used as a measure of the unsharpness of an image produced by this imaging system. In practice, however, the point spread function of an imaging system is very difficult to measure. For the experiment described in Figure 2.7A, the size of the circular hole must be chosen very carefully. If the circular hole is too large, the picture formed in the detector becomes the image of the circular hole. On the other hand, if the circular hole is too small, the image formed becomes the image of the X-ray focal spot. In either case, the image cannot be used to measure the PSF of the imaging system.

Theoretically, the point spread function is a useful concept in estimating the sharpness of an image. Experimentally, the point spread function is difficult to measure because of constraints just noted. To circumvent this difficulty in determining the point spread function of an imaging system, the concept of the line spread function is introduced.

2.5.1.2 Line Spread Function (LSF)

Let us replace the circular hole with a long narrow slit in the lead plate and repeat the experiment. The image formed on the image receptor becomes a line of a certain width with nonuniform gray level distribution. The gray level value is high in the center of the line, decreasing toward both sides until it assumes the gray level of the background. The shape of this gray level distribution is called the line spread function (LSF) of the imaging system. Theoretically, a line spread function can be considered to be a line of continuous holes placed very close together. Experimentally, the line spread function is much easier to measure than the PSF. Figure 2.7B illustrates the concept of the line spread function of the system.

2.5.1.3 Edge Spread Function (ESF)

If the narrow slit is replaced by a single step wedge such that half the imaging area is lead and the other is air, then the gray level distribution of the image is the edge spread function (ESF) of the system. For an ideal imaging system, any trace perpendicular to the edge of this image would yield a step function

$$\text{ESF}(x) = 0 \qquad -B \le x < x_0 \tag{2.10}$$
$$\phantom{\text{ESF}(x)} = A \qquad x_0 \le x \le B$$

where x is the direction perpendicular to the edge, x_0 is the location of the edge, $-B$ and B are the left and right boundaries of the image, and A is a constant. Mathematically, the line spread function is the first derivative of the edge spread function given by the equation

$$\text{LSF}(x) = \frac{d[ESF(x)]}{dx} \tag{2.11}$$

It should be observed that the edge spread function is easy to obtain experimentally, since only a sharp-edged lead plate is required to set up the experiment. Once the image has been obtained with the image receptor, a gray level trace perpendicular to the edge yields the edge spread function of the system. To compute the line spread function of the system, simply take the first derivative of the edge spread function. Figure 2.7C depicts the experimental setup used to obtain the edge spread function.

2.5.1.4 Modulation Transfer Function (MTF)

Let us now substitute for the lead plate a line pair phantom with different spatial frequencies, and repeat the preceding experiment. In the image receptor, an image of the line pair phantom will form. From this image, the output amplitude (or gray level) of each spatial frequency can be measured. The modulation transfer function of the imaging system, along the line perpendicular to the line pairs, is defined as the ratio between the output amplitude and the input amplitude expressed as a function of spatial frequency

$$MFT(u) = (\text{output amplitude/input amplitude})_u \qquad (2.12)$$

where u is the spatial frequency measured in the direction perpendicular to the line pairs. Mathematically, the MTF is the magnitude (see Eq. 2.2) of the Fourier transform of the line spread function of the system given by the following equation:

$$MTF(u) = |\mathscr{F}[LSF(x)]| = \left| \int_{-\infty}^{\infty} [LSF(x) \exp(-i2\pi xu)]dx \right| \qquad (2.13)$$

It is seen from Eq. (2.12) that the MTF measures the modulation of the amplitude (gray level) of the line pair pattern in the image. The amount of modulation determines the quality of the imaging system. The MTF of an imaging system, once known, can be used to predict the quality of the image produced by the imaging system. For a given frequency u, if $MTF(v) = 0$ for all $v \geq u$, then the imaging system under consideration cannot resolve spatial frequency equal to or higher than u. The MTF so defined is a one-dimensional function: it measures the spatial resolution of the imaging system only in a certain direction. Extreme care must be exercised when the MTF is used to describe the spatial resolution of the system; the direction of the measurement must also be specified.

Notice that the MTF of a system is multiplicative; that is, if an image is obtained by an imaging system consisting of n components, each having its own MTF_i, then the total MTF of the imaging system is expressed by the following equation.

$$MTF(u) = \prod_{i=1}^{n} MTF_i(u) \qquad (2.14)$$

It is obvious that a low MTF value in any given component will yield an overall low MTF of the complete system.

2.5.1.5 Relationship Between ESF, LSF, and MTF

The MTF obtained as described in Section 2.5.1.4 is sometimes called the high contrast response of the imaging system, because the line pair pattern or the edge source used is a high contrast phantom. By "high contrast," we mean that the object (lead) and the background (air) offer high radiographic contrast. On the other hand, MTF obtained with a low contrast phantom constitutes the low contrast response of the system. The MTF value obtained with a high contrast phantom is always larger than that obtained with a lower contrast phantom for a given spatial frequency.

With this background, we are ready to describe the relationship between the edge spread function, the line spread function, and the modulation transfer function. Let us set up an experiment to obtain the MTF of a digital imaging system composed of a light table, a television camera, and a digital chain that converts the video signal into digital signal and forms the digital image. The experimental steps are as follows:

1. Cover half the light table with a sharp-edged, black-painted metal sheet. Such an object is called an *edge source.*
2. Obtain the digital image of the edge source with the imaging system, as shown in Figure 2.8A. Then the ESF(x) has a gray level distribution (as shown in Fig. 2.8B), which is obtained by taking the average value of several lines (a–a) perpendicular to the edges. Observe the noise characteristic of the ESF(x) in the figure.
3. The line spread function (LSF) of the system can be obtained by taking the first derivative numerically from the edge spread function (ESF) (Eq. 2.10), which is indicated by the arrows in Figure 2.8B. The resulting LSF is depicted in Figure 2.8C.
4. To obtain the MTF of the system in the direction perpendicular to the edge, a 1-D FFT (Eq. 2.7) is applied to the line spread function shown in Figure 2.8C. The magnitude of this 1-D FFT is then the MTF of the imaging system in the direction perpendicular to the edge. The result is shown in Figure 2.8D.

This completes the experiment to obtain the MTF from the ESF and the LSF. In practice, we can take 10% of the MTF values as the minimum resolving power of the imaging system. In this case, the MTF of this imaging system is about 1.0 cycle/mm.

2.5.1.6 Relationship Between the Input Image, the MTF, and the Output Image

Let $A = 1$, $B = \pi$, and $x_0 = 0$, and extend the edge spread function described in Eq. (2.10) to a periodic function with period 2π (Fig. 2.9A). This periodic function now can be expressed as a Fourier series representation, or more explicitly, as a sum of infinitely many sinusoidal functions, as follows:

$$ESF(x) = \frac{1}{2} + \frac{2}{\pi} \left(\sin + \frac{\sin 3x}{3} + \frac{\sin 5x}{5} + \frac{\sin 7x}{7} + \cdots \right) \qquad (2.15)$$

The first term, ½, in this Fourier series is the DC term. Subsequent terms are sinusoidal, and each is characterized by an amplitude and a frequency.

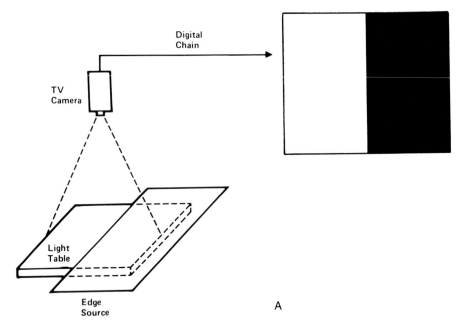

Figure 2.8 Relationship between the ESF, the LSF, and the MTF. (A) The experimental setup: the imaging chain consists of a light table, a TV camera, and a digital chain; the object is a one-step wedge. (B) The ESF (arrows) by averaging several lines through a–a. (C) The LSF. (D) The MTF.

If the partial sum of Eq. (2.15) is plotted, it is apparent that the partial sum will approximate the periodic step function more closely as the number of terms increases (Fig. 2.9B). We can also plot the amplitude spectrum or the spatial frequency spectrum shown in Figure 2.9C, which is a plot of the amplitude against the spatial frequency (Eq. 2.15). From this plot we can observe that the periodic step function $ESF(x)$ can be decomposed into infinite components, each of which has an amplitude and a frequency. To reproduce this periodic $ESF(x)$ exactly, it is necessary to include all the components. If some of the components are missing or have diminished amplitude values, the result is a diffused edge. A major concern in the design of an imaging system is to avoid having missing components or diminished amplitudes.

The MTF of a system can be used to predict the missing or modulated amplitudes. Consider the lateral view image of a plastic circular cylinder taken with a perfect X-ray imaging system. Figure 2.10A shows the optical density trace perpendicular to the edges of the circular cylinder in the image. How will this trace look if the X-ray image is digitized by the video camera digital system described in Section 2.5.1.5?

To answer this question, we first take the Fourier transform of this perfect trace, which gives its spatial frequency spectrum (Fig. 2.10B). If this frequency spectrum is multiplied by the MTF of the imaging system shown in Figure 2.10C, frequency

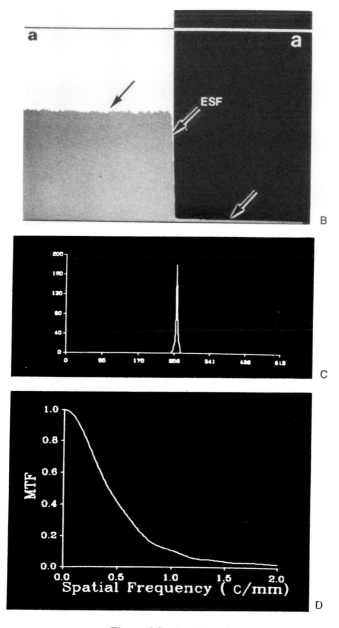

Figure 2.8 (*continued*)

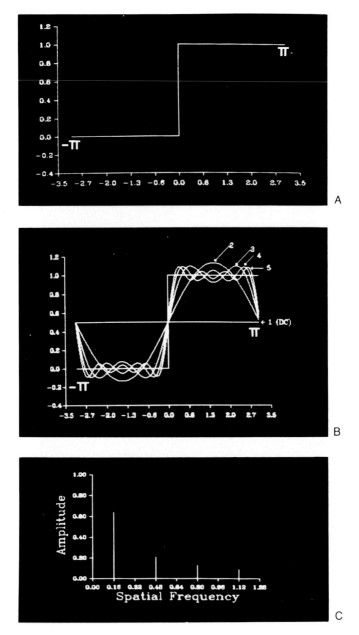

Figure 2.9 Sinusodial functions representation of a step function. (A) The step function. (B) Partial sums of sinusodial functions; numerals correspond to the terms described in Eq. (2.15). (C) Amplitude spectrum of the step function.

by frequency, the result is the output frequency response of the trace (Figure 2.10D) obtained with this digital imaging system. It is seen from Figure 2.10B and 2.10D that there is no phase shift; that is, all the zero crossings are identical between the input and the output spectra. The output frequency spectrum has been modulated to compensate for the imperfect video camera digital imaging system. The inverse Fourier transform of this modulated output frequency spectrum (Fig. 2.10D) is the expected trace of the image due to the imperfection of the video camera digital imaging system. Figure 2.10E shows the expected trace. Figure 2.10F is the super-position of the perfect and the expected traces. It is seen that both corners in the expected trace lose their sharpness.

This completes the description of how the concepts of point spread function, line spread function, edge spread function, and modulation transfer function can be used to measure the unsharpness of an image. The concept of using the MTF to predict the unsharpness due to an imperfect system has also been introduced.

2.5.2 Measurement of Noise

MTF is often used as a measure of the quality of the imaging system, although by definition it is only a measure of a single optical characteristic of an imaging system, namely, the ability to reproduce fine details. It provides no information regarding the effect of noise and radiological contrast on the image. Since both these parameters affect detail visibility only, high modulation transfer values do not necessarily result in a good diagnostic quality image if the noise level is high. The study of the noise that arises from quantum statistics, electronic noise, and film grain represents another measure on the image quality. To study the noise, we need the concept of the power spectrum, or Wiener spectrum, of noise produced by an imaging system. Let us make the assumption that all the noise N is random and does not correlate with the signals S that form the image; then the signal-to-noise power ratio spectrum, or the signal-to-noise power ratio $P(x,y)$, of each pixel is defined by

$$P(x,y) = \frac{S^2(x,y)}{N^2(x,y)} \tag{2.16}$$

Figure 2.11 illustrates signal and the associated random noise in a line trace on an image of uniform background.

A high signal-to-noise ratio (SNR) means that the image is less noisy. A common method increasing the SNR (i.e., reducing the noise in the image) is to take many images of the same object and average them. This, in a sense, minimizes the contribution of the random noise to the image. If M images are averaged, then the average signal-to-noise power ratio $P(x,y)$ becomes

$$\bar{P}(x,y) = \frac{M^2 S^2(x,y)}{M \, N^2(x,y)} = M \, P(x,y) \tag{2.17}$$

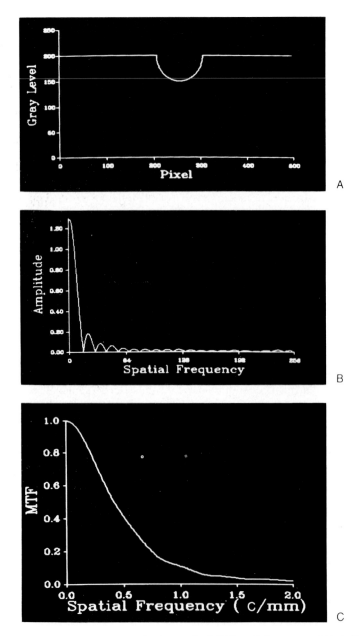

Figure 2.10 Relationship between the input, the MTF, and the output. (A) A line profile from a lateral view of a circular cylinder from a perfect imaging system. (B) The spatial frequency spectrum of (A). (C) MTF of the imaging system described in Figure 2.8D. (D) The output frequency response (*B* X *C*). (E) The predicted line trace from the imperfect imaging system obtained by an inverse Fourier transform of (D). (F) Superposition of (A) and (E) showing the rounding of the edges (arrows) due to the imperfect imaging system.

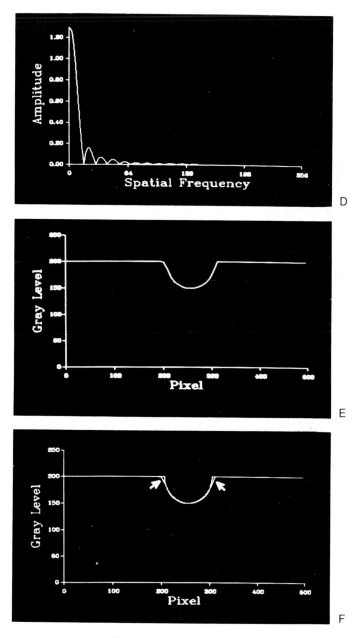

Figure 2.10 *(continued)*

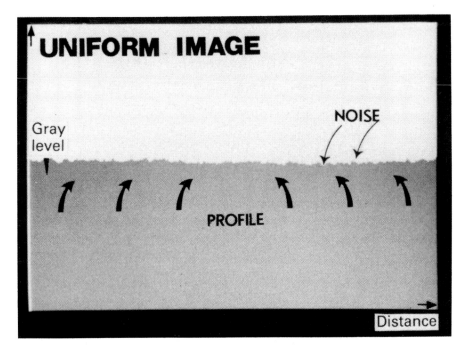

Figure 2.11 Example demonstrating signal and noise in a line trace on a uniform background image (white). The small variation along the profile is the noise. If there had been no noise, the line trace would have been a straight line.

The signal-to-noise ratio is the square root of the power ratio

$$SNR(x,y) = \sqrt{\bar{P}(x,y)} = \sqrt{M}\sqrt{P(x,y)} \qquad (2.18)$$

Therefore, the signal-to-noise ratio increases by the square root of the number of images averaged.

Equation (2.18) indicates that it is possible to increase the signal-to-noise ratio of the image by this averaging technique. The average image will have less noise and a smoother visual appearance. For each pixel, the noise $N(x,y)$, defined in Eq. (2.16), can be approximated by using the standard deviation between the average image and the image under consideration.

Figure 2.12 illustrates how the signal-to-noise ratio of the imaging system is computed. Take a chest X-ray image, digitize it with an imaging system M times, and average the results. If we assume that the signal is the average image $f(x,y)$ (Fig. 2.12B), and the noise of each pixel (x,y) can be approximated by the standard deviation between f_i and f, where f_i is a digitized image, and $1 \le i \le M$, then the signal-to-noise ratio for each pixel can be computed by using Eqs. (2.16) and (2.18). Figure 2.12 shows a digitized image $f_i(x,y)$, the average image $f(x,y)$ with $M = 16$, and the difference image between $f_i(x,y)$ and $f(x,y)$. The difference image (Fig. 2.12C) shows a faint image of the chest, demonstrating that the noise in the imaging system is not random.

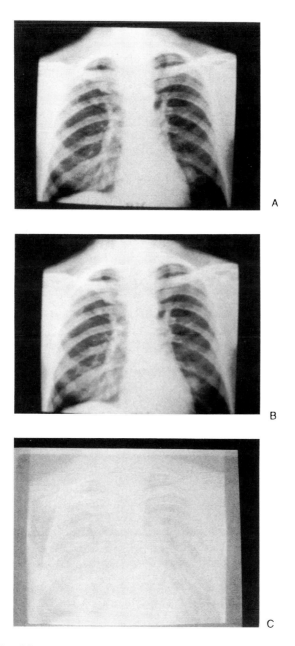

Figure 2.12 The differences in a digitized X-ray chest image before and after averaging. (A) Chest X-ray film digitized with a TV camera. (B) Digital image of the same chest X-ray film digitized 16 times and then averaged. (C) Subtraction of (B) from (A).

CHAPTER

3

Image Acquisition I: Conventional Projection Radiography

3.1 Principles of Conventional Projection Radiography

Conventional projection radiography accounts for 70% of the total number of diagnostic imaging procedures. Therefore, to transform radiology from a film-based to a digital-based operation, we must understand conventional projection radiographic procedures and methods of digitizing radiographic films. This chapter discusses these two topics.

3.1.1 Some Standard Procedures Used in Conventional Projection Radiography

Conventional X-ray imaging procedures are used in all subspecialties of a radiology department, including neuroradiology, emergency, pediatric, mammography, chest, genitourinary, gastrointestinal, cardiovascular, and musculoskeletal. Although the detailed procedures differ within each subspecialty, the basic procedures can be summarized as follows:

1. Check patient X-ray requisition for anatomical area of interest for imaging.
2. Set patient in position for X-ray examination, and set the X-ray collimator to adjust for the size of the exposed area.
3. Select a proper film–screen cassette.
4. Place cassette in the holder located behind or on the examination table under the patient.
5. Determine X-ray exposure factors for obtaining the best quality image with minimum exposure.

6. Expose the patient to obtain a latent image on the film–screen cassette.
7. Process the exposed film through a film processor.
8. Retrieve the developed film from the film processor.
9. Inspect the radiograph through a light box for proper exposure or other errors (e.g., patient movement).
10. Repeat steps 3–9 if the image on the film is unacceptable for diagnosis. Always keep in mind that the patient should not be subjected to unnecessary additional exposure.
11. Submit the film to a radiologist for review.
12. Remove the patient from the table after the radiologist has determined that the quality of the radiograph is acceptable for diagnosis.
13. Release the patient.

Figure 3.1 shows a standard setup of a conventional radiographic procedure room and a diagnostic area. The numbers in the figure correspond to the preceding steps.

3.1.1.1 The Effect of kVp, mA, and mAs Settings on the Appearance of a Radiograph

The radiographic image consists of structural patterns of various shades of gray. The degree of difference in shades of gray between selected areas on the images is referred to as the *image contrast*. Image contrast, in turn, is a function of the following parameters:

subject contrast
film contrast
x-ray scatter
film fog level

Subject contrast is defined as the relative difference in X-ray intensity transmitted through an anatomical structural or an object compared to other surrounding structures. It is affected by the inherent physical properties of the object under consideration—for example, effective atomic number, density, and object thickness. Subject contrast is also affected by extrinsic conditions: kVp, mA, and mAs settings, which are controlled by the X-ray examination procedure.

This section discusses these extrinsic conditions and their effect on the appearance of a radiographic image. The properties of film contrast and fog level, the characteristic curve of an X-ray film, and the effects of scatter are discussed in subsequent sections.

Before we consider the X-ray transmitted through an object, let us review the effects of kVp, mA, and mAs on the X-ray fluence (number of photons/unit area) incident on the surface of the object. X-ray fluence can be broken down into two components: the quantity (intensity of number) of X-ray photons and the quality (energy spectrum) of the X-ray photons. The quantity of the X-ray fluence incident on the subject is approximately proportional to:

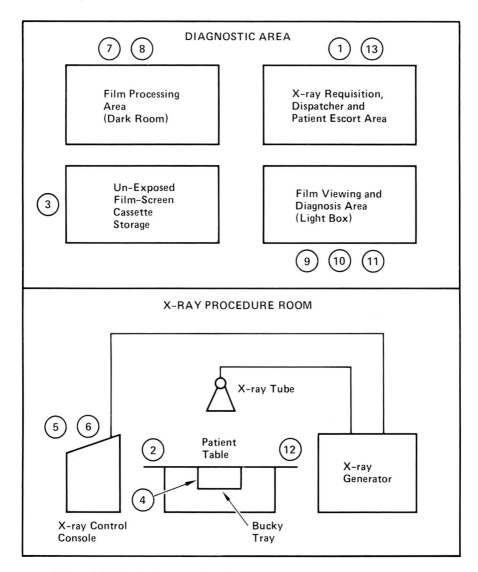

Figure 3.1   Standard setup of a radiographic procedure and diagnostic area.

the square of the X-ray tube kilovolt potential difference $(kVp)^2$
the X-ray tube current, in milliamperes (mA)
the X-ray exposure time, in seconds (s)

Subject contrast results when the fraction of photons absorbed in one area of the object is different from that absorbed in adjacent areas. The fraction of photons absorbed is called the absorption coefficient A and is a function of two variables—

the property of the material with which the photons interact and the energies of the interacting photons:

$$A = (Z,E) \tag{3.1}$$

where Z is the atomic number of the material and E is the X-ray photon energy.

For example, the absorption coefficients of bone and soft tissue plotted as a function of energy diverge at lower X-ray energies and then converge at higher energies. This implies that a radiograph at a lower kVp will have a greater contrast between the bone and soft tissue than a radiograph of the same area acquired at a higher kVp. In general, a low kVp technique will produce a higher contrast image and a high kVp technique will produce a lower contrast image. However, most photons from an exposure taken at a low energy setting (low kVp) will be absorbed by the patient, hence will not penetrate through the patient. As a result, they cannot contribute to the formation of the image.

The tube current (mA), the time of exposure (s), or the product of the two (milliampere-seconds: mAs) will contribute to the number of photons entering and leaving the patient. Therefore these are the factors determining the degree of darkness on the film. A low mAs setting may not have enough X-ray photons to form a good image (underexposed), and a high mAs setting may overexpose the film. If we increase the mAs in a procedure, an increased number of X-ray photons will reach the film-screen. This will result in an increase in the exposure to this film, causing a darker appearance of the image. Thus, the darkening of the film is affected by both the kVp and the mAs.

3.1.1.2 Methods of Reducing X-Ray Scatter

So far the discussion of radiographic image contrast has been oversimplified because scattered radiation has not been considered. When X-ray photons travel through the patient, they are scattered, and the result is a radiograph with relatively low image contrast. Scattered X-ray photons tend to blur an image, since the actual location of the photon is misrepresented. For example, in chest radiography, the contribution to the film exposure from scattered X-ray photons can be equal to or greater than from the primary photons.

Scattered radiation is a primary cause of poor image quality in radiology. Methods of removing scattered X-rays generally result in increased patient exposure. Factors affecting the amount of scatter include kVp, patient thickness, and X-ray field size, which can be defined as follows:

1. *kVp:* the amount of scattered photons contributing to the image is a function of kVp because (a) higher kVp results in greater percentage of Compton scattering interaction versus photoelectric interaction and (b) higher energy photons undergoing Compton scattering tend to scatter more in the forward direction (onto the image receptor or film–screen).
2. *Patient thickness:* an increase in patient thickness increases the probability of Compton interaction before the photon can exit the patient.

3. *Field size:* the larger the X-ray field size, the greater the amount of scatter will be (plateau reached at approximately 30 cm × 30 cm field). The X-ray field size is an important factor for controlling scatter radiation. Smaller field sizes have the advantage of reducing patient dose.

There are several methods of minimizing the scattered photon contribution to the image; among these is the use of a radiographic grid. Invented by Gustave Bucky in 1913, the radiographic grid is still the most effective way to minimize scatter. The physical construction consists of lead foil strips separated by X-ray transparent spacers. The lead absorbs the scattered X-ray photons, thus degrading radiographic image contrast.

Several parameters are used to characterize a radiographic grid: the grid ratio, the focal range, the number of lines per millimeter, and mass of lead per unit area. The grid ratio is defined as the ratio of the height of the lead strips to the distance between them. An increase in this ratio decreases the amount of scattered photons reaching the film–screen cassette, hence increases the image contrast.

The focal range is the range of distances between the X-ray focal spot and grid, at which point the divergence of the X-ray beam matches the lead strip divergence. Using the grid outside the recommended focal range results in fewer primary photons reaching the film–screen cassette. A higher value on lines/mm and/or mass of lead/area in the grid reduces the amount of scatter; but at the same time, the procedure will require a higher exposure.

3.1.2 Image Receptor
3.1.2.1 Screen–Film Combination

The X-ray photons exiting the patient carry with them the information necessary to make an image; the problem is that they cannot be visualized by the human eyes. This information must be converted into a latent image, which in turn can be transformed into a visual image.

The common image receptor used in diagnostic radiology is the film–screen combination consisting of a double-emulsion, radiation-sensitive film between two intensifying screens housed inside a lighttight cassette (Fig. 3.2). The X-ray film consists of a transparent (polyethylene terephthalate) plastic substrate called the base, which is coated on both sides by an emulsion of silver halide crystals suspended with a gelatin medium. A slight blue tint is commonly incorporated in the base to give the radiograph a pleasing appearance. A photographic emulsion can be exposed to X-rays directly, but it is more sensitive to light photons of much less energy (≈ 2.5–5 eV).

The intensifying screen, which is made of a phosphor (e.g., crystalline calcium tungstate), is more sensitive to the diagnostic X-ray energy (20–90 keV). The X-ray photons exiting the patient impinge onto an intensifying screen, and the visible light given off by the screen exposes the film. X-ray photons that are not absorbed by the front screen in the cassette can be absorbed by the back screen. The light emitted from this second screen then exposes the emulsion on the back side of the film. The

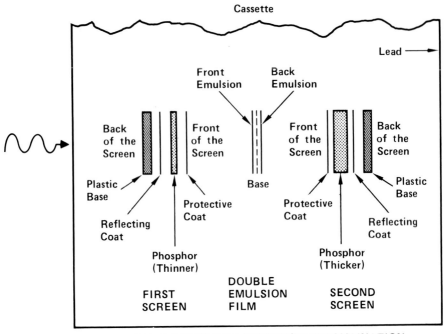

PHYSICAL SET UP OF A SCREEN/FILM COMBINATION

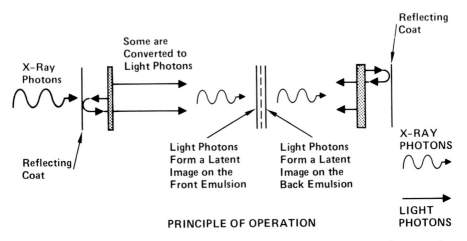

PRINCIPLE OF OPERATION

Figure 3.2   Schematic of a film–screen cassette and the formation of a latent image on the film. (Distances between materials are used for illustration purposes, materials are actually in contact with each other.)

double-emulsion film thus can effectively reduce the patient exposure by half. With the film–screen as the image detector, the patient receives much lower exposure than is the case when film alone is used. Image blur due to patient motion can also be minimized with a shorter exposure time.

Calcium tungstate phosphor was used in most screens until about 1971. New technology with rare earth phosphors has resulted in a more sensitive screen. Figure 3.2, which presents a sectional view of the film–screen cassette, also shows its interaction with X-ray photons.

Formation of Latent Image

The formation of the latent image on the film, called the *photographic effect,* is not well understood. The Gurney–Mott theory, summarized here, is an accepted, though incomplete, explanation of the latent image formation, which remains a topic of research.

The visible light photon output from the intensifying screen is absorbed by the photographic emulsion primarily by the photoelectric interaction of light photons with atoms of the silver halide crystals. These crystals consist of silver (Ag^+), bromine (Br^-), and iodine (I^-) ions, with about 90–99% silver bromide and 10–1% silver iodide suspended in the emulsion. Each crystal (grain) is about $1–2$ μm in size. When X-ray film is exposed to light photons, electrons from the bromide ion are given enough energy to escape the ion. The free electrons move through the crystal and are trapped in one of the crystal defects called a *sensitivity speck.* The crystal has other defects called *point defects,* which are responsible for photographic sensitivity. Point defects consist of silver ions that migrate through the crystal. When one silver ion mates with an electron in a sensitivity speck, the ion becomes a neutralized metallic silver atom.

$$Ag^+ + e^- \rightarrow Ag \tag{3.2}$$

This process can be repeated in another crystal, in the same crystal within the same sensitivity speck, or in a different speck. More than one silver atom can exist within a sensitivity speck. A sensitivity speck is called a *latent image center* if it contains at least two silver atoms. Any crystal within the emulsion can have more than one latent image center, and this process of latent image formation can occur within any crystal in the emulsion.

Development of X-Ray Film

The development process of an exposed X-ray film consists of the following steps.

Developer. The basic reaction of the developer is to change the remaining silver ions, within a single crystal (grain), into silver atoms. Developers act as a supply of electrons, which become entrapped inside a sensitivity speck in the emulsion. Once within a sensitivity speck, the migrating silver ions can attach and reduce to a silver atom, as described in Eq. (3.2). This is the same physical phenomenon that occurs in crystals during exposure to light or X-ray photons. The speed of this reaction depends on the number of silver atoms within a latent image center and the number of latent image centers formed during exposure to light or X-ray photons. Therefore, time is a fundamental factor in the development process. Development should be discontinued when the ratio between the number of exposed, developed crystals to the number of unexposed, undeveloped crystals reaches a maximum.

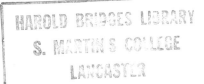

Fixing.   The fixing step removes remaining undeveloped silver halide crystals. If film is not fixed properly, it will appear cloudy because the remaining silver halide crystals act to disperse light.

Washing.   Washing removes developing and fixing agents from the emulsion.

Drying.   Drying removes water from the emulsion.

Film Optical Density

The number of developed crystals per unit volume in the developed film will determine the fraction of light that can be transmitted through the unit volume. This transmission of light is referred to as the optical density of the film in that unit volume. Technically, the optical density (OD) is defined as the logarithm base 10 of 1 reciprocal transmittance of a unit intensity of light:

$$OD = \log_{10}\left(\frac{1}{\text{transmittance}}\right) \tag{3.3}$$

$$= \log_{10}\left(\frac{I_0}{I_t}\right)$$

where I_0 = light intensity before transmission through the film
          I_t = light intensity after transmission through the film

The film optical density is used to represent the degree of film darkening due to X-ray exposure.

Characteristic Curve of X-Ray Film

The relationship between X-ray exposure and film optical density is called the *characteristic curve* or the *H and D curve* (after F. Hurter and V. C. Driffield, who first published such a curve in England in 1890). The logarithm of relative exposure is plotted instead of the exposure itself, partly because it compresses a large linear segment to a manageable logarithm scale, which makes analysis of the curve easier. An idealized curve (Fig. 3.3) shows three linear segments.

The first linear region, the toe, is called the based density or the base-plus-fog level (usually OD = 0.12–0.20). For very low exposures, the film optical density remains at the fog level and is independent of exposure level. Next is a linear segment over which the optical density and the logarithm of relative exposure are linearly related (usually between OD 0.3 and 2.2). In the third segment, the shoulder corresponds to high exposures or overexposures: in this case, most of the silver halide converted to metallic silver (usually OD 3.2). The film becomes saturated, and the optical density is no longer a function of exposure level.

The characteristic curve is usually described by the following parameters:

the film gamma
the average gradient
the film latitude
the film speed

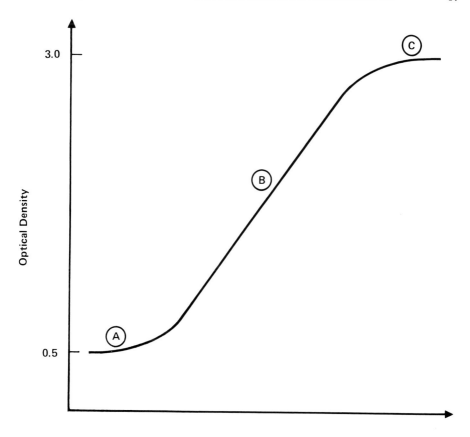

LOG RELATIVE EXPOSURE ON FILM

Figure 3.3   Relationship between logarithm of relative X-ray exposure and film optical density plotted as a curve, the characteristic curve or the H and D curve; see text for discussion of points A–C.

The film gamma (γ) is the maximum slope of the characteristic curve, and is described by the formula:

$$\gamma = \frac{D_2 - D_1}{\log_{10}E_2 - \log_{10}E_1} \tag{3.4}$$

where D_2 = highest OD value within the steepest portion of the curve (B in Fig. 3.3)
D_1 = lowest OD value within the steepest portion of curve
E_2 = exposure responsible for D_2
E_1 = exposure responsible for D_1

The average gradient of the characteristic curve is the slope of the characteristic curve calculated between optical density 0.25 and 2.00 above base plus fog level for radiographic films. This optical density range of 0.25–2.00 is considered acceptable for diagnostic radiology. For example, assuming a base and fog level of 0.15, the range of acceptable optical density is therefore 0.40–2.15. The average gradient can be represented by the following formula:

$$\text{average gradient} = \frac{D_2 - D_1}{\log_{10}E_2 - \log_{10}E_1} \tag{3.5}$$

where D_2 = 2.00 + base and fog level
             D_1 = 0.25 + base and fog level
             E_2 = exposure responsible for D_2
             E_1 = exposure responsible for D_1

The film latitude describes the range of exposures used in the average gradient calculation. Thus, as described in Eq. (3.5), the film latitude is equal to $\log_{10}E_2 - \log_{10}E_1$.

The film speed (unit: 1/roentgen) can be defined as follows:

$$\text{speed} = \frac{1}{E} \tag{3.6}$$

where E is the exposure (in roentgens) required to produce a film optical density of 1.0 above base and fog. Generally speaking

1. The latitude of a film varies inversely with film contrast, film speed, film gamma, and average gradient.
2. Film gamma and average gradient of a film vary directly with film contrast.
3. Film fog level varies inversely with film contrast.
4. Faster films require less exposure to achieve a specific density than slower films.

Large-Latitude Film

A film may have a latitude value that does not cover the range of exposures required in a certain imaging application. Therefore, a film with a larger latitude may be required. Large-latitude film can be helpful in imaging of the thorax area because X-ray photons passing through the mediastinum are attenuated to a much greater extent than those passing through the lungs.

If the range of exposures within an area to be imaged is too wide for the entire linear portion of the film response, pertinent image information will fall into the toe and shoulder of the characteristic curve. The results is an inaccurate portrayal, since the information in the toe and shoulder regions has low contrast resolution. The solution is to use a film that has a linear region that covers a much wider range of exposures. Such a medium is referred to as large- or wide-latitude film.

3.1.2.2 Image Intensifier Tube

Another image receptor used very often in projection radiography is the image intensifier tube. The image intensifier tube is particularly useful for fluorographic

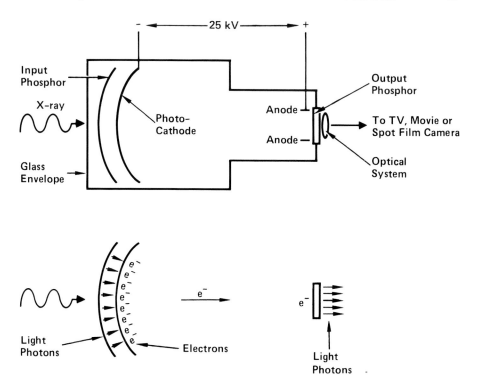

Figure 3.4   Schematic of the image intensifier tube and the formation of an image on the output screen.

procedures, which allow imaging of moving structures and dynamic processes in real time. Although X-ray films exposed close together in time can provide some information about these structures and processes, the use of an image intensifier can maximize the information available from the study and minimize the X-ray exposure to the patient. An image intensifier tube is shown schematically in Figure 3.4.

The X-rays, exiting the patient, enter the image intensifier tube through the glass envelope and are absorbed in the input phosphor intensifying screen. The input screen converts X-ray photons to light photons. The light emitted from the screen next strikes the light-sensitive photocathode, causing the emission of photo-electrons. These electrons are then accelerated across the tube (by approximately 25,000 V) and strike the output screen. In this way, the variance of the X-ray pattern caused by the attenuation of the patient is converted into a variance of electron density. This stream of electrons is focused and converges upon another screen called the output phosphor. At the time the electrons are absorbed by the output phosphor, the image information carried by the electron stream is once again converted to light of greater brightness than the light output from the input phosphor, hence the term image intensifier. This brightness gain in an image intensifier is the product of two gains:

- *Minification gain:* the light intensity increases by a factor equal to the ratio of the areas between the input and output phosphors. The minification gain for an image intensifier with a 10-inch-diameter input phosphor and a 1-inch-diameter output phosphor is 100.
- *Flux gain:* each light photon emitted by the input phosphor will result in the generation of many light photons exiting the output phosphor. On average, this gain of light photons is about 50.

Therefore the brightness gain for this image intensifier is approximately $100 \times 50 = 5000$.

Image intensifiers are generally listed by the diameter of the input phosphor, ranging from 4.5 to 14 inches. The light from the output phosphor is then coupled to an optical system for detection using a movie camera, a TV camera, or a spot film camera.

3.2 X-Ray Film Scanner

Since 70% of the radiographic procedures still use film as an output medium, it is necessary to investigate methods to convert images from films into digital format. This section discusses film scanners of different types: video camera, drum scanner, solid state camera, and laser scanner. For a summary of operating characteristics, see Table 3.1, at the end of Section 3.2.4.

To understand the specification and operational procedure of these scanners, it is necessary to use the concept of sampling. As described in Chapter 2, when a radiographic film is digitized, the shades of gray in the film are quantized into a two-dimensional array of nonnegative integers called pixels or samples. The gray level values of these pixels must represent the radiographic image favorably, to allow us to reconstruct completely the original image from them. The well-known sampling theorem states that:

> If the Fourier transform of the image $f(x,y)$ vanishes for all u,v where $|u| \geq 2f_N$, $|v| \geq 2f_N$, then $f(x,y)$ can be exactly reconstructed from samples of its nonzero values taken $\frac{1}{2}f_N$ apart or closer. The frequency $2f_N$ is called the Nyquist frequency.

The theorem implies that if the samples are taken more than $\frac{1}{2}f_N$ apart, it will not be possible to reconstruct completely the images from these samples. The difference between the original image and the image reconstructed from these samples is caused by aliasing error. The aliasing artifact creates new frequency components in the reconstructed image, which are called moiré patterns. Examples of moiré patterns created by the laser scanning on radiographic films are given in later sections.

3.2.1 Video Scanning System

A video scanner system consists of three major components: a scanning device (video camera) that scans the X-ray film, an analog/digital converter that converts the video signals from the camera to gray level values, and an image memory to store the digital signals from the A/D converter.

3.2.1.1 Video Camera

The television camera is a well-known technology. The device (Fig. 3.5) consists of a camera tube, focusing and deflecting coils, an optical system, and the associated electronics. The camera tube is a cylindrical glass envelope containing an electron gun (cathode) at one end and a target and faceplate at the other (anode). The tube is surrounded by a yoke containing magnetic focus and deflecting coils. The faceplate is coated on the inside with a thin transparent metal film called the signal plate, which is charged to about $+25$ V.

Next is a thin layer of photoconductive material that forms the target. The name varies depending on the type of photoconductor used as the target material, for example, vidicon,* Saticon, Newvicon, plumbicon, image-orthicon. Behind the target is a positively charged (250 V) fine wire mesh.

Consider what happens when the camera is turned on with the lens cap on (no light) and an electron beam from the cathode is attracted to the anode. The beam scans the target line by line from left to right and top to bottom, reaches the bottom of the target, and retraces its path by moving back to the top, repeating the scanning pattern. During the scan, electrons decelerate after passing through the wire mesh and are deposited on the inside of the target. The photoconductor, at this point, appears as many capacitors with negative charges inside and positive charges (metal film) outside (adjacent to the faceplate) (see Fig. 3.5, A).

When the cap of the camera lens is opened and light strikes the photoconductor, photoelectrons pass through the photoconductor and neutralize the positive charge on the metal film. As a result, electrons at the inside of the target plate are expelled and an electron image is formed on the back of the target (Fig. 3.5, B). Depending on the amount of light striking the target, electrons are present in the dark areas and proportionally absent in the light areas.

Meanwhile, the electron beam of the camera continuously scans the target. It replaces the lost electrons and restores the uniform surface charge. As the electrons are replaced, a current flows in the external target circuit. This current is proportional to the number of electrons required to restore the uniform charge, and therefore to the light intensity at that point. It is also proportional to the electron beam velocity, which in turn determines the time available for the charge to flow. Current variations in the target circuit produce video signals representing the image (Fig. 3.5, C).

The standard video signal is the EIA (Electronic Industries Association) RS 170, which has 525 video lines. This standard video signal consists of synchronization signals, blanking (retracing of the electron beam), and the actual waveform of the current, which forms the image. If this video signal is connected to a TV monitor, it will appear as a video image. The 1050-line system (i.e., a video image consisting of 1050 lines) is also used for film digitizing.

---

* In this book, the term "vidicon" often designates the camera itself.

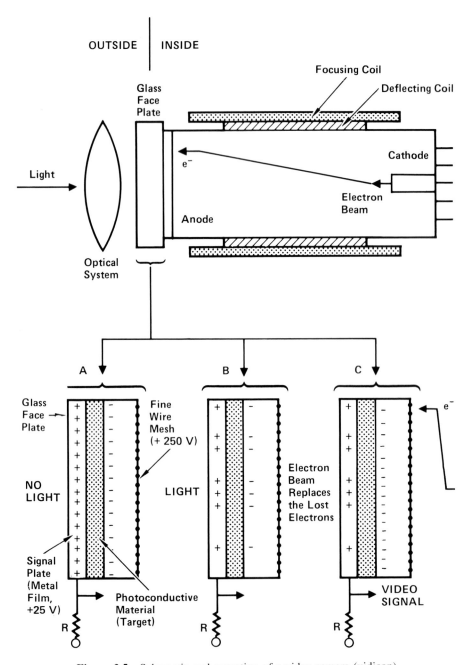

Figure 3.5 Schematic and operation of a video camera (vidicon).

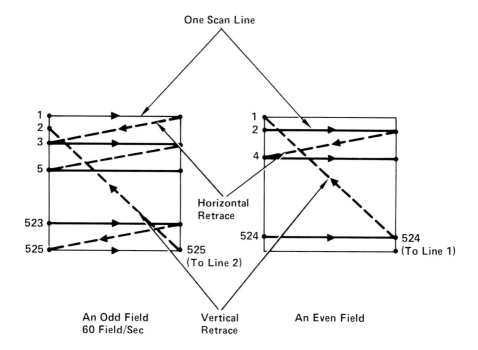

INTERLACED SCANNING — FOR MINIMIZING FLICKERING

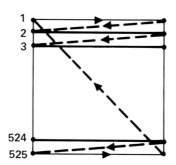

PROGRESSIVE SCANNING — FOR PULSED MODE DIGITAL FLUOROGRAPHY

Figure 3.6 Some terminology used in video scanning.

3.2.1.2 Terminology Used in Video Scanning

This section discusses the terminology used in video scanning based on the nomen-clature of the Radio-Electronics-Television Manufacturers Association (RETMA). Figure 3.6 illustrates some of these terms.

A *TV Frame* consists of consecutive video scanning lines that compose the image. The most popular standard is 525 lines per frame. A *TV field* is half a TV frame and consists of alternate scanning lines in a frame. Thus, an even field consists of all even lines in a frame and an odd field consists of all odd lines. Another important term is *interlaced scanning*. In a 2:1 interlaced scan, the electron beam first scans all odd lines in an image and then all even lines. The procedure is then repeated. That is, the interlaced scan first produces an odd field and then an even field, and so forth. Using this terminology, a 2:1 interlaced scan produces 262½ lines per field.

Thus, the specifications 2:1 interlace $^{525}/_{60}$ means that the electron beam scans an image with 2:1 interlace, the total number of lines in the frame is 525, and each field consists of 262½ lines and is scanning with the speed of $^{1}/_{60}$ second per field. An interlaced scan is used to minimize perceived flicker or individual flash of light detected by the eyes when the scan speed is less than 50 fields per second. It is a tradeoff between accepting a lower spatial resolution (field) and avoiding perceived flickering (60 field/s).

Progressive scanning is a mode in which the electron beam scans every consecutive line instead of every other line. Progressive scanning is used in most high resolution display systems. It is clear that in progressive scanning, the electron beam scans every line of the image, whereas in the interlaced mode the electron beam scans every other line.

Bandpass (*bandwidth*) is the frequency range of an imaging system that the electronic components or the video scanning system is designed to transmit. For example, in a 525-line system, the highest resolution the system can handle is 262½ line pairs in the horizontal scanning direction. The highest frequency signal this video scanning system has to carry per second is 4,134,375 (262.5 × 525 × 30). Therefore, to transmit the signal accurately, the electronic components in this scanning system should have a bandpass of at least 4.13 MHz. In practice, the requirement for a 525-line system is about 4.5 MHz.

Finally, we come to the *Kell factor*. In a television scanning system, the vertical spatial resolution of a 525-line system is about 370 lines, which is less than the horizontal spatial resolution (525 pixels or 262½ line pairs). The ratio between the vertical resolution and the number of scan lines of the system is called the Kell factor, which in this case is about 0.7 ($^{370}/_{525}$).

3.2.1.3 Analog-to-Digital (A/D) Conversion

To digitize an X-ray film with a video camera, it is necessary to convert the video signal obtained from the camera into digital numbers. This procedure is called analog-to-digital (A/D) conversion. Most A/D converters today are real-time devices; this means that they can digitize 30 frames of video signals in one second. Consider the 525-line system with a bandwidth of 4.5 MHz: to achieve real-time operation, the minimum A/D conversion time per pixel is about 220 nanoseconds (ns).

Most of the A/D converters for video scanning are 8-bit units; this means that the entire range of the video signals can be converted to 256 gray levels. Because of the inherent characteristics of the video signals, however, it is difficult to obtain meaningful gray levels of more than 128. As a result, the video digitization gives only about 7 bits of true information. This low density resolution capability means that video scanning should not be used to digitize X-ray films that require more than 128 gray levels. For example, it will not be adequate to use a video camera to digitize a full-scale chest X-ray film and hope that it can preserve all the optical density information of the chest X-ray. The advantages of a video camera are low cost and high speed: it can digitize an X-ray film to $512 \times 512 \times 8$ bits in $\frac{1}{30}$ second.

3.2.1.4 Digital Image of an X-Ray Film from Video Scanning

The last component in a complete video digitizer, the image memory, generally is attached to the A/D converter in the electronic circuitry. While the electron beam continues scanning the target and the video camera gives out video signals, the A/D converter also continuously converts the video signal to gray levels. Each gray level value is then stored in the image memory as a pixel. When the electron beam finishes a complete scan, the image memory will have a $525 \times 525 \times 8$ image. Since the electron beam and the A/D converter continue scanning and digitizing the film concurrently even after a complete frame has been formed, the gray level value in the image memory is continuously updated until either the scanning or the digitizing process stops.

The image stored in the image memory is the digital representation of the X-ray film obtained by using the video camera. If the image memory is connected to digital-to-analog conversion circuitry, which again connects to a TV monitor, this image can be displayed on the monitor (which is the video image) or as soft copy (i.e., an X-ray film). The image memory can be connected to an image processing system or a computer with a peripheral storage device for long-term image archive. Figure 3.7 shows a block diagram of a film scanner. The digital chain is a standard component of all film scanners.

3.2.2 Drum Scanner

The drum scanner is a mechanical device that consists of a rotating drum, a light source, and a photodetector. An X-ray film is wrapped around a drum and clamped to it, to ensure that the film adheres exactly to the cylindrical surface of the drum. For the transmission type of scanning, the light source inside the drum transmitted through the film attached to the transparent drum is measured by a photodetector located outside the drum and converted to a gray level value. Most drum scanners can measure a small area (12.5–400 μm) and convert the optical density in the film to more than 256 levels. A drum scanner can be used to obtain high spatial resolution digital images from X-ray films.

The disadvantages of a drum scanner are slow scanning speed and the difficulty of aligning the X-ray film in the drum. A typical digitizing speed is from about 35,000 to 60,000 pixels per second. An example of a drum scanner is the System P-1000 photoscan by Optronics International, Inc. (Chelmsford, MA). The digital image from the drum scanner can be transferred directly to a host computer or output to a magnetic tape for off-line storage.

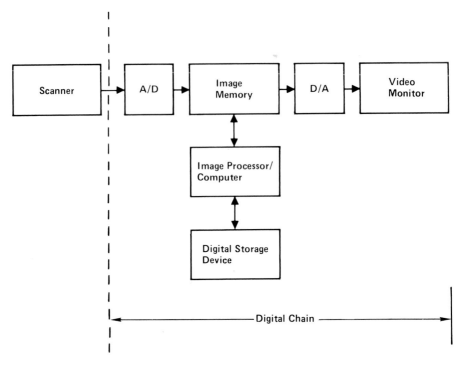

Figure 3.7 Block diagram of a film scanner.

3.2.3 Solid State Camera

A solid state imaging scanner made of charge-coupled devices (CCDs) can be used as film digitizer. Its quality is comparable to or better than that of the TV camera as described in Section 3.2.1.1. Just like the vidicon, a solid state camera consists of three major components: a photodetector, the associated circuitry, and an image memory. When a light box is used to illuminate an X-ray film, the transmitted light photons through the X-ray film are detected by the photodetector, which converts the light photons to electrons. The associated circuitry carries the electric signals to an A/D converter and forms a digital image in the image memory. Photodetectors of two types are used as the image sensor: photodiode arrays and CCDs.

3.2.3.1 Photodiode

A photodiode is a solid state p-n junction that generates electrons when exposed to light. During operation, the junction is reverse-biased and exhibits a high imped-ance. The top layer of the device is made very thin, to permit light to penetrate the junction. Impinging photons release electron–hole pairs. In the depletion layer, where the electron field is strong, these mobilized carriers do not recombine but migrate under the influence of the field to create a current in the external circuit.

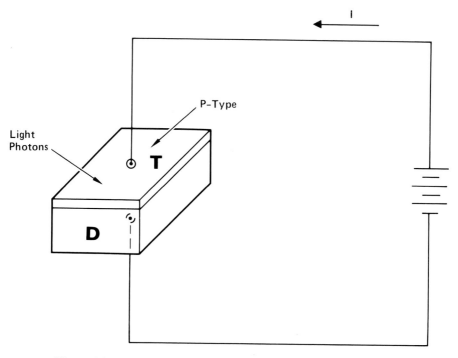

Figure 3.8 Scheme of a photodiode: top layer, T; depletion layer, D.

This current is proportional to the light photon flux. Since the reverse-biased junction presents a high impedance, the current is controlled by light intensity and is relatively independent of the external applied voltage. The depletion layer is made comparatively thick, to capture long wavelength photons. The operation of a photodiode is depicted in Figure 3.8.

3.2.3.2 Charge-Coupled Device

Like the transistor, the charge-coupled device (Fig. 3.9) is a derivative from the concept of semiconductor electronics. As a result of advances in transistor technology, computer memory components are available with thousands of memory elements on a single chip of silicon. Charge-coupling is making possible comparably sized memory components with tens of thousands of memory cells per silicon chip at approximately the same cost.

Charge-coupling is the collective transfer of units of mobile electric charge called *packets*. By means of the external manipulation of voltages, the packets stored within a semiconductor storage element can move to a similar adjacent storage element. The quantity of the stored charge in a packet can vary widely, depending on the applied voltages and on the capacity of the storage element. The amount of electric charge in each packet can represent information. A charge-coupled device possesses at least three components: input, charge-coupling, and output. The use of

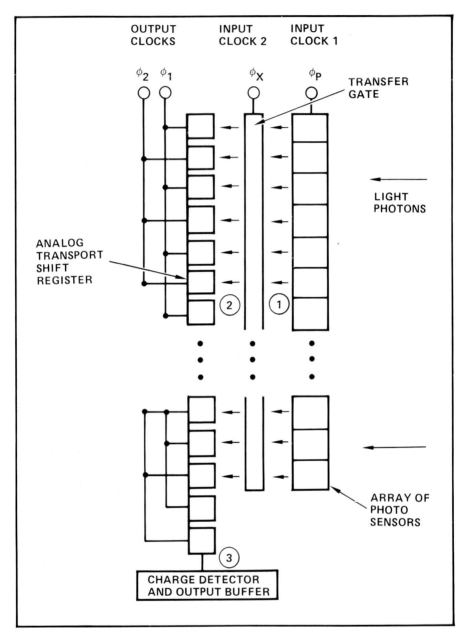

Figure 3.9 CCD linear array sensor: (1) electrons from the photoelectric effect representing the image data are transferred to a transfer gate by a charge coupling (clock ϕ_p); (2) the electrons are further transferred from the transfer gate to a parallel CCD analog transport shift register (clock ϕ_x); (3) one line of image data is transferred to an output buffer serially (clocks ϕ_1, ϕ_2).

CCDs as imaging sensors for digitizing X-ray films is made possible by the following series of events.

Generally, CCDs are fabricated from silicon, and when light photons fall on arrays of densely packed silicon substrate, the photons are absorbed at these photo sites through the photoelectric effect. The result is the generation of electrons in a quantity proportional to the amount of incident light photons. If the pattern of the incident light photons is a focused light image from an optical system viewing an illuminated X-ray film, the charge packets created in these photo site arrays will be a faithful reproduction of the X-ray image. This "electro-optic" creation of electrons represents an input to the CCD.

The packets of electrons generated by the light can be moved to a point of detection (see points 1, 2, and 3 in Fig. 3.9), just as in a shift register, and converted to an electrical signal representative of the X-ray image incident on the device. This signal can be digitized to form a digital image or converted to a standard RS 170 video format and displayed on a TV monitor.

3.2.3.3 Scanning Methods

There are three types of solid state camera: line scan, linear motion, and area scan. Both line scan and linear motion cameras use a solid state linear array as the image sensor, whereas the area scan camera uses a rectangular array. The line scan camera has a stationary photodiode array, and during the scanning, the X-ray film moves across the field of the image sensor. The line-scanning method is very similar to laser scanning, described in Section 3.2.4. The Reticon (EG&G, Sunnyvale, CA) is an example of this type of line scanning using a solid state sensor; it uses up to 4096 photodiodes, with center-to-center distance between photodiodes of about 15 μm.

In the case of the linear motion camera, both the camera and the X-ray films are stationary but the linear array inside the camera moves across the field of view. Figure 3.10 shows the movement of the linear array inside the camera. One commercial linear motion camera is the EIKONIXSCAN 78/99 by Eikonix (Bedford, MA), which can digitize an X-ray film to a 1728 × 2048 × 12 image. Another is the digitizing camera model 322 by Datacopy (Palo Alto, CA), which utilizes 1728 CCD sensors, producing an image up to 1728 × 2592 × 8.

The third type of solid state camera, the area scan camera, has less spatial resolution than the linear array camera but scans with much faster. At present, area sensors do not have sufficient spatial resolution for digitizing X-ray films to diagnostic quality.

3.2.4 Laser Scanner

The principle of laser scanning is as follows. A rotating polygon mirror system is used to guide a collimated low power (5 mW) laser beam (usually helium–neon) to scan across a line of the radiograph in a light tight environment. The radiograph is advanced and the scan is repeated for the second line, and so forth. The optical density of the film is measured from the transmission of the laser through each small

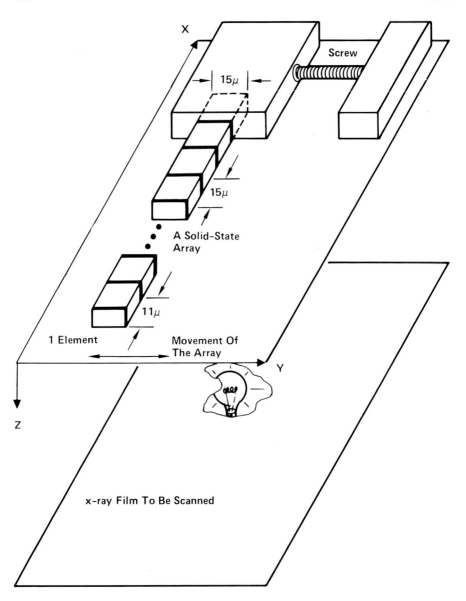

Figure 3.10 Schematic of a solid state linear array inside a linear motion camera. The movement of the array in the y direction is controlled by a lead screw–stepping motor system. The precision of the stepping motor is about 0.75 um. The dimensions of the photodiode array are given. The X-ray film is placed below the linear array and above the light source, perpendicular to the z direction.

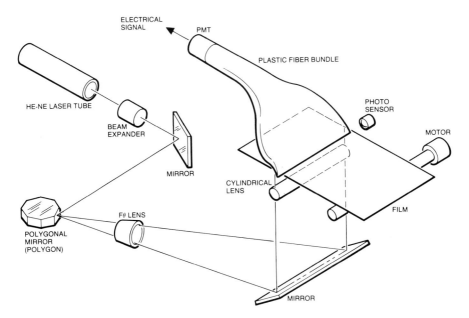

Figure 3.11 Schematic of a laser film scanner.

area (e.g., 175 μm × 175 μm) of the radiograph using a photomultiplier tube (PMT) and a logarithmic amplifier. This electric signal is sent to a digital chain, where it is digitized to 8–12 bits from the A/D. The data are then sent to a computer, which provides a storage device for the image. The scan process can be described as a repetition of the following sequential steps:

1. Laser beam scans one line of the radiograph.
2. Photomultiplier detects light transmission one pixel at a time.
3. Amplifier and signal conditioners perform analog signal processing.
4. Analog-to-digital converter digitizes signal to 8–12 bits.
5. Data controller mediates data transmission to computer.
6. Mechanical transport system moves the film to the next scan line.

Figures 3.11 and 3.12 show the schematic and the block diagram of a laser scanner system. Table 3.1 compares the four different types of film scanner: video, drum, solid state, and laser.

3.3 Digitization

3.3.1 Parameters Affecting the Quality of Digitization

Before a film scanner is ready for use in clinical environments, it is important to evaluate its specifications and to verify the quality of the digitized image. This

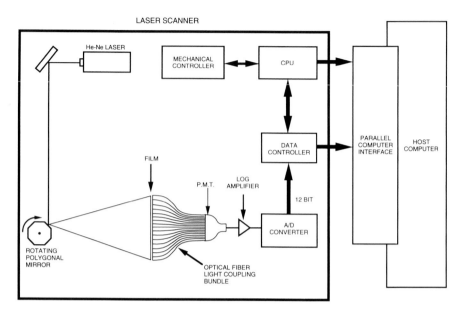

Figure 3.12   Block diagram of a laser film scanner interfacing to a host computer.

section describes some standard tests used routinely to evaluate the quality of a film scanner. The laser scanner described in Table 3.2 is used as an example.

3.3.1.1 Optical Density Versus Gray Level Value

The mapping of optical density to gray level for the laser scanner can be measured by scanning a calibrated Kodak 310-ST-252 photographic step wedge (composed of silver halide particles suspended in a gelatin) and recording the optical density of each step and the resulting digital output value. The quoted accuracy of the step wedge is the larger of ± 0.02 optical density or 2% of the optical density value. The table consists of 21 optical density steps ranging from 0.06 OD to 3.09 OD. A rectangular region consisting of 2000 pixels used for averaging the digital output value for each step should be sufficient.

Figure 3.13, the optical density to gray level transfer curve for the scanner, shows that the digitization of optical density is highly linear over the step wedge range (0.06–2.50 OD). It has a range from 500 to 3500 gray levels over this optical density range. Linearity in this range (0.06–2.50 OD) covers essentially most diagnostic films produced in today's radiology departments.

3.3.1.2 Accuracy of the Laser Scanner Digitization

It is difficult to measure the accuracy of the digital representation of an optical density value because there is no film that is perfectly uniform in optical density and

Table 3.1 Comparison of Film Scanners Specifications

Specification	TV Camera	Solid State (linear motion) Camera	Rotating Drum	Laser Scanner
Pixel size	Variable, depends on the distance between film and camera	Variable, depends on the distance between film and camera (from 3.7 μm to 176 μm)	Adjustable from 25 μm to 400 μm	50–200 μm (laser spot size)
Matrix size	512 $\times$ 512 1024 $\times$ 1024	Variable, 1728 $\times$ 2048 1720 $\times$ 2592	Variable	Variable, 2000 $\times$ 2400
A/D (maximum bits per pixel)	8	8–12	8–12	8–12
Data rate	5–20 MHz (8 bits)	200 kHz to 2 MHz (dependent on bits per pixel)	35–60 kHz (8 bits)	230 kHz (12 bits)
Time to scan one 14 in. $\times$ 17 in. X-ray film	1/30 second (512, 8 bits) 2/15 second (1024, 8 bits)	60 seconds	120 seconds (1024, 8 bits)	75 seconds (2000, 12 bits)
Image quality	Fair	Good	Excellent	Excellent
Adjustments required	Minimum	Yes	Yes	Minimum
Possibility of improvement	Limited	Yes	Limited	Yes
Price	Low	Low	High	High
Easy to use	Yes	Needs occasional calibration	Difficult to adjust alignment and to insert film	Yes

Source: Summary from manufacturers' specifications which can be changed from time to time. The reader should check the performance of the digitizer as suggested in Section 3.3.

Table 3.2 Specifications of a Laser Scanner

Film size supported	14 $\times$ 17, 14 $\times$ 14, 12 $\times$ 14, 10 $\times$ 12, 8 $\times$ 10 (in. $\times$ in.)
Pixel size	From 50 μm to 200 μm
Sampling distance	50, 75, 100, 125, 150, 170, 200 μm
Optical density range	0–2, 0–4
Bits/pixel	12 bits
Hardware interface	SCSI, DR11_W*
Laser power	5 mW
Scanning speed	200 lines/s

* SCSI, small computer systems interface; DR11_W is a parallel iterface protocol.

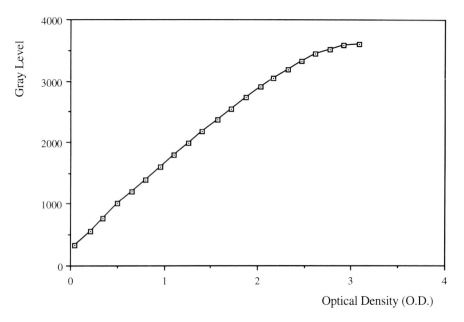

Figure 3.13 Relationship between the input film optical density and gray level values of a laser scanner; linearity is maintained up to OD 2.5.

free of noise. To measure the nonuniformity (overall constancy) and noise (local constancy), we can use 10 × 10 pixel area blocks of the Kodak step wedge. The 10 × 10 areas should be large enough for statistical accuracy and small enough to avoid any nonuniformities presented on the step wedge.

Field uniformity can be measured by scanning the calibrated step wedge at five different locations along the scan direction. These locations correspond to various degrees of offset from the center of the scanning field. The scanning line should cover a distance of 14 inches. The 500 data points from each step (100 points from each location) can then be used to calculate the root mean square (rms) fluctuation from a constant input to the system. Figure 3.14 summarizes the overall conversion accuracy of the scanner.

Field nonuniformities parallel to the scan direction arise mainly from fluctuations in the laser output intensity, nonuniformities in the fiber-optic light coupling, and quantum noise in the light detection system. Nonuniformities perpendicular to the scan direction arise from longer term drift of the laser intensity and from lower frequency noise and drift in the detection electronics. The overall flat field response of the system is the combined responses in the parallel and perpendicular directions.

Noise values can be determined by scanning 10 × 10 square pixel area blocks and calculating the standard deviation of the resultant gray level values. The standard deviation from the five different locations along the scan direction can be averaged.

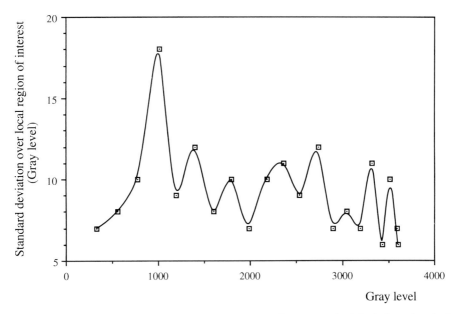

Figure 3.14 Flat field response: plot showing change in the standard deviation of optical density over the density range of a laser scanner. Data are accumulated over the entire imaging field (global variations). In general, the standard deviation is less than 1%.

3.3.1.3 Contrast Frequency Response of the Scanner

The laser scanner's frequency response can be tested by scanning a high precision microlithographed line pair (lp) pattern consisting of alternate and equally spaced dark and light stripes at different spatial frequencies. One such pattern (USAF 1951) was developed by the U.S. Air Force. The dark and light areas correspond to optical densities 0.05 and 3.40, respectively. The average gray level for the dark and light stripes can be obtained from the digitized image, and the contrast frequency response (CFR) can be calculated for each frequency. The CFR parallel to the scan direction can be determined from line pair patterns oriented perpendicular to the beam traversal direction and the perpendicular CRF from line pair patterns oriented parallel to the scanning laser beam. These values indicate the degree to which contrast depends on spatial frequency and are given by:

$$\text{CFR}(f) = \frac{D_{\max}(f) - D_{\min}(f)}{D_{\max}(f)} \tag{3.7}$$

where
$D_{\max}(f)$ = digital value of dark stripe
$D_{\min}(f)$ = digital value of light stripe
f = Spatial frequency of the stripes

The laser scanner has a "full width at half-'maximum'" spot size of 50 μm in the scanning direction and 50 μm perpendicular to the scan direction. The sampling distance in both directions is 50 μm.

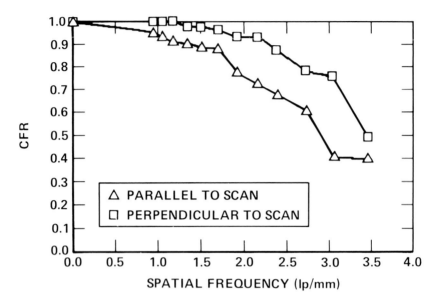

Figure 3.15 Contrast frequency response (CFR) of a laser scanner in both the parallel and perpendicular scan directions.

Figure 3.15 shows the contrast frequency response curves for the laser scanner in directions parallel and perpendicular to the scan direction. The response drops to 0.5 at a frequency of 2.9 cycles/mm in the direction parallel to scan direction and 3.5 lp/mm in the direction perpendicular to the scan. To measure the linearity of the scanner, we count the number of pixels in one millimeter from the left of the film to the right and from the top to the bottom. Figure 3.16 shows the results.

3.3.2 Aliasing Artifacts

3.3.2.1 Practical Consideration

Aliasing artifacts are low spatial frequency components introduced to the digitized image as a result of undersampling during digitization. They appear most often when a high resolution digitization device like a laser scanner is used on X-ray films with patterns of certain types.

Films produced by today's radiology departments can be categorized into four classes, depending on how the film was obtained:

1. Conventional X-ray films obtained without a grid.
2. Digital images (CT, MRI) printed by a laser film printer.

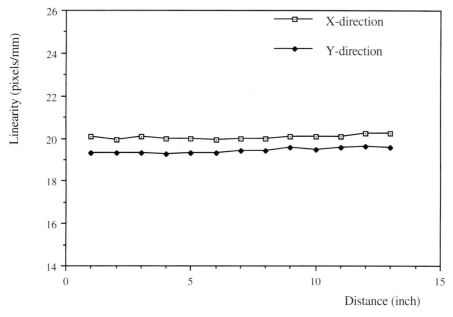

Figure 3.16 Linearity of the scanner. The number of pixels per millimeter is counted from the left of the film to the right, and from the top to the bottom.

3. Conventional X-ray films obtained with a grid.
4. Films produced by a video multiformat camera.

Normally, digitized images obtained from films with a low resolution scanner (e.g., a video camera) do not contain any noticeable aliasing artifacts. This is because the low modulation transfer function (MTF) of the scanner filters out much of the high frequency content of the image, with the result that frequencies above the Nyquist frequency are negligible. Category 1 X-ray films obtained without a grid and category 2 films produced by a laser film printer, when digitized with a high resolution laser scanner, may or may not contain aliasing artifacts, depending on the frequency contents of the image. In almost all cases, the artifacts will be weak and not visually prominent.

Care must be exercised, however, when digitizing category 3 X-ray films with a grid and category 4 films produced by a multiformat camera. Close examination of these two categories reveals a structured background of periodic line patterns superimposed on the image. For films produced with a grid, the background pattern consists of the septa of the grid used, while for films obtained with a multiformat camera, they are the raster video scan lines. Table 3.3 shows some typical line pattern frequencies produced by grids and multiformat cameras on film obtained from various imaging modalities.

To examine the effect of these high spatial frequency background line patterns on

Table 3.3   Some Moiré Patterns Observed in
Digitized Images of X-Ray Films
Obtained Using the Grid and Films
Produced with Multiformat Cameras

X-Ray Film with Grid (lead strips/mm)		Multiformal Camera (scan line pair/mm)		
80 lines/in.	100 lines/in.	DSA	CT	MRI
3.1*	4.0*	2.7	3.4	5.7

*   Without a magnification factor. With a magnification factor, the value
should be lower.

the digitized image, let us assume that these films are digitized with the laser
scanner with a spot size of 100 μm and a sampling distance x of 175 μm. The
sampling theory states that these background periodic lines will produce moiré
patterns because of aliasing, unless the following condition is satisfied:

$$\Delta x = 175 < \frac{1}{2f} \qquad\qquad (3.8)$$

where Δx is the sampling interval and f is the frequency of the background line
pattern.

To avoid moiré patterns for the case of the laser scanner, the highest allowable
frequency would be 2.86 cycles/mm. Examination of the frequency values in Table
3.3 reveals that images containing background line patterns with frequencies above
2.8 cycles/mm (CT and MRI images produced by the multiformat camera and the
X-ray image obtained using a grid) will contain moiré patterns when digitized, since
Eq. (3.8) is violated.

Figure 3.17 shows some examples. The four digitized images in the left-hand
column come from films with background line patterns obtained from four different
modalities (see also Table 3.3). The display contrast and the brightness of each
digitized image were adjusted to highlight the moiré patterns, which depend on the
frequency and contrast of the line patterns, the orientation of the line patterns with
respect to the scanning direction, and the MTF of the scanner.

To minimize the occurrence of distracting moiré patterns in the resultant image,
the film should be scanned with the background line patterns oriented perpendicular

Figure 3.17   Some examples of moiré patterns on images digitized with a laser scanner; all
films have background periodic line patterns. (1) Arteriogram: moiré patterns (slanted vertical
lines) appear on both left and right images. (2) MRI: moiré pattern (woven horizontal lines)
on left image only. (3) CT: moiré pattern (horizontal lines) on left-hand image only; the level
and window settings on the left-hand image are adjusted to highlight the moiré pattern in the
background. (4) Digital subtraction arteriography (no moiré pattern seen): left-hand image,
line patterns oriented parallel to scan direction (scanner resolved lines well), moiré patterns
are more severe; right-hand image line patterns oriented perpendicular to scan direction
(scanner does not resolve lines as well), moiré patterns are less severe.

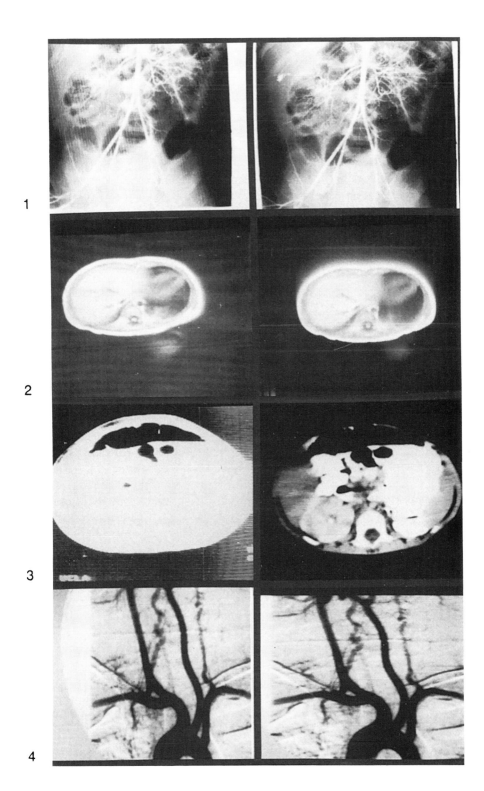

to the direction in which the resolution of the scanner is worst. This is because more of the high frequency components due to the periodic line patterns will be filtered out, and therefore the spectral content above the Nyquist frequency of the scanner will be diminished. In this case, the resolution is worse in the direction parallel to the scan direction. This is a tradeoff between higher resolution and the avoidance of aliasing artifacts.

The right-hand column in Figure 3.17 shows the corresponding images digitized with the scanning beam traversing perpendicular to the background line patterns, that is, in the direction perpendicular to the direction in which the scanner's MTF is lowest. It can be seen that the presence of moiré patterns due to aliasing has been minimized.

The appearance of moiré patterns due to inadequate sampling of images with high frequency components has been documented for many digitizing systems. Examples shown in Figure 3.17 are some interesting cases from diagnostic radiology.

3.3.2.2 Sampling Artifacts Arising from Grid Patterns

In this section, we will use the Fourier transform method to derive the relationship between a sample (or digitized) image and the original image with a grid pattern. This functional relationship is based on three parameters: the laser spot size of the digitizer, the sampling distance, and the angle between the grid lines and the direction perpendicular to the laser beam scanning direction. We will compare the theoretical results with digitized X-ray films with grid lines based on the amplitude and the frequency of the aliasing artifacts by varying these three parameters.

Theoretical Model

The projectional image of an object with a grid pattern for the local approximation can be written as follows:

$$f(x,y) = f_{img}(x,y) + g_{img}(x,y) \tag{3.9}$$

where $f_{img}(x,y)$ is an image without the grid pattern and $g_{img}(x,y)$ is the grid pattern image. Since our interest is in the grid line aliasing artifacts, we will consider only the grid line image $g_{img}(x,y)$.

An ideal stationary antiscatter grid is made of transmissive material (e.g., aluminum) interspersed with an opaque material (e.g., lead) in an alternating pattern of period T (see Fig. 3.18). The Fourier series of an one-dimensional periodic function $g_{img}(x + T) = g_{img}(x)$ is

$$g_{img}(x) = a_0 + \sum_{n=1}^{\infty} a_n \cos(2\pi n f_0 x + \phi_n) \tag{3.10}$$

where a_0, a_n and ϕ_n are constants, $f_0 = 1/T$ is the grid frequency. The frequency spectrum of the grid is discrete, with the frequencies f_0, $2f_0$, $3f_0$, ... Conventional X-ray imaging systems normally have cutoff frequencies about 5 lp/mm. If the grid

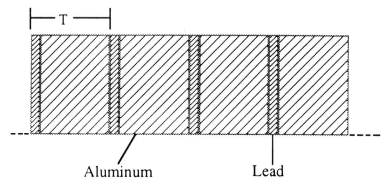

Figure 3.18   Cross-sectional view of an antiscatter grid; T is the distance between two lead strips.

frequency f_0 used is from 2.5 lp/mm to 4 lp/mm, the harmonic frequencies $2 f_0$, $3 f_0, \ldots,$ will be larger than the cutoff frequencies of these imaging systems. Only the fundamental frequency f_0 will be left on the film. Even if the cutoff frequency of an X-ray image system is greater than 5 lp/mm, the amplitudes of the higher harmonic components of the grid lines will still be less than that of the fundamental frequency because the MTF of the X-ray image system is subject to high frequency attenuation. To the first-order approximation, we will consider only the fundamental frequency. If we ignore the dc component a_0 and tilt the film so that the grid lines have an angle θ with respect to the x axis (Fig. 3.19). The grid lines on the film can be written as follows:

$$g_{\mathrm{img}}(x,y) = A\cos[2\pi(f_0 \sin \theta x - f_0 \cos \theta y) + \phi_1] \qquad (3.11)$$

The x axis is defined such that when $\theta = 0^0$ the grid lines lie along the x direction; A is a constant and ϕ_1 is a phase factor.

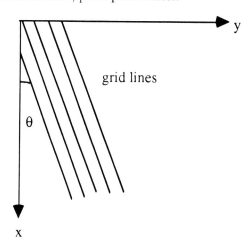

Figure 3.19   The coordinates of grid line orientation; θ is the angle between the grid lines and the x axis.

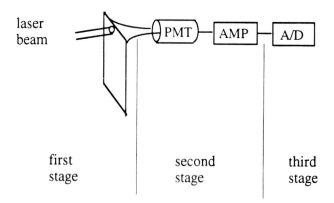

first stage   second stage   third stage

Figure 3.20 Simplified schematic laser film digitizer and the three stages of the digitizing process.

A simplified digitization process of a laser film digitizer is shown in Figure 3.20. A laser beam scans the film in the horizontal (y) direction and the film moves in the vertical (x) direction. After each horizontal scan, the film is advanced one step and the laser beam scans the next line. This process continues until the entire film has been scanned. A photomultiplier tube (PMT) receives the transmitted light beam and converts the light signals to the electrical signals. The electrical signals go through amplifiers (AMP) and then to an analog-to-digital converter (A/D). For simplicity, we consider the digitization as a three-stage process. In the first stage, a laser beam scans through the film. In the second stage, the PMT and the amplifiers function along the scanning direction as a low pass filter, which we call the PMT-AMP component. In the third stage, the A/D converter samples the signals.

In the first stage, the intensity of the light transmitted through the film is proportional to the average light passing through the area where the laser spot scans. This corresponds to averaging the image with a finite focal spot, such that

$$g_{avg}(x,y) = \iint g_{img} (x + \alpha, y + \beta) \, w(\alpha,\beta) d\alpha \, d\beta \tag{3.12}$$

where $g_{avg}(x,y)$ is the smoothed grid image and $w(\alpha,\beta)$ is the intensity distribution of the laser spot.

Taking the Fourier transforms of both sides of Eq. (3.12), we obtain

$$G_{avg}(u,v) = G_{img}(u,v)W^*(u,v) \tag{3.13}$$

where $G_{avg}(u,v)$ and $G_{img}(u,v)$ are the Fourier transforms of $g_{avg}(x,y)$ and $g_{img}(x,y)$, respectively; $W^*(u,v)$ is the conjugate of the Fourier transform of $w(x,y)$.

In the second stage, featuring the PMT-AMP component, the light signals are converted to electrical signals and then go through the amplifiers. We assume that this part of the system is linear and affects the signals in the scanning direction (y direction) only. If the frequency response of this component is $S(v)$, the signal spectrum after this stage is

$$G(u,v)= G_{avg}(u,v)S(v) \tag{3.14}$$
$$= G_{img}(u,v)W^*(u,v)S(v)$$

In the third step, the A/D converter converts analog values to discrete values. Discrete sampling in the frequency domain, according to sampling theory, is given by

$$G_s(u,v) = \frac{1}{d_x d_y} \sum_{m=-\infty}^{\infty} \sum_{n=-\infty}^{\infty} G(u - mf_x, v - nf_y) \tag{3.15}$$

where $G_s(u,v)$ is the Fourier transform of the sampled image, d_x and d_y are sampling distances in the x and y directions, respectively, and $f_x = 1/d_x$ and $f_y = 1/d_y$ are the corresponding sampling frequencies.

To obtain the final analytical results, let's go back to $G(u,v)$ in Eq. (3.14). The Fourier transform of the grid image $g_{img}(x,y)$ (Eq. 3.11) is

$$G_{img}(u,v) = \frac{A}{2} \, [e^{j\phi_1}\delta(u - f_0 \sin \theta, v + f_0 \cos \theta) \tag{3.16}$$

$$+ \, e^{-j\phi_1}\delta(u + f_0 \sin \theta, v - f_0 \cos \theta)]$$

Substituting Eq. (3.16) ito Eq. (3.14), we obtain

$$G(u,v) = \frac{A}{2} \, [e^{j\phi_1}\delta(u - f_0 \sin \theta, v + f_0 \cos \theta) \tag{3.17}$$

$$+ \, e^{-j\phi_1}\delta(u + f_0 \sin \theta, v - f_0 \cos \theta)]W^*(u,v)S(v)$$

$$= \frac{A}{2} \, [e^{j\phi_1}\delta(u - f_0 \sin \theta, v + f_0 \cos \theta)W^*(f_0 \sin \theta, -f_0 \cos \theta)$$

$$\times \, S(-f_0 \cos \theta) + e^{-j\phi_1}\delta(u + f_0 \sin \theta, v - f_0 \cos \theta)$$

$$\times \, W^*(-f_0 \sin \theta, f_0 \cos \theta)S(f_0 \cos \theta)]$$

If we assume that the laser spot intensity has a Gaussian distribution, we can write

$$w(x,y) = B \, \exp\left[-\frac{2(x^2 + y^2)}{a^2} \right] \tag{3.18}$$

where B is a normalized constant and a is a constant that determines the size of the laser spot. The Fourier transform of $w(x,y)$ is

$$W(u,v) = \exp\left[-\frac{(a\pi)^2}{2} (u^2 + v^2) \right] \tag{3.19}$$

If the PMT-AMP component pulse response is real, its Fourier transform $S(v)$ is conjugate symmetric, that is:

$$|S(f_0 \cos \theta)| = |S(-f_0 \cos \theta)| \tag{3.20}$$

$$\text{and} \qquad \angle S(f_0 \cos \theta) = -\angle S(-f_0 \cos \theta) = \eta(f_0, \theta)$$

where $\angle$ represents the phase angle and $\eta(f_0, \theta)$ is used here for simplicity. Substituting Eqs. (3.19) and (3.20) into (3.17), we obtain

$$G(u,v) = \frac{A}{2} \exp\left[-\frac{(a\pi)^2}{2}(f_0^2) \right] |S(f_0 \cos \theta)| \tag{3.21}$$

$$\times [e^{j\phi_1 - jn(f_0,\theta)}\delta(u - f_0 \sin \theta, v + f_0 \cos \theta)$$

$$+ e^{-j\phi_1 + jn(f_0,\theta)}\delta(u + f_0 \sin \theta), v - f_0 \cos \theta)]$$

To reconstruct the sampling image, we begin by substituting Eq. (3.21) into (3.15), multiplying Eq. (3.15) by a square reconstruction filter $H(u,v)$

$$H(u,v) = d_x d_y \qquad |u| < f_x/2, |v| < f_y/2$$

$$= 0 \qquad \text{elsewhere}$$

and taking an inverse Fourier trnasform. Thereupon, the sampled grid line image becomes

$$g_s(x,y) = A \exp\left[-\frac{(a\pi)^2}{2} f_0^2 \right] |S(f_0 \cos \theta)| \tag{3.22}$$

$$\times \sum_{m=-M}^{M} \sum_{n=-N}^{N} \cos[2\pi(f_0 \sin \theta - mf_x)x$$

$$+ 2\pi(-f_0 \cos \theta + nf_y)y + \phi_1 - \eta(f_0,\theta)]$$

Here M, N are determined so that when $|m| < M$ and $|n| < N$,

$$|f_0 \sin \theta - mf_x| < \frac{f_x}{2} \tag{3.23}$$

$$|f_0 \cos \theta - nf_y| < \frac{f_y}{2}$$

$$f_{mn} = [(f_0 \sin \theta - mf_x)^2 + (f_0 \cos \theta - nf_y)^2]^{1/2} \tag{3.24}$$

Equation (3.22) is the summation of many cosine terms. Each cosine term represents a single-frequency moiré pattern with the spatial frequency f_{mn}, a phase factor $\phi_1 - \eta(f_0,\theta)$, and a tilt of angle φ with respect to the x direction, where

$$\tan \varphi = \frac{f_0 \sin \theta - mf_x}{f_0 \cos \theta - nf_y} \tag{3.25}$$

The final digitized grid pattern image $g_s(x,y)$ should be the superposition of all these cosine terms. The aliasing frequency is defined as f_{mn}, which is a function of the sampling frequency and angle θ. When the aliasing frequency f_{mn} is close to zero, the contribution of the first two terms inside the cosine in Eq. (3.22) becomes very small, and the phase factor $\phi_1 - \eta(f_0,\theta)$ contributes significantly to the aliasing artifacts. In this case, the aliasing appearance is a slow varied background. The background level is dependent on the phase factor. Otherwise, the phase factor does not affect the amplitude and has no effect on the visibility of the moiré pattern in most cases. The aliasing amplitude

$$A \exp\left[-\frac{(a\pi)^2}{2}f_0^2\right]|S(f_0 \cos\theta)| \tag{3.26}$$

decreases exponentially with the laser spot size a and depends on the angle θ.

Experiments

To verify the theoretical model, let us use two X-ray films, one from a chest anthropomorphic phantom (Radiology Support Devices, Inc., Long Beach, CA) and the other from an 8.25 cm uniform plastic block, with a 1.5 mm focal spot size X-ray tube at 90 kV(p), 15 mAs, and 152 cm FFD (focus-to-film distance). Let us use a Fuji AW film cassette with medium 200 screen and Kyokko GM-1 films. Both films are then exposed with an antiscatter grid (MXE, Inc., Culver City, CA: 14 in. × 17 in., 4 lp/mm; grid ratio, 6:1) and digitized with a Lumiscan 100 scanner (Lumisys, Sunnyvale, CA) with different laser spot sizes (50, 70, 105, and 210 μm) and sampling distances (200, 250, 300, and 350 μm) at different θ angles (0°, 5°, and 10°). The images with the uniform plastic block and the grid pattern are used to calculate the frequencies and amplitudes of the artifacts. The 2-D Fourier transforms of these images are calculated first and are found to have a well-defined pattern close to a single frequency. The frequency and the amplitude of each image can be calculated from the Fourier spectrum.

Theoretical Calculations

We plot the relationships between the aliasing frequency and the sampling frequency, the aliasing frequency and the film angle tilted, and the aliasing amplitude and the laser spot size by using Eqs. (3.22), (3.23), (3.24), and (3.25). It is easy to prove that there is only one pair of (m, n) that satisfies Eq. (3.23) for each sampling frequency, with the result that the aliasing artifacts are always a single frequency. The indices m and n representing the aliasing frequency in these equations can be selected depending on the sampling conditions.

The effects of the sampling distance on the aliasing frequency, illustrated in Figure 3.21, can be calculated from Eq. (3.24). In these calculations, we assume that $d_x = d_y$, to ensure that the digital imaging has the same magnification in the x and y directions, and θ is kept constant for each curve. The grid frequencies in Figure 3.21 are 4 and 3 lp/mm respectively. For each grid frequency, three angles (0°, 5°, 10°) were used to calculate the aliasing frequency. Note that when the sampling frequency is equal to or half or one-third of the grid frequency, the aliasing frequency is the minimum. The aliasing frequency oscillates with the sampling frequency until the sampling frequency reaches Nyquist frequency.

Figure 3.22 demonstrates the variation of the aliasing frequency with the angle θ. The curves were calculated from Eq. (3.24), where angle θ was varied but f_x and f_y were kept constant. In Figure 3.22A, the sampling frequency and the grid frequency are equal for each curve; they are different in Figure 3.22B. The increase in aliasing frequency with angle can be explained as follows. When the film is tilted a small angle, the apparent grid frequency in the y direction decreases, whereas the grid

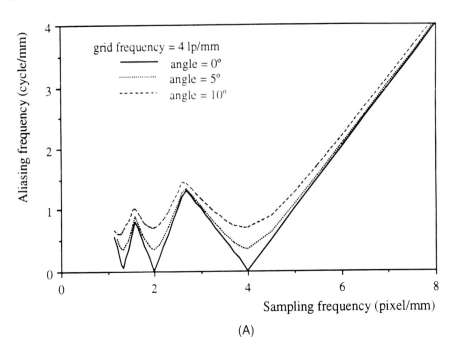

(A)

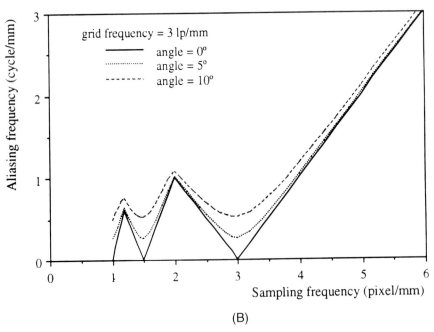

(B)

Figure 3.21 Effect of sampling frequency on aliasing frequency. Aliasing frequency is at a minimum when the sampling frequency equals the fractions of the grid frequency: (A) grid frequency 4.0 lp/mm; (B) grid frequency 3.0 lp/mm.

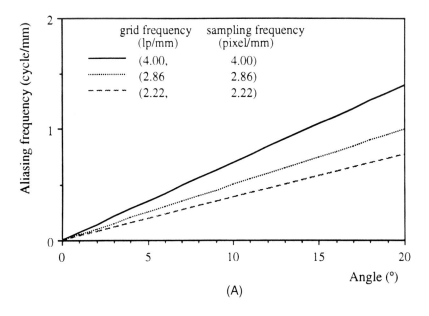

(A)

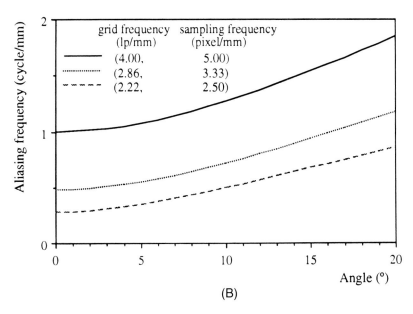

(B)

Figure 3.22   Effect of the angle between the grid lines and the direction perpendicular to the scanning direction on the aliasing frequency: (A) sampling frequency = grid frequency; (B) sampling frequency ≠ grid frequency.

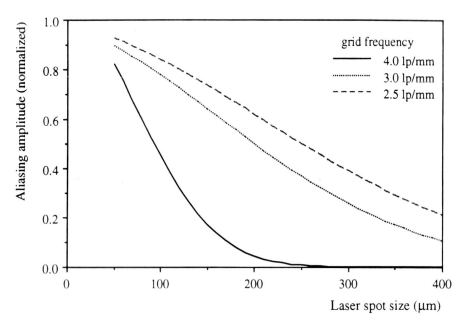

Figure 3.23 Effect of laser spot size on aliasing amplitude.

frequency in the x direction increases (Fig. 3.19). Because the grid frequency in the x direction increases from zero, we assume that there is no aliasing problem in this direction. As the angle increases, the grid frequency in the y direction $f_0 \cos\theta$ decreases. Since the sampling frequency f_y was kept constant, the aliasing frequency $|f_0 \cos\theta - f_y|$ increases.

Figure 3.23 shows the effect of the laser spot size on the amplitude of the aliasing artifact, assuming that all other parameters remain unchanged. From Eq. (3.26) we notice that the spot size a does not affect the aliasing frequency, but strongly influences the amplitude. As the laser spot size a increases, the amplitude decreases. This is because the laser spot is behaving like a low pass filter. The larger the laser spot, the narrower the pass band. If the grid frequency is fixed, the amplitude of the grid frequency is reduced as the filter becomes narrower (i.e., as the laser spot size increases).

Comparing Theoretical and Experiment Results

We calculate the frequencies and the amplitudes of aliasing artifacts of the film with a grid pattern and compare them with the theoretical results. The experimental and the theoretical results of the sampling frequency on the aliasing frequency are shown in Figure 3.24. The grid frequency used for the theoretical curve was 3.82 lp/mm, which is different from 4 lp/mm, the nominal number of the grid frequency. This difference may be attributed to many factors, including error in the calibration of the laser scanner, and the degree of accuracy of the grid frequency given. The true grid frequency (3.82 lp/mm) was calculated from the Fourier spectrum of the

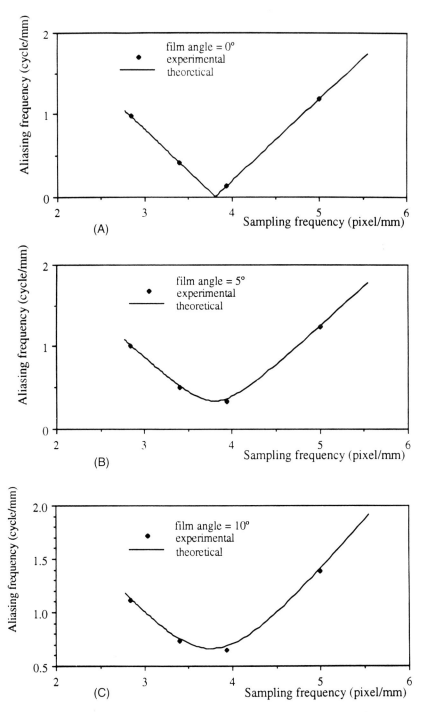

Figure 3.24 Comparison of theoretical and experimental results of aliasing frequency versus sampling frequency for a grid frequency of 3.82 lp/mm and three different film angles: (A) 0°, (B) 5°, and (C) 10°. The minimum aliasing frequency occurs when the sampling frequency is 3.82 pixels/mm.

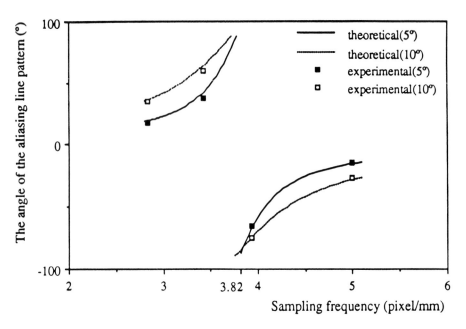

Figure 3.25 Comparison of the theoretical and experimental results of the angle of the aliasing patterns versus the sampling frequency for a grid frequency of 3.82 lp/mm. Note the sudden change of the angle when the sampling frequency is above and below 3.82 pixels/mm; this corresponds to the orientation change of the moiré pattern.

digitized image, which was obtained by sampling the film with 100 μm (10 pixel/mm). The experimental results are very close to the theoretical results. The tilted angle φ of the aliasing pattern with respect to the x direction also was calculated from the frequency components f_x and f_y obtained from the digitized images. These results, together with the theoretical results from Eq. (3.25) are shown in Figure 3.25. Note the change of the orientation of the angle of the aliasing line when the sampling frequencies are above and below the grid frequency 3.82 lp/mm. (see also related digital images Figs. 3.28, 3.29).

The effects on the aliasing amplitude of varying the laser spot size of the digitizer are shown in Figure 3.26; these results do not fit well with the theoretical curve. The reason for this discrepancy is that we assume the laser spot is Gaussian, but the true laser spot may not be strictly circular symmetric Gaussian.

Figure 3.27 shows a chest phantom film with a grid line pattern (4 lp/mm) that is hardly visible in this image. The region in the square including the left lung and mediastinum is digitized with different parameters to allow an appreciation of the visual effect of the moiré pattern (Figs. 3.28 and 3.29). The laser spot size used in Figure 3.28 is 105 μm; it is doubled in Figure 3.29. The moiré pattern, which appears on most of the images when the sampling spot size is 105 μm (Fig. 3.28), is hardly seen on the images with 210 μm sampling spot size because of the decreasing amplitude of this pattern. This effect can be explained from Figure 3.26, as we

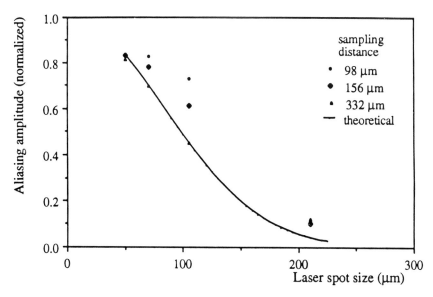

Figure 3.26 Comparison of theoretical and experimental results of the aliasing amplitude versus laser spot size. The high amplitude value is responsible for the visualization of the aliasing artifacts.

notice that the amplitude of the moiré pattern sampled with 105 μm is about four to five times larger than that of 210 μm.

In both Figures 3.28 and 3.29, the sampling distances are 200, 254, 293, and 352 μm from the first to the fourth column, and the angles are 0°, 5°, and 10° from the first to the third row, respectively. With a 105 μm spot size, when the sampling distance equals to 254 μm (the second column), which is the closest to the grid interval 262 μm (3.82 lp/mm), the aliasing frequency is the smallest—that is, the distance between the lines is largest—and the artifact appears stronger. As the sampling distance moves away from the grid interval, the aliasing frequency increases and the line pattern becomes closer, and the artifacts are less prominent (the first and the fourth columns). The aliasing frequency also increases with the increase of the angle (comparing each column from the top to the bottom).

The visibility of the aliasing artifacts is dependent on three factors: the amplitude of the aliasing in Eq. (3.22), the frequency response of the display, and human visual sensitivity. The amplitude of the aliasing artifacts is independent of the sampling frequency but may depend on the orientation of the grid line pattern. The effect of the angle θ on the amplitude depends on the bandwidth of the PMT–AMP frequency response $S(v)$. If the cutoff frequency of $S(v)$ is high enough, θ will not affect the amplitude. The amplitude is always the minimum when $\theta = 0°$. Generally speaking, the smaller the amplitude, the less dominant the aliasing artifacts. Rather than discussing various display systems in detail, we assume a system that functions as a low pass filter. The human visual response varies with grid frequency; it has been

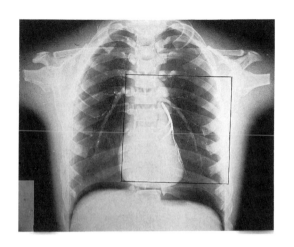

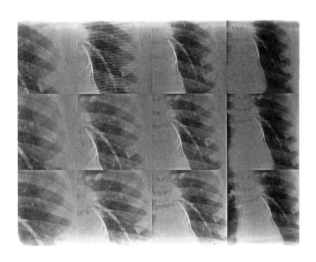

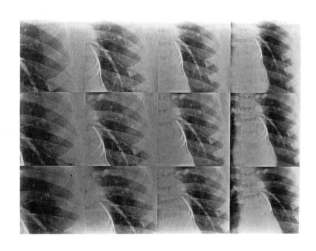

reported that the highest response of human eyes is around $1-2$ lp/mm, decreasing on both sides.

It is also observed from Figure 3.28 that the orientation of the moiré pattern depends on the specific set of digitizing parameters. (Note: the images shown here are in the anatomical position, which is rotated $90°$ clockwise with respect to the digitizing position.) This relationship can be explained by Eq. (3.25) and from Figure 3.25. The images in the first row have aliasing patterns almost parallel to the x direction. The second-row images were digitized with the film tilted $5°$, and the angles of aliasing patterns vary from $-70°$ to $35°$. In the third row, the images were digitized with the film tilted $10°$, and the angles of the aliasing patterns vary from $-80°$ to $55°$. These angles can be predicted from Eq. (3.25). Note that the digitized images taken at different sampling distances shown in Figures 3.28 and 3.29 seem to have different magnifications. This is because all digitized images are 512×512 pixels; they will be the same size when displayed on the screen regardless of sampling distances. Since a smaller area on the film is covered when a smaller sampling distance is used, however, the images appear to have different magnifications in the two cases.

Discussion

We have presented a mathematical model to explain the aliasing artifacts (moiré pattern) caused by digitizing of an X-ray film with a grid pattern. The model includes three parameters: laser spot size (of the digitizer), sampling distance, and angle between the grid lines and the sampling direction. The results derived from this model compare favorably with experimental values.

The results of this work show that the digitization process cannot totally eliminate aliasing artifacts by using this system without losing the imaging resolution. But a proper choice of the digitization parameters will minimize the visibility of the aliasing artifacts and allow future processing to remove artifacts.

We recommend that during the digitization process, the film be positioned such that the grid lines are perpendicular to the scanning direction. This way it becomes possible to utilize the high frequency attenuation characteristic of the digitizer

---

Figure 3.27   Chest phantom film with a scarcely visible grid line pattern. The square is the digitization region.

Figure 3.28   Digital images digitized with a 105 μm focal spot size at different sampling distances and angles. Images in rows 1–3 from top to bottom were digitized with the film tilted $0°$, $5°$, and $10°$ respectively. Images in columns 1–4 from left to right were digitized with sampling distances of 200, 254, 293, and 352 μm, respectively. The aliasing artifacts are most prominent at 254 μm and 293 μm. Some aliasing artifacts are seen at 200 μm with $0°$ and $5°$. Observe the abrupt change of the moiré pattern orientation in column 2.

Figure 3.29   Digital image digitized with a 210 μm focal spot size at different sampling distances and angles. Images in rows 1–3 from top to bottom were digitized with the film tilted $0°$, $5°$, and $10°$ respectively. Images in columns 1–4 from left to right were digitized with sampling distances of 200, 254, 293, and 352 μm, respectively. For this large focal spot size, no appreciable aliasing artifacts are seen regardless of sampling distance and tilted angle.

PMT–AMP component to reduce the amplitude of the grid lines. The amplitude of the aliasing artifacts is independent of the sampling frequency. We cannot reduce the aliasing amplitude by varying the sampling frequency. If the Nyquist frequency condition cannot be satisfied, we must select a sampling frequency from Figure 3.21 which will give a higher aliasing frequency: since the display system functions as a low pass filter, the high frequency attenuation characteristic of the display system will render the aliasing artifacts less prominent. Besides, a digital image can be postprocessed. The high frequency aliasing artifacts can be removed more easily than the low frequency components because the original image is dominated by low frequency components. Once the sampling distance has been selected, the laser spot size should be selected to be the same as the sampling distance.

Since it is difficult to remove the grid line aliasing artifacts in the digitizing process, it is preferable to remove them from the digitized image. One method is to implement the Fourier transform and search for the sharp peaks, which subsequently can be filtered out.

This model also explains two phenomena that had been puzzling us during the past several years. First, why do aliasing artifacts appear to be more prominent under certain digitization conditions? Second, why does the orientation of the moiré pattern change abruptly when there is only a slight change in the digitization conditions? Figure 3.28 allows us to understand the characteristics of the moiré pattern under various digitization conditions. Results from this model can serve as guides in the minimization of aliasing artifacts using current generation digitizers and in the design of the next generation of film scanners.

3.3.2.3 Sampling Artifacts: A Systematic Approach

We have discussed the sampling artifact based on laser spot size, sampling distance, and angle between the grid lines and the scanning direction. These three parameters are all related to the sampling theory. However, a mathematical explanation using the Nyquist sampling theorem, which considers only the spatial frequency of the original film image and the sampling interval, is not adequate. It is also necessary to incorporate the frequency transfer characteristics between the image and various components of the laser film scanner. In addition, we need to understand how sensitive the human observer is to this artifact. Next we will design a model, with parameters including the spatial frequency characteristics of various components in a scanner as well as the human observer response, to explain characteristics of the sampling artifact.

3.4 Spatial Frequency Characteristics of the Laser Film Scanner

3.4.1 Component Analysis

The schematic diagram of a scanner depicted in Figure 3.30 shows the path of transmitted laser light as it passes through the film and is processed by many stages whose components include the following:

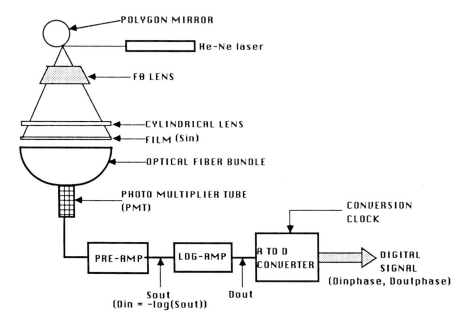

Figure 3.30 Schematic diagram of the KFDR-S laser film scanner (Konica Corporation, Japan).

fiber bundle,
laser beam optical system: photomultiplier tube (PMT),
preamplifier

logarithic amplifier (log-amp)
A/D converter

The most important components affecting the frequency response characteristics of the laser scanner are the laser beam and the logarithmic amplifier. The other components are also important, but their frequency bandwidth is high enough (compared to the 1 MHz sampling clock rate used by most scanners) to render them negligible for the purposes of this study.

3.4.1.1 *Laser Beam Optical System*

The laser spot profile has a Gaussian distribution with the form:

$$p(x) = \exp\left(- 2\frac{x^2}{w^2} \right) \tag{3.27}$$

where x is the radial distance from the center of the spot and w is the beam width (radial distance at which intensity drops off by $1/e^2$).

Therefore the transmitted light signal s_{out} through the film can be obtained by convolving the laser profile equation with the image pattern $s_{in}(x)$ (Fig. 3.31). Thus,

$$s_{out}(x) = \int p(\xi)\, s_{in}(x + \xi)d\xi \tag{3.28}$$

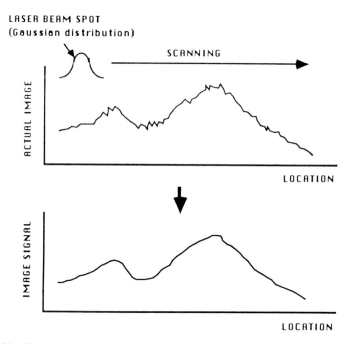

Figure 3.31 The image signal is the result of the convolution between the laser beam and the actual image.

The modulation transfer function (MTF) of the optical system (before the PMT in Fig. 3.30) can be obtained from the Fourier transform of $p(x)$, $P(u)$:

$$\text{MTF}_{\text{opt}}(u) = P(u) = \int \exp\left(-2\,\frac{x^2}{w^2}\right) \exp(-2\pi jux)\, dx \qquad (3.29)$$

3.4.1.2 Frequency Characteristics of Logarithmic Amplifier

The light signal is converted into an electrical signal by the PMT. After the PMT the signal is conditioned using a preamp and a log-amp. As mentioned earlier, since the frequency transform characteristics of the preamp is fast enough to handle the image data from the PMT, we concentrate on the frequency response of the log-amp.

The MTF characteristics of the log-amp can be obtained by measuring the maximum and the minimum level of the input signal, $D_{\text{in/max}}$ and $D_{\text{in/min}}$, and the corresponding maximum and the minimum level of the output signal, $D_{\text{out/max}}$ and $D_{\text{out/min}}$, at various input frequencies u (cycles/mm).

$$\text{MTF}_{\text{amp}}(u) = \frac{D_{\text{out/max}}(u) - D_{\text{out/min}}(u)}{D_{\text{in/max}}(u) - D_{\text{in/min}}(u)} \qquad (3.30)$$

where $D_{\text{in/max}}(u) = -\log[S_{\text{out/min}}(u)]$, $D_{\text{in/min}}(u) = -\log[S_{\text{out/max}}(u)]$.

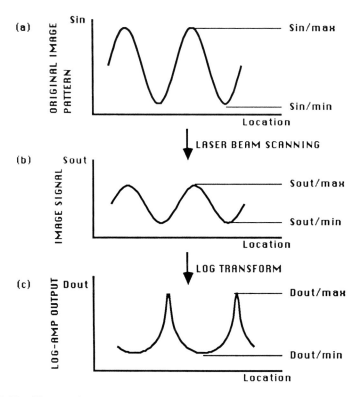

Figure 3.32 Change of the waveform at each stage in the laser film scanner (see also Fig. 3.30): (a) original image pattern on the film, (b) input for the log-amp, (c) output from the log-amp.

3.4.1.3 Image Signal Before A/D Converter

Thus far we have considered the degradation of the original film image due to the laser spot profile and the frequency response characteristics of the analog signal conditioning electronics. Figure 3.32 shows this situation. A pure sinusoidal film image about to be digitized with the film scanner appears in Figure 3.32a. After the sine wave pattern has been scanned with the laser and converted into an electrical signal, the original sine pattern becomes degraded, as shown in Figure 3.32b. The waveform is essentially the same before and after the preamp stage because the preamp has a wide bandwidth. The signal is then converted into optical density information by the log-amp (Fig. 3.32c). If the averages of S_{in} and S_{out} are equal to a constant K_s, which is the case in Figure 3.32, we can write:

$$S_{in/max} + S_{in/min} = S_{out/max}(u) + S_{out/min}(u) = K_s \qquad (3.31)$$

Here, $S_{in/max}$ and $S_{in/min}$ are constants because these are the maximum and minimum of the original sine wave pattern.

The system $\text{MTF}_{\text{opt}}(u)$ (Eq. 3.29), which includes the optical system and the preamp, can be measured by:

$$\text{MTF}_{\text{opt}}(u) = \frac{S_{\text{out/max}}(u) - S_{\text{out/min}}(u)}{S_{\text{in/max}} - S_{\text{in/min}}} \tag{3.32}$$

And, from expressions (3.31) and (3.32), the following can be obtained:

$$S_{\text{out/max}}(u) = \tfrac{1}{2}[\text{MTF}_{\text{opt}}(u)(S_{\text{in/max}} - S_{\text{in/min}}) + K_{\text{s}}] \tag{3.33a}$$

$$S_{\text{out/min}}(u) = K_{\text{s}} - S_{\text{out/max}}(u) \tag{3.33b}$$

Similarly, if we assume

$$D_{\text{in/max}}(u) + D_{\text{in/min}}(u) = D_{\text{out/max}}(u) + D_{\text{out/min}}(u) = \tag{3.34}$$

$$-\log[S_{\text{out/min}}(u) + S_{\text{out/max}}(u)] = K_{\text{d}}$$

then from Eqs. (3.30) and (3.34) we obtain:

$$D_{\text{out/max}}(u) = \frac{1}{2}\{\text{MTF}_{\text{amp}}(u)[D_{\text{in/max}}(u) - D_{\text{in/min}}(u)] + K_{\text{d}}\} \tag{3.35a}$$

$$D_{\text{out/min}}(u) = K_{\text{d}} - D_{\text{out/max}}(u) \tag{3.35b}$$

3.4.2 The Effects of Sampling

Thus far we have analyzed the frequency transform characteristics of the analog signal before the A/D conversion. Now we turn to the effects of the sampling interval. Since the frequency response characteristics of the digitized signal depend on the in-phase and out-of-phase sampling conditions of the A/D converter, digitizing artifacts will be seen.

3.4.2.1 In-Phase and Out-of-Phase Sampling

It can be shown that the sampling values for the in-phase and out-of-phase sampling conditions depend on the signal spatial frequency u (cycles/mm) and the sampling interval a (mm) (see Fig. 3.33).

- in-phase sampling

$$\text{inphase}(u) = \sin(ua\pi) \qquad\qquad \text{for } \frac{1}{3a} \le u \le \frac{1}{2a} \tag{3.36a}$$

$$\text{inphase}(u) = \begin{array}{ll} \sin(nua\pi) & (\theta \ge 0) \\ \sin^2(nua\pi) & (\theta < 0, |\theta| \le \theta_t) \\ \sin(n-1)ua\pi & (\theta < 0, |\theta| \ge \theta_t) \end{array} \qquad \text{for } 0 \le u < \frac{1}{3a} \tag{3.36a$'$}$$

where $\theta = \dfrac{1}{au} - 2n$, θ_t satisfies $\cos^2(\pi ua/2)\theta_t = \cos\{\pi ua(1 - |\theta_t|/2)\}$, and n is number of sample points within $1/2u$ (i.e., $n = 1$ when $1/3a \le u \le 1/2a$).

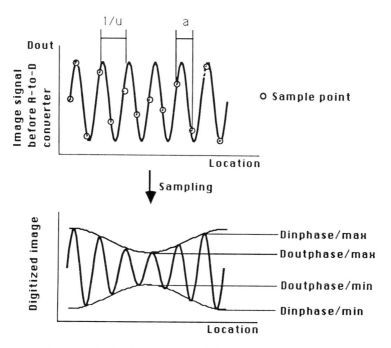

Figure 3.33   In-phase and out-of-phase sampling conditions.

- out-of-phase sampling

$$\text{outphase}(u) = \sin(nua\pi)\cos(ua\pi)\left(1 - \frac{1}{2}\left|\frac{1}{au} - 2n\right|\right) \tag{3.36b}$$

The overall frequency response for the in-phase and out-of-phase sampling conditions can be obtained by combining Eqs. (3.36a), (3.36a′), and (3.36b) with (3.35a) and (3.35b). Note that $D_{\text{out/max}}(u)$ given in Eq. (3.35a) can be decomposed into two terms; the first will be affected by the location of the sampling, whereas the second is a constant (K_d) and will not be affected. Thus,

- in-phase sampling

$$D_{\text{inphase/max}}(u) = \frac{1}{2}\left\{\text{inphase}(u)\ \text{MTF}_{\text{amp}}(u)\ \log\left[\frac{S_{\text{out/max}}(u)}{S_{\text{out/min}}(u)}\right] + K_d\right\} \tag{3.37a}$$

Similarly,

$$D_{\text{inphase/min}}(u) = -\frac{1}{2}\left\{\text{inphase}(u)\ \text{MTF}_{\text{amp}}(u)\ \log\left[\frac{S_{\text{out/max}}(u)}{S_{\text{out/min}}(u)}\right] - K_d\right\} \tag{3.37b}$$

- out-of-phase sampling

$$D_{\text{outphase/max}}(u) = \frac{1}{2}\left\{\text{outphase}(u)\ \text{MTF}_{\text{amp}}(u)\ \log\left[\frac{S_{\text{out/max}}(u)}{S_{\text{out/min}}(u)}\right] + K_d\right\} \tag{3.38a}$$

$$D_{\text{outphase/min}}(u) = -\frac{1}{2}\left\{\text{outphase}(u)\,\text{MTF}_{\text{amp}}(u)\,\log\left[\frac{S_{\text{out/max}}(u)}{S_{\text{out/min}}(u)}\right] - K_{\text{d}}\right\} \tag{3.38b}$$

where $S_{\text{out/max}}(u)$ and $S_{\text{out/min}}(u)$ are given in Eqs. (3.33a) and (3.33b) and $D_{\text{out/max}}(u)$ and $D_{\text{out/min}}(u)$ satisfy the conditions:

$$D_{\text{outphase/max}}(u) \leq D_{\text{out/max}}(u) \leq D_{\text{inphase/max}}(u) \tag{3.39a}$$

$$D_{\text{inphase/min}}(u) \leq D_{\text{out/min}}(u) \leq D_{\text{outphase/min}}(u) \tag{3.39b}$$

3.4.2.7 Contrast Difference Due to Sampling

If we define the constrast of the image C as

$$C = \frac{\text{maximum level} - \text{minimum level}}{\text{maximum level} + \text{minimum level}} \tag{3.40}$$

we can use this parameter to measure the performance of the system. Substituting Eqs. (3.37) and (3.38) into Eq. (3.40), we obtain the equations for the in-phase contrast and the out-of-phase contrast:

$$C_{\text{inphase}}(u) = \frac{D_{\text{inphase/max}}(u) - D_{\text{inphase/min}}(u)}{D_{\text{inphase/max}}(u) + D_{\text{inphase/min}}(u)} \tag{3.41a}$$

$$= \frac{1}{K_{\text{d}}}\left\{\text{Inphase}(u)\text{MTF}_{\text{amp}}(u)\,\log\left[\frac{S_{\text{out/max}}(u)}{S_{\text{out/min}}(u)}\right]\right\}$$

$$C_{\text{outphase}}(u) = \frac{D_{\text{outphase/max}}(u) - D_{\text{outphase/min}}(u)}{D_{\text{outphase/max}}(u) + D_{\text{outphase/min}}(u)} \tag{3.41b}$$

$$= \frac{1}{K_{\text{d}}}\left\{\text{Outphase}(u)\text{MTF}_{\text{amp}}(u)\,\log\left[\frac{S_{\text{out/max}}(u)}{S_{\text{out/min}}(u)}\right]\right\}$$

We can also define the contrast of the artifact seen on the digitized image as follows:

$$C_{\text{artifact}}(u) = \frac{D_{\text{inphase/max}}(u) - D_{\text{outphase/min}}(u)}{D_{\text{inphase/max}}(u) + D_{\text{outphase/min}}(u)} \tag{3.42}$$

$$= \frac{[\text{inphase}(u) + \text{outphase}(u)]\text{MTF}_{\text{amp}}(u)\,\log\left[\dfrac{\alpha + \text{MTF}_{\text{opt}}(u)\beta}{\alpha - \text{MTF}_{\text{opt}}(u)\beta}\right]}{[\text{inphase}(u) + \text{outphase}(u)]\text{MTF}_{\text{amp}}(u)\,\log\left[\dfrac{\alpha + \text{MTF}_{\text{opt}}(u)\beta}{\alpha - \text{MTF}_{\text{opt}}(u)\beta}\right] - 2\log\left[\dfrac{\alpha^2 - \text{MTF}_{\text{opt}}(u)^2\beta^2}{4}\right]}$$

where $\alpha = S_{\text{in/max}} + S_{\text{in/min}}$ and $\beta = S_{\text{in/max}} - S_{\text{in/min}}$.

3.4.3 Results

3.4.3.1 Contrast Frequency Response

The contrast frequency responses given in Eqs. (3.41a) and (3.41b) were computed using variable sampling intervals and laser spot sizes. The sampling intervals used

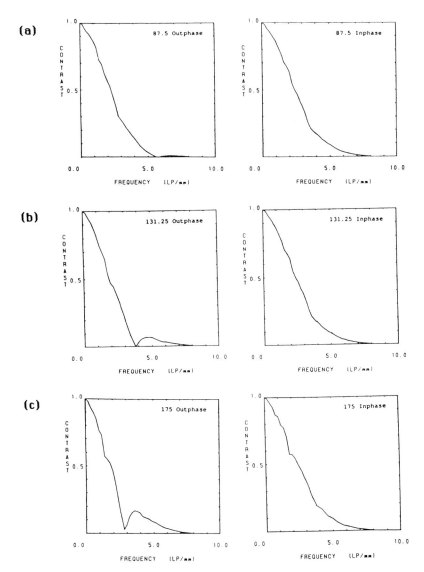

Figure 3.34 Results of contrast frequency responses for in-phase (right-hand column) and out-of-phase (left-hand column) conditions for sampling interval of (a) 87.5 μm, (b) 131.25 μm, and (c) 175 μm.

were 87.5, 131.3, and 175.0 μm, corresponding to the pixel sizes in a typical film scanner. Figure 3.34 shows the results.

Sampling artifacts will be seen at frequencies above the zero crossing on the out-of-phase contrast frequency response curves. For example, given a sampling interval of 175.0 μm, moiré patterns may be seen in the resulting digitized image if the film image contains spatial frequencies higher than 2.7 cycles/mm. Similarly, arti-

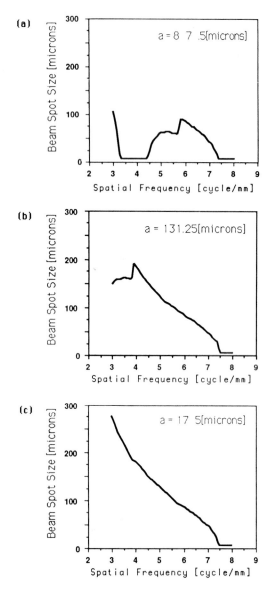

Figure 3.35 The spot size required to avoid sampling artifacts for sampling intervals of (a) 87.5 μm, (b) 131.25 μm, and (c) 175 μm.

Figure 3.36 Experimental results to verify the curves in Figure 3.35. Sampling interval used was 175 μm, and spatial frequency of the grid is 6 lp/mm. Laser beam spot size: (A) 135 μm, (B) 95.0 μm, and (C) 87.0 μm. In (c), which corresponds to the condition underneath the curve, sampling artifact is visible (see text for details).

facts will be seen on a digitized image if the original film has frequency components higher than 3.8 cycles/mm for a sampling interval of 131.3 μm, and higher than 5.6 cycles/mm for a sampling interval of 87.5 μm. High frequency information on medical radiographs often is manifested in the form of period line patterns from antiscatter grids and from TV raster lines.

From Figure 3.34 the artifact can be understood as the difference of the amplitudes between the in-phase contrast and the out-of-phase contrast. That is, a human observer will recognize the envelope shown in Figure 3.33 as a digitizing artifact.

3.4.3.2 Digitizing Artifact

In designing a radiological film scanner, as we discussed in Section 3.3.2.2, it is necessary to adjust the sampling interval and the spot size to avoid digitizing artifacts to which a human observer would be sensitive. The minimum detectable contrast that can be noticed by a human observer has been studied by many groups and has been documented as about 0.03 optical density. The results of this analysis of receiver operating characteristics showed a contrast level of 0.015 optical density. Substituting this value on the left-hand side of Eq. (3.42), we derived the relationship between beam width w in Eq. (3.27), which is embedded in $S_{out/max}(u)$ in Eqs. (3.29), (3.33a), and (3.33b), and spatial frequency u, in which no artifacts will be observed. Figure 3.35 shows the relation between beam width and spatial frequency at sampling intervals of 87.5, 131.25, and 175.0 μm. Parameter values selected in the area underneath the curve in each figure represent conditions in which digitizing artifacts will be visualized by a human observer. For example, in Figure 3.35a the sampling interval is 87.5 μm, and if the spatial frequency of the grid is 5 lp/mm, then the beam spot size should be larger than 75 μm to avoid the artifact. In essence, using a larger beam spot size to avoid digitizing an artifact is equivalent to applying a low pass filter to the digitized image.

To verify Figure (3.35), which relates laser spot size, image frequency content, and observer sensitivity to sampling artifacts, we scanned film images obtained with antiscatter grids using conditions above the curve, on the curve, and underneath the curve. Laser spot sizes of 135.0, 95.0, and 87.0 μm were used, with a sampling interval of 175 μm. Figure 3.36 shows uniformly exposed X-ray film with a grid pattern of 6 lp/mm (72% aluminum, 28% lead) that has been scanned by laser beams of three different spot sizes. Figure 3.36A shows the result corresponding to the scanning condition above the curve (i.e., no scanning artifact). In, Figure 3.36B, representing the condition corresponding to points on the curve, a scanning artifact is barely visible. Figure 3.36C, which corresponds to the condition below the curve, does show a scanning artifact.

3.5 Summary

The contrast on a digitized image can be studied by analyzing each stage in the laser film digitizer, including the optical system, the signal processing chain, and the sampling intervals. A relationship between the spatial frequency and the laser beam spot size was derived based on the definition of image contrast and the minimum optical density resolution that the human eye can detect. This relationship can be used as a guideline to avoid digitizing artifacts in designing laser scanners and other types of radiological digitizing device.

CHAPTER

4

Image Acquisition II: Imaging Plate and Digital Radiography

As discussed earlier, 70% of radiographic procedures are conventional projection radiographic examinations. For a radiology department move from film-based to digital-based operation, however, it is essential to derive new imaging acquisition systems that can directly convert to digital format most of the radiographic examinations performed.

This chapter discusses two approaches. The first is to utilize existing equipment in the radiographic procedure room and change only the image receptor component. Two technologies, imaging plate and digital fluorography, belong to this approach. This method does not require any modification of the procedure room and is therefore more easily adopted for daily clinical practice. The second approach is to redesign the conventional radiographic procedure equipment, including the geometry of the X-ray beams and the image receptor. This method is therefore more expensive to adopt, but it offers special features that would not otherwise be available in the conventional procedure.

Imaging plate technology was introduced in the late 1970s and early 1980s. Growth in the field has been stimulated by the work of researchers at Xerox Medical Systems (xeroradiography, electronic scanning of selenium plate), Image Systems Division/3M (electroradiography), M.D. Anderson Hospital, Texas (laser scanning of selenium plate), Fuji Photo Film Company, Ltd. (laser-stimulated luminescence phosphor plate), and Philips Medical Systems (electrophoretic devices).

An imaging plate (IP) system consists of two components: an imaging plate to store the latent image and a scanning mechanism to extract the latent image from the plate to form a digital image. In the past, the development of plate technology has been hindered by the low spatial resolution and signal-to-noise ratio of the IP compared to the X-ray film, as well as the difficulty of display and storing the IP images. At the present time, most of these technological problems have been resolved. The remaining obstacle is the initial investment cost, which is still very substantial.

4.1 Laser-Stimulated Luminescence Phosphor Plate Technology

Use of the laser scanner to digitize X-ray films was discussed in detail in Chapter 3. Reading a laser-stimulated luminescence phosphor plate entails scanning principles similar to those used in the laser scanner. Instead of scanning an X-ray film, however, the laser is used to scan an image receptor called a *laser-stimulated luminescence phosphor plate* (or imaging plate, IP). An imaging plate system, commonly called computed radiography (CR), consists of two components: the imaging plate and the scanning mechanism. This section describes the physics of the imaging plate, specifications of the system, system operation, and some clinical considerations.

4.1.1 Principle of the Laser-Stimulated Luminescence Phosphor Plate

The imaging plate consists of a support coated with a photostimulable phosphorous layer made of europium-activated barium fluorohalide compounds [BaFX:Eu^{2+} (X = Cl, Br, I)]; in physical size it is similar to a conventional radiographic screen. After the X-ray exposure, the photostimulable phosphor crystal is able to store a part of the absorbed X-ray energy in a quasi-stable state. Stimulation of the plate by a helium–neon laser beam having a wavelength of 633 nm leads to emission of luminescence radiation, the amount of which is a function of the absorbed X-ray energy.

The luminescence radiation stimulated by the laser scanning is collected through a focusing lens and a light guide into a photomultiplier tube, which converts it into electrical signals. Figure 4.1 shows the physical principle of the laser-stimulated luminescence phosphor imaging plate. The size of the imaging plate, in inches, can be 8 × 10, 10 × 12, 14 × 14, or 14 × 17.

4.1.2 A Computed Radiography System Block Diagram and Its Principle of Operation

The imaging plate is housed inside a cassette just like a film–screen system. Exposure of the imaging plate to X-ray irradiation results in the formation of a latent image on the plate (similar to the latent image formed in a film–screen receptor). The exposed plate is then processed through a computed radiographic system for extracting the latent image—analogous to the development of exposed film by a film developer.

There are four major components in the computed radiographic system: the

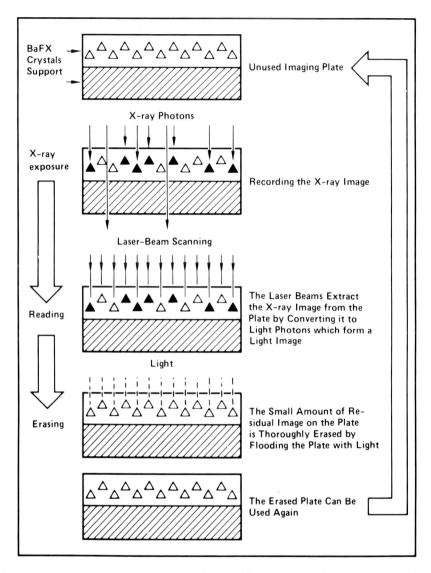

Figure 4.1 Physical principle of laser-stimulated luminescence phosphor imaging plate.

image reader, the image processor, the image storage devices, and the image re-corder. The output of this system can take the form of a printed film or a digital image—the latter can be stored in a digital storage device and displayed on a video monitor. Figure 4.2 shows the first commercial computed radiographic system (FCR-101), introduced in 1987, and the latest system, the AC-II and the FCR-9000, all manufactured by Fuji Medical Systems, Japan. Note the difference in size be-tween these two systems after eight years of development. Figure 4.3 shows the principle of operation, describing how the image plate actually moves inside the CR system based on the FCR-101. Although the current system takes up much less floor

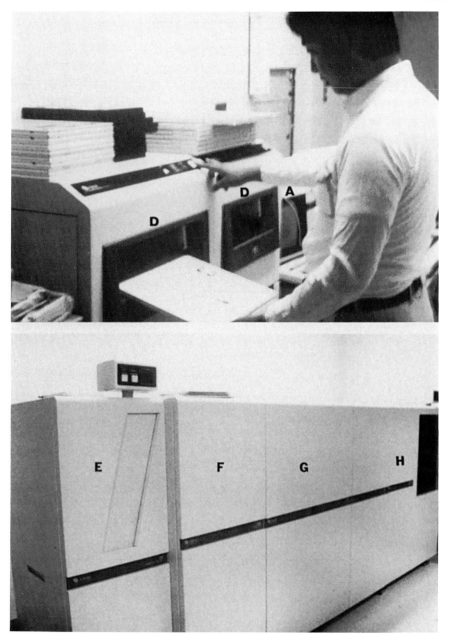

Figure 4.2 An early computed radiography system, the FCR-101 (see text for key to letters), and two recent systems, the AC-II and the FCR-9000.

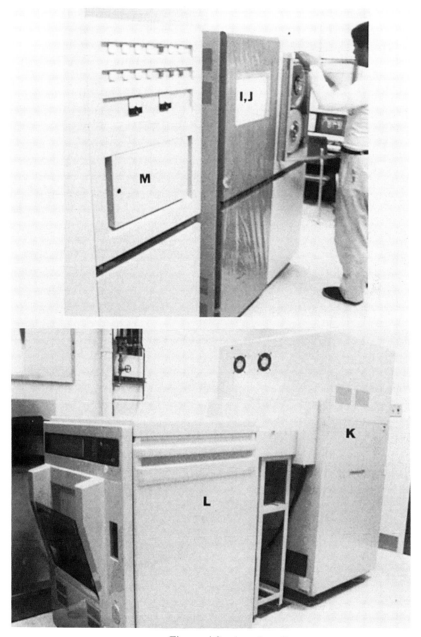

Figure 4.2 (*continued*)

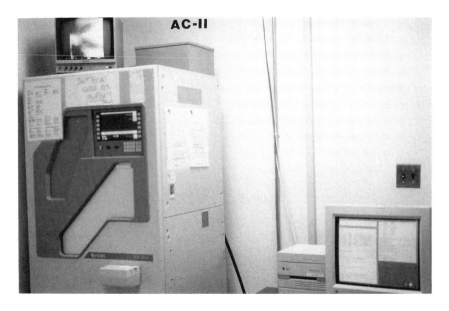

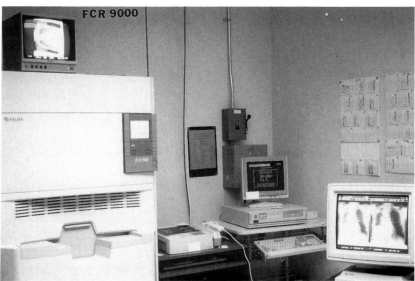

Figure 4.2 (*continued*)

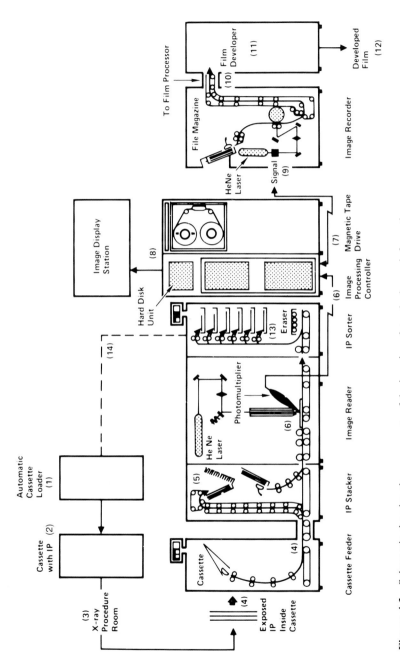

Figure 4.3 Schematic showing the movements of the imaging plate, the image information, and the film inside an early CR system; see text for key to numbers.

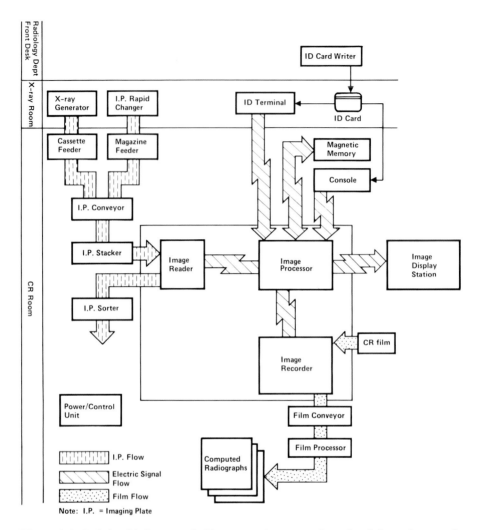

Figure 4.4 Relationship between the X-ray procedure room, the patient information recording component (front desk), and the CR system.

space, the principle of operation remains very similar. Also, the current system no longer uses a magnetic tape drive for storage. Figure 4.4 shows the connections between the exposure of the imaging plate in the X-ray procedure room, the patient information reader, and the CR system.

The following steps for using the CR system correspond to the numbers shown in Figure 4.3.

1. An erased imaging plate is loaded automatically into a cassette.
2. The cassette with the imaging plate inside is placed under the patient for an exposure (see step 4 in Fig. 4.3).

3. An exposure is made in the X-ray procedure room, and the cassette is sent to the CR room for processing.
4. The cassette is fed into the cassette feeder in a lighttight environment and the plate is dropped into the IP conveyor.
5. The IP conveyor delivers the plate into an IP stacker, which queues exposed plates to be processed.
6. The conveyor delivers an imaging plate to the image reader, and the luminescence radiation stimulated by the laser scanning is collected and fed into the image processor.
7. The image processor processes the electronic signals, performs analog-to-digital conversion, formats the signals to an image, enhances the image contrast, and transmits the digital image to an image recorder and a storage device.
8. The processed image is stored in the image memory and can be sent to a computer disk or magnetic tape for permanent storage. It can also be displayed on a video monitor through a linkage to an image display station.
9. The processed digital image can also be sent to an image recorder, which writes the image on a film with a laser printer.
10. The exposed film is sent to a conveyor, which carries it to a standard film developer.
11. The film developer develops the film, treating it like a conventional exposed X-ray film.
12. The image on the film is then the hard copy of the exposed image.
13. The processed image plate is sent through the conveyor to an IP sorter, which sorts it according to size, and the plate is erased by flooding it with high intensity light.
14. The plate can be inserted into a cassette loader and reused.

The CR system also has an automatic patient recording component that transmits patient information, from an ID card the size of a conventional credit card, through an ID terminal to the system database (see Fig. 4.4). Selected information from this ID card is merged with the image and is printed on top of the film or displayed with the image on the video monitor for identification purposes.

We have described the operation of a removable IP plate CR system. There are also nonremovable IP systems in which several plates circulate inside the system but no cassette is used. Two configurations are possible: the standing type (patient in an upright position) and the recumbent type (patient supine or prone). During the exposure, the conveyor transports an IP to the proper position aligned with the region of interest of the patient. After the exposure, the conveyor transports the exposed IP to the IP reader for scanning and carries an unexposed plate to the proper position for a possible second exposure. Nonremovable IP systems are good for special procedure rooms (e.g., for chest examination) because less time is needed to load and unload the cassette. In addition, since the mechanical handling necessitated by loading and unloading is minimized, the chances of breaking the IP are reduced. The disadvantage of the nonremovable IP system is that it requires modifications to the procedure room.

4.1.3 Description of System Components

The major components of a computed radiographic system are described in Sections 4.1.3.1–4.1.3.10.

4.1.3.1 ID Card Writer

The ID card writer (Fig. 4.2, A) is a unit for writing on, reading, and erasing plastic cards with a magnetic strip carrying patient identification data. The cards may be erased and reused many times; a fresh card is used for each patient who undergoes an X-ray procedure.

4.1.3.2 ID Terminal

In the ID terminal (Fig. 4.2, B), the ID card encoding the patient data is read and displayed. The operator can input patient information and radiographic procedure via functional keys of the terminal. The patient and examination data are correlated with the number of the imaging plate, which is obtained by scanning the plate with a bar code reader. These data are transferred to the main processor. Several ID terminals may be connected to one CR system. In the current system, a direct interface of the ID terminal with the radiology information system (RIS) is possible. Patient information can be transmitted directly from the RIS, minimizing typographical errors.

4.1.3.3 Console and Automatic Cassette Loader

The console (Fig. 4.2, C) is the main user interface with the system. It contains an image monitor and a control monitor. Interactive elements are a mode switch for routine or manual operation, functional keys for special procedures, and a magnetic card reader for input of patient data. The cassette loader (Fig. 4.2, D) is used to load an imaging plate automatically into a cassette.

4.1.3.4 Cassette Feeder

The cassette feeder (Fig. 4.2, E) is a module for manual insertion of a cassette with an exposed IP. The cassette feeder is provided with appropriate mechanisms for unloading the cassette, conveying the imaging plate to the IP stacker, and returning the empty cassette to the user.

4.1.3.5 Image Plate Stacker

The IP stacker (Fig. 4.2, F) temporarily stores imaging plates from the cassette feeder and sends imaging plates one by one to the image reader based on a command from the image processing controller. The stacker has two functions: to feed the imaging plates in first-in, first-out order, and to move an IP to a bypass conveyor line, through which imaging plates received last can be fed to the reader by priority. This bypass function is important because it allows the system to process IPs from emergency patients in timely fashion.

4.1.3.6 Image Reader and Image Plate Sorter

The image reader (Fig. 4.2, G) has a precision laser spot scanning mechanism for prereading and main readings. Prereading scans the plate at a selected sampling area to determine the optical density range of the plate, which in turn is used for automatic gain control for the main reading. During the main reading, the laser spot extracts image information from the plate as light signals. The light signals are converted to electrical signals, digitized, and transmitted to the image processing controller. The automatic gain control feature in the image reader, by which X-ray image information recorded on the imaging plate can be read with the optimum sensitivity, ensures that even when the X-ray exposure varies, the gray levels of the output image are always kept in a proper region.

The IP sorter (Fig. 4.2, H) serves to erase the residual image on the imaging plate after reading and to sort and store the imaging plates by size and type. The IP sorter includes conveyor parts, two erase zones, and trays for different sizes of imaging plates.

4.3.1.7 Image Processing Controller and Image Storage Devices

The image processing controller (Fig. 4.2, I) consists of a microprocessor for giving accurate instructions to each component of the system and controlling system operations of all kinds, and a high speed image processor for the computation of various algorithms capable of processing images in accordance with the purpose of a given diagnosis. The image processing controller has magnetic disk storage for temporary recording of image information, operation, and test programs. Image storage devices (Fig. 4.2, J) consist of magnetic tape drives and magnetic and optical storage devices.

4.3.1.8 Image Recorder

The image recorder (Fig. 4.2, K) converts image information from digital signals to analog signals and then feeds the analog signals, as input signals, to the optical modulator. Controlling a laser beam by these input signals, the image recorder writes the image onto a CR film. The image recorder houses a super precision laser beam scanning mechanism and a high precision film conveying mechanism that sends the film on which the image information has been recorded in succession to the film processor. The image recorder includes a film supply unit for loading the films under daylight conditions. The image recorder is provided with a counter, which indicates the number of films that have been processed.

4.1.3.9 Film Processor and Power/Control Unit

The film processor, similar to a standard film processor as described in Chapter 3, is a module (Fig. 4.2, L) in which the film that has been exposed in the image recorder is developed. The power/control unit (Fig. 4.2, M) supplies the electric power to the CR system. The power switch for each equipment device is sequentially turned on and off.

4.1.3.10 Plate Conveyor and Film Conveyor; Image Display Station

The plate conveyor and film conveyor (Fig. 4.3) is a system of mechanical parts that transport the plate from the cassette feeder to the IP sorter, and the exposed film from the image recorder to the film processor. In the design of current CR systems, this component becomes very compact to preserve space and to reduce the number of moving parts, minimizing the possibility of mechanical failures. The digital image can be sent to a display station (Fig. 4.4) for soft copy display.

4.1.4 Specifications of the Image Reader and Recorder

The principles of the image reader and image recorder in the CR system are similar to those applicable to the laser scanner, discussed in Chapter 3, and the laser printer, to be mentioned in Chapter 9. The only difference between the image scanner and the laser reader is that the laser scanner scans an X-ray film, whereas the image reader scans the imaging plate. The laser printer and the image recorder are almost identical, since both write digital images onto single emulsion films.

Table 4.1 shows the specifications of the image reader and the recorder. A comparison of Tables 3.2 and 9.4 indicates that the characteristics of laser scanner and image reader, and of laser printer and image recorder, are quite similar. In general, the digital image generated by the image reader is $2000 \times 2000 \times 8$ bits or higher, depending on the size of the film and the sampling raster.

Table 4.1   Specification of the Image Reader and Recorder
in a Computed Radiographic System

	Reader	Recorder
Image format	43.2 cm × 35.6 cm	21.4 cm × 17.6 cm
	35.6 cm × 35.6 cm	17.6 cm × 17.6 cm
	30.5 cm × 25.4 cm	20.1 cm × 16.7 cm
	20.3 cm × 25.4 cm	20.0 cm × 25.1 cm
Sampling raster	5–10 pixels/mm	10 pixels/mm
Laser spot size	100 μm	120 μm
Gray levels	8 bits (A/D)	10 bits (D/A)
Speed	90 seconds for	90 seconds for
	43.2 cm × 35.6 cm	21.4 cm × 17.6 cm
Laser power	15 mW	0.1 mW

4.1.5 Operating Characteristics of the Scanning Laser-Stimulated Luminescence System

A major advantage of the CR system compared to the conventional film–screen system is that the imaging plate is linear and has a large dynamic range between the X-ray exposure and the relative intensity of the stimulated phosphors. Hence, under similar X-ray exposure conditions, the image reader is capable of producing images with density resolution comparable or superior to those from the conventional film–screen system. Since the image reader automatically adjusts the amount of exposure received by the plate, over- or underexposure within a certain limit would not affect the appearance of the image. This useful feature can best be explained by the two examples given in Figure 4.5.

In quadrant A of Figure 4.5, example I represents a plate exposed to a higher relative exposure level but a narrower exposure range (10^3–10^4). The linear response of the plate after laser scanning yields a high level but narrow light intensity (photostimulable luminescence, PSL) range of 10^3–10^4. These light photons are

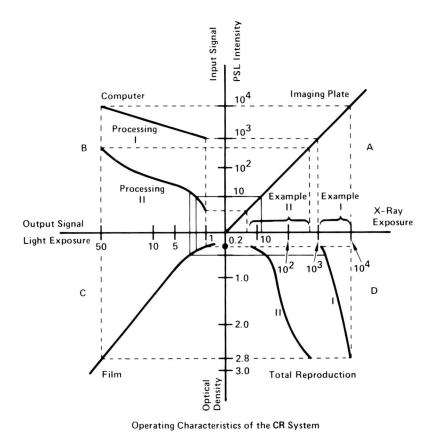

Operating Characteristics of the CR System

Figure 4.5 Two examples illustrating the operating characteristics of the CR system.

converted into electric output signals representing the latent image stored in the image plate. The image processor senses a narrow range of electrical signals and selects a special lookup table (top linear curve in quadrant B, Fig. 4.5), which converts the narrow dynamic range (10^3–10^4) to a large light relative exposure of 1 to 50. If a large-latitude film is used that covers the dynamic range of the light exposure from 1 to 50, as shown in quadrant C (see discussion on large-latitude film in Section 3.1.2.1), these output signals will register the entire optical density range from OD 0.2 to OD 2.8 on the film. The total system response, including the imaging plate, the lookup table, and the film subject to this exposure range is depicted as curve I in quadrant D. The system–response curve, relating the relative exposure on the plate and the OD of the output film, shows a high gamma value and is quite linear. This example demonstrates how the system accommodates a high exposure level but a narrow exposure range.

Returning now to quadrant A in Figure 4.5, consider example II, in which the plate receives a lower exposure level but wider exposure range. The CR system automatically selects a different lookup table in the image processor to accommodate this range of exposure, with the result that the output signals again spans the entire light exposure range from 1 to 50. The system–response curve is shown as curve II in quadrant D. The key in selecting the correct lookup table is the range of the exposure: it has to span the total light exposure of the film, namely from 1 to 50. It is noted that in both examples, the entire useful optical density range for diagnostic radiology is utilized.

If a conventional film–screen combination system was used, exposure in example I in Figure 4.5 would utilize only the higher optical density region of the film, whereas in example II it would utilize the lower region. Neither case would utilize the full dynamic range of optical density in the film. From these two examples it is seen that the CR system allows the utilization of the full optical density dynamic range, regardless of whether the plate is overexposed or underexposed. The same effect will be achieved if the image recorder is not used to produce a hard copy of the digital image formed from the output signal. That is, the digital image produced from the image reader and the image processor will also utilize the full dynamic range of the 10-bit digital number. The principle of the laser scanner system discussed in Chapter 3 can be applied to the rationalization of these phenomena, as well.

4.1.6 Some Clinical Applications

The CR system is an excellent method of converting conventional projection radiographic images into digital format. It does not require recording the image on film first and later digitizing it through a scanner. Instead, the image is stored as a latent image in the imaging plate, whereupon the laser reader reads the latent image from the plate and converts it into digital form directly. The imaging plate can be erased and reused. In addition, it has some other clinical applications, including the following:

1. Since the CR system can automatically adjust for under- or overexposure, acceptable diagnostic images can be produced at exposures that would have provided unacceptable, or at least marginal, radiographs if conventional film–screen techniques had been used. This characteristic is important for intensive care units and emergency room applications, since it is often difficult to obtain radiographs of proper exposure in the clinical environment.
2. The large latitude in the digital image allows excellent visualization of both soft tissue and bone detail.
3. Because of the wide dynamic range of the system, it is possible to reduce the X-ray dose to patients based on the information required. For example, in a screening procedure (e.g., scoliosis assessment and follow-up of fracture alignment), 5–10% of the conventional dose will produce acceptable images—a substantial benefit to the patient.
4. It is possible to virtually eliminate the need for repeat examinations due to exposure errors, especially for the portable radiographic units. Figure 4.6 shows a series of skull films taken with different exposures comparing the conventional film–screen and the CR techniques.

4.2 Digital Fluorography

Digital fluorography is another method that can produce a digital X-ray image without substantial changes in the radiographic procedure room. The technique does, however, require an add-on unit in the conventional fluorographic system.

Recall that fluorography is the procedure of displaying fluoroscopic images on a video monitor using an image intensifier coupling with a video camera (see Section 3.1.2.2). This technique is used to visualize the motion of body compartments (e.g., blood flow, heart beat) and the movement of a catheter, as well as to pinpoint a body region for making a film image for subsequent detailed diagnosis. Each exposure required in a fluorographic procedure is very minimal compared with a conventional X-ray procedure.

Digital fluorography is considered to be an add-on system because a digital chain is added to an existing fluorographic unit. This method utilizes the established X-ray, image intensifier, video scanning, and digital technologies. The output from a digital fluorographic system is a sequence of digital images displayed on a video monitor.

Digital fluorography has an advantage over conventional fluorography in that it gives a larger dynamic range image and can remove uninteresting structures in the images by performing digital subtraction.

Other names used for digital fluorography are digital subtraction angiography and digital subtraction arteriography (both abbreviated as DSA), digital video angiography (DVA), intravenous videoarteriography (IVA), computerized fluoroscopy (CF), and digital video subtraction angiography (DVSA).

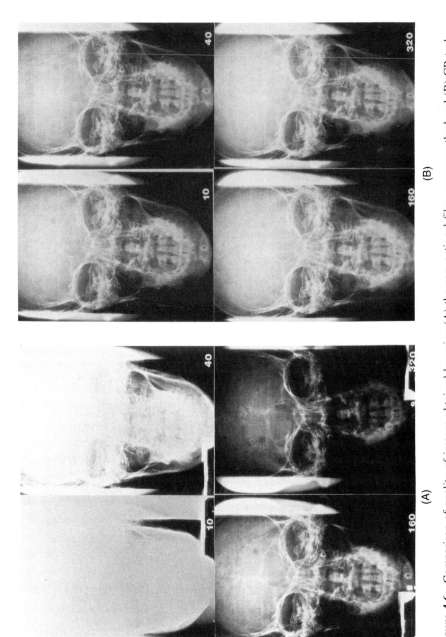

(A)

(B)

Figure 4.6 Comparison of quality of images obtained by using (A) the conventional film–screen method and (B) CR techniques. Exposures were 70 kV(p); 10, 40, 160, and 320 mA·s on a skull phantom. It is seen that in this example the CR technique is almost dose independent.

Source: Courtesy of Dr. S. Balter.

4.2.1 Description of System Components

A complete digital fluorographic system consists of four major components; the numbered items in the list that follows correspond to numbered areas in Figure 4.7.

1. *X-ray source.* The X-ray tube itself and a grid to minimize scattering were described in Section 3.1.1. The X-ray source also includes a collimator.
2. *Image receptor.* The image receptor used in a digital fluorographic system is an image intensifier tube; its function was described in Section 3.1.2.2
3. *Video camera plus optical system.* The light from the image intensifier goes through an optical system, which allows the video camera to be adjusted for focusing. The amount of light going into the camera is controlled by means of a light diaphragm. The operating procedure of the TV camera was described in Section 3.2.1.1. The type of camera used in digital fluorography is usually a plumbicon or a CCD. The scanning mechanism can either be interlaced or progressive, and the camera matrix size can be from 512 to 1024 pixels per line.
4. *Digital chain.* The add-on unit is the digital chain, which consists of an A/D converter, image memories, image processor, digital storage, and video display. The A/D converter, the image memory, and the digital storage can handle $512 \times 512 \times 8$ bit images at 30 frames per second, or $1024 \times 1024 \times 8$ bit images at 7.5 frames per second. A digital storage disk that can accommodate such high speed data transfer, which is essential for cardiac imaging, is called a *real-time digital disk* or a storage array. Figure 4.8 illustrates a digital fluorographic system showing a 14-inch image intensifier and a plumbicon camera. Table 4.2 shows the spatial resolution limitation of a digital fluorographic system and some measurements obtained from the system shown in Figure 4.8. As this table indicates, the spatial resolution of the DSA is limited by the size of the digital image, not by the image intensifier tube.

4.2.2 Operational Procedure

A digital fluorography imaging session proceeds as follows.

1. The patient is positioned according to conventional fluorographic procedure.
2. Mask images without contrast material injection are taken.
3. An intravenous or intra-arterial bolus injection of a contrast medium is administered, either manually or through a power injector.
4. The X-ray source is turned on and digital frames are obtained with the proper imaging mode (see Section 4.2.3).
5. Frames within a bolus injection cycle are selected and stored in the digital disk.
6. Another bolus injection is administered if necessary, and the cycle is repeated.
7. A sequence (or sequences) of digital images showing the contrast medium flowing through a region of interest is obtained.
8. Any such sequence of images can be enhanced with the mask images described in Section 4.2.4.

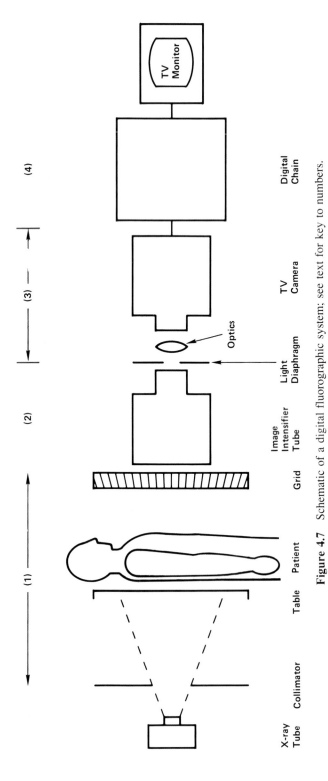

Figure 4.7 Schematic of a digital fluorographic system; see text for key to numbers.

Table 4.2 Spatial Resolution of a Digital Fluorographic System Without Geometric Magnification

Image Intensifier Mode (in.)	Image Intensifier Resolution (lp/mm)	Nyquist Resolution Limitation for DSA (lp/mm)		Measured Resolution: Fig. 4.8 (lp/mm)	
		512 System	1024 System	512 System	1024 System
14				0.85	0.90
9	3	1.1	2.2		
6	4	1.5	3.0	1.5	1.75
4.5	5	2.1	4.2		

4.2.3 Imaging Mode

"Imaging mode" refers to the timing of radiographic events between the emission of X-ray energy and data acquisition (see Fig. 4.9).

In the *pulsed mode*, the X-ray output is pulsed from one to four times (or higher)

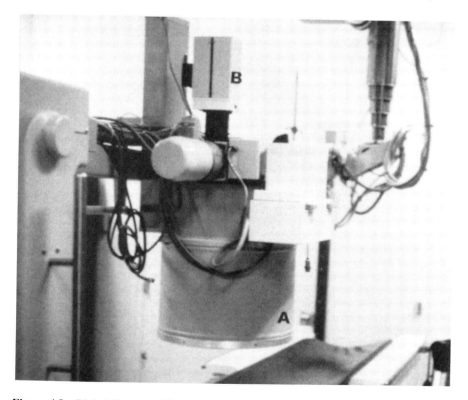

Figure 4.8 Digital fluorographic system with (A) a 14-inch image intensifier and (B) a 1024-bit plumbicon camera attached to a digital chain.

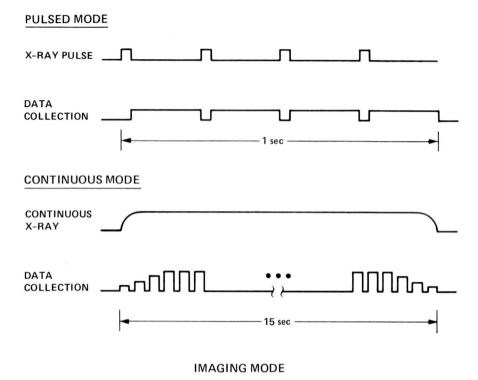

Figure 4.9 Two imaging modes in digital fluorography: pulsed and continuous.

per second, and an image is formed after the end of the first pulse and before the second. This mode is characterized for high milliamperes and is used for detailed vascular and conventional radiographic examinations.

In the *continuous mode*, the X-ray flux is continuous for greater than 15 seconds and an image is formed during each 33 ms interval. This mode is characterized by low milliamperage and is used for cardiac and vascular examinations.

4.2.4 Processing Mode

"Processing mode" refers to the method of enhancing the image data, once acquired. In the case of digital fluorography, the goal is to enhance the contrast appearance in the vascularity. The processing method is based on the general linear filtering technique shown in Eq. (4.1):

$$P = \sum_{i=1}^{n} W_i P_i \tag{4.1}$$

where P_i = a sequence of n images acquired during a fluorographic procedure
           i = the time when the image is acquired

W_i = the weighted factor for each pixel of P_i
P = the filtered image or the resultant image after the processing

The set of weighted factors W_i is subject to the constraint

$$\sum_{i=1}^{n} W_i = 0 \qquad\qquad (4.2)$$

This constraint is necessary to guarantee that all the background materials will be subtracted. It is seen that to ensure that this condition is satisfied, some W_i will have to be negative. The selection of weighted factor W_i is based on the characteristics of the contrast material bolus flowing through a region of interest (e.g., blood vessels in the region). Figure 4.10A is a typical plot of contrast material bolus flowing through an artery following intravenous contrast material administration.

Four techniques are available for processing the images; the choice depends on the method of selecting the W_i.

1. *Conventional DSA mask subtraction.* This technique is commonly used in the pulsed mode. One image, the mask, is taken before the injection of contrast medium and then is subtracted from an image with maximum contrast material. Figure 4.10B shows an example, in this case, $W_9 = +1$, $W_3 = -1$ and the rest of $W_i = 0$. W_3 is the image without contrast, and W_9 is the image with the maximum contrast. This subtraction would give an image that shows only the contrast material in the blood vessel.

2. *Integrated remasking.* Because a lower exposure is used in integrated remasking, each acquired image obtained in a continuous mode contains more noise than those obtained in the pulsed mode. One method of minimizing the noise is to use averaging (see Section 2.5.2). In the example shown in Figure 4.10C, five frames before contrast injection (all with $W_i = -1$) and five after (all with $W_i = 1$) are averaged. As a result, the filtered image P will have less noise. Integrated remasking is best performed retrospectively in selecting the best set of images for averaging.

3. *Matched filtering.* Matched filtering is based on the technique commonly used in electrical engineering to detect a signal of known shape that is contained in a noisy waveform. The signal to be detected in the case of DSA, the characteristic curve of the bolus flow after contrast injection, is embedded in a sequence of noisy images. To start the matched filtering technique, the characteristic curve of the bolus flow is obtained retrospectively using the gray level values from a fixed region of interest in the complete sequence of images. The x axis is shifted upward until the positive area of the curve equals the negative area (see Fig. 4.10D). The amount of shifting defines a new shifted x axis.

The new ordinates of the curve with respect to the shifted x axis are then used as the weighted factor for the corresponding images in the sequence. This assignment of weighted factors will maximize the effects of the bolus contrast with a minimum amount of noise. It is noted that any W_i so selected can be manually deleted if frame P_i contains unacceptable noisy image data.

Figure 4.11 uses the example of an intracranial aneurysm to compare the results

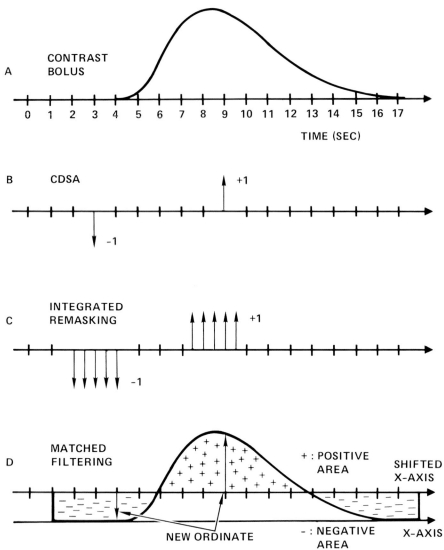

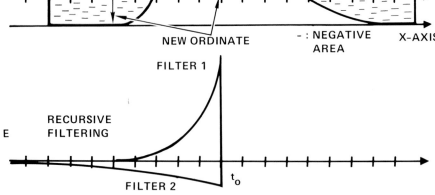

Figure 4.10 (A) The characteristic curve of the contrast bolus flow and four image processing techniques for digital fluorography: (B) conventional DSA mask subtraction, (C) integrated remasking, (D) matched filtering, and (E) recursive filtering.

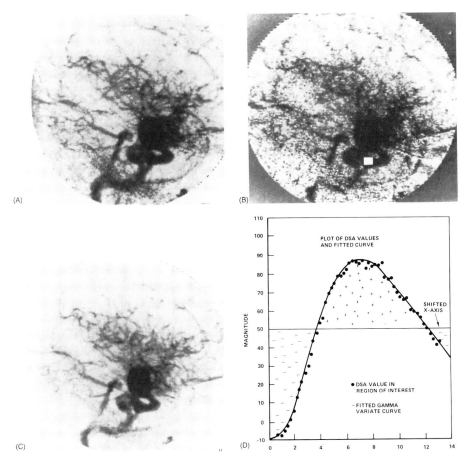

Figure 4.11   (A) Lateral projection of an intracranial aneurysm acquired using simple (non-integrated) remasking with conventional DSA technique. Technique: 90 kV(p), 1000 mA, 71 ms; one image per second for 16 seconds. (B) One image from 38-image sequence acquired for matched filtering. Technique: 85 kV(p), 23 mA continuous for 16 seconds; 8-frame video integration. Noise level of all images in the sequence was high. This image corresponded to peak opacification of the internal carotid arteries. Region of interest (white square) is used to generate plot of DSA values and form matched filter. (C) Matched filter result. This image was judged superior to (A) in iodine signal-to-noise ratio, although patient exposure was less than one-third that of the standard DSA run used for (A). (D) Plot of DSA values in the region of interest shown in (B) as a function of time. Smooth curve is plot after a gamma curve fitting to the data points.

Source: Courtesy of Dr. S. Riederer.

obtained from a conventional DSA and an image obtained through the matched filtering technique. In this case, the shape of the characteristic bolus curve is computed retrospectively by measuring the gray level values in the artery of interest (Fig. 4.11B: square white region). The horizontal line in Figure 4.11D is the shifted x axis, which separates the positive area with the negative area. Clearly, in this case, the matched filtering technique (Fig. 4.11C) yields a better quality subtracted image than the conventional DSA (Fig. 4.11A).

4. *Recursive filtering.* Recursive filtering is occasionally used to process DSA images because of the characteristics of video scanning. As applied to video image processing, "recursive" means that the image formed during the exposure of some frame is a combination of the image presently being read from the video camera and images formed during earlier frames. By repeating this logic for many successive frames, an event is observed, density from contrast medium in the current frame being contributed by that in several preceding frames. For this reason, this filtering technique is used when the video camera is very laggy or sticky.

Figure 4.10E illustrates a simple recursive technique using two filters: filter 1 is the result of adding three images frames, whereas filter 2 is the result of subtracting eight image frames. It is noted that filter 2 is equivalent to the integrated masked images in the conventional DSA. It is also seen that the area under the curve defined by filter 1 should equal the area above the curve by defined filter 2.

Among these four techniques, conventional DSA mask subtraction is used mostly for pulsed imaging modes; integrated remasking and matched filtering are generally selected for the continuous imaging mode. Table 4.3 compares the four

Table 4.3 Comparison of Four DSA Postprocessing Techniques*

	Conventional DSA	Integrated Remasking	Matched Filtering	Recursive Filtering
Imaging mode	Pulsed	Pulsed/continuous	Pulsed/continuous	Continuous
Images acquired per second	1	4–30	4–30	30
Current used	300–1000 mA	Pulsed, 75–250 mA; continuous, 10–30 mA	75–250, pulsed 10–30, Continuous	10–30
Required minimum video SNR	500:1	250:1/100:1	250:1/100:1	100:1
Number of images in a single DSA run	15	60[†]	60[†]	60[‡]
Operator intervention required	Small	Moderate	Moderate	Small
Effective integration time	≈30 ms	≈1–5 s	≈5 s	≈8 s
Signal-to-noise ratio of DSA image[§]	1	1–2	≈ 2.0	≈ 1.7

* Values shown are assumed for an intravenous angiographic study of the extracranial carotid arteries.

† Even with continuous exposure, images may be summed in groups of seven or eight prior to storage.

‡ Assuming equal patient exposure for each, and a 15-second examination.

§ Although 30 frames/second is possible, storage of filtered sequences at a lower rate (≈4 s) is sufficient and will not sacrifice image quality.

techniques based on an intravenous angiographic study of the extracranial carotid arteries.

4.3 Low-Scattering Digital Radiographic System

Both imaging plate technology and the digital fluorographic system can be run without changing the X-ray source, after only minimal modifications to the image detector system. The low-scattering digital radiographic systems discussed in this section—the line scan and flying-spot scanning techniques—require substantial modifications in the configuration of both the X-ray source and the detector system.

4.3.1 Line Scan Technique

In the line scan technique, the X-ray source is first collimated with a lead slit. The linear X-ray beam is transmitted through the patient and detected by a linear detector array (see Fig. 4.12). The collimated X-ray source and the detector array form a functional unit which defines a vertical beam. An image is obtained by moving the

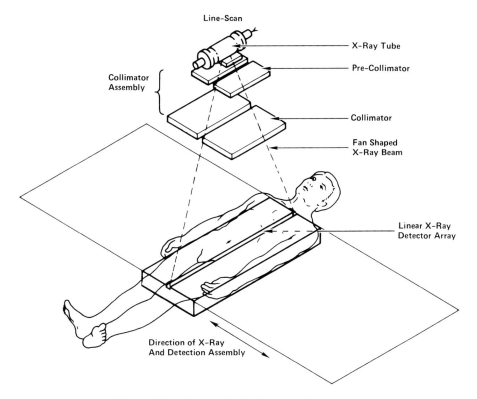

Figure 4.12   Schematic of a line scanning system.

Table 4.4 Specifications of a Prototype
Digital Line Scan Chest
Unit Image

Field size	20 in. × 20 in.
Image matrix	1024 × 1024
Pixel size	0.5 mm × 0.5 mm
Resolution	1.0 lp/mm
Gray scale	256 levels (8 bits)
Scan time	4 seconds
Maximum skin exposure	35 mR

unit transversely across the patient. In the vertical direction (i.e., longitudinal to the detector array), the sampling distance is defined by the detector-to-detector spacing, while in the horizontal direction it is determined by the distance between two sets of detector readings.

An example of the line scan technique is a prototype digital chest unit developed by Picker International. The detector array in this system consists of 1024 photodiodes coupled to a gadolinium oxysulfide screen. The separation between diodes is 0.5 mm, resulting in a total array length of 51.2 cm (20 in.). Also, the horizontal pixel dimension, 0.5 mm, is the same as the longitudinal dimension. Therefore, in both directions, the spatial resolution is 1.0 lp/mm. Table 4.4 gives the specifications of this prototype chest unit.

4.3.2 Flying-Spot Scan Technique

In the flying-spot scan technique (see Fig. 4.13), the X-ray source (a) is first collimated with a slit (b), which is further collimated into a pencil beam (d) by a rotating disk with radial slits (c) perpendicular to the beam. The pencil beam scans horizontally from left to right across the patient while the disk rotates, and the attenuation is measured by a system of solid state scintillators and photomultiplier tubes (e). The crystals are large enough to intercept a whole plane of X-rays formed by (b) independent of the rotational position of the disk.

Therefore, regardless of the position of the disk, the detector can measure the X-ray transmission through the slit. The continuous rotation of the disk allows measurements of adjacent points along the same transverse plane. In practice, the disk rotates about 1800 rpm; an independent optical system determines this rotational position as a function of time. The output of the detector as a function of time can then be correlated with the disk's rotational position to give the X-ray transmission as a function of position within the X-ray plane. This generates a one-dimensional transverse line through the subject. To generate the second dimension, the X-ray tube, collimator, rotating disk, and detector, functioning as a unit, translates the beam through to the patient (two arrows in Fig. 4.13). The detector output is then sent to a digital chain to form a digital image.

The advantage of flying-spot scanning is the low dosage to the patient because of the minimal amount of scattering as the X-ray source is collimated to a pencil beam.

FLYING-SPOT SCAN

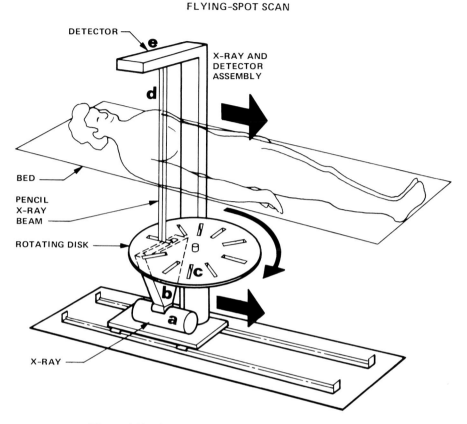

Figure 4.13 Schematic of a flying-spot scanning system.

There are two principal disadvantages. First, the utilization of the X-ray energy is low, since most X-ray photons are blocked by the collimators and, as a result, the X-ray source tends to have a short life. Second, a low signal-to-noise ratio, which is due to the low photon counts per pixel, in turn yields a noisier image.

Table 4.5 summarizes some characteristics of three of the digital radiographic systems discussed thus far: digital fluorography, line scan, and flying-spot scan.

4.4 Dual-Energy Imaging

In the discussion of digital subtraction angiography (DSA), we mentioned integrated masking, a technique based on temporal mask subtraction. The term "temporal" reflects the correspondence of the time axis of each image in the imaging sequence to the time axis of the characteristic curve of the contrast bolus in the blood. Therefore, the filtering techniques developed for images obtained from DSA are based on the characteristics of the bolus injection curve.

Table 4.5 Characteristics of Three Digital Radiographic Systems

Characteristic	DSA/DF	Line Scan	Flying Spot
Camera S/N	1000:1		
Detector	Plumbicon camera	Phosphor screen + 1024 photodiodes	Scintillator + PMT
Image matrix	512 or 1024	512 or 1024	512 or 1024
Display matrix	512 or 1024	512 or 1024	512 or 1024
Density resolution	8 bit	8 bit	8 bit
Spatial resolution	2 lp/mm	1–2 lp/mm	1.6 lp/mm
Frame/second	30	0.25	0.25
Energy range	50–90 kV(p) 25–150 mA	80–130 kV(p) (max) 110 mA	135 kV(p) 200 mA
Dosage		35 mR	0.5 mR

The *dual-energy imaging mode* (developed by Alvarez and Macovski, 1976) is another image processing mode that can enhance resultant images by manipulating two images obtained at two different X-ray energy levels. This technique can be applied to images obtained from conventional projection radiography, computed radiography, digital fluorography, or the new low-scattering scanning systems. The same principle can also be used in computerized tomography as discussed in Chapter 5.

4.4.1 Concept of Aluminum (AL) and Plastic (PL) Component Images

Consider an object of interest consisting of two materials M_1, and M_2 each with thickness X_1 and X_2 respectively. This object is exposed to an X-ray beam I_0 as shown in Figure 4.14. The dual-energy theory states that the X-ray image of each material is composed of an aluminum (AL) and a plastic (PL) component. The AL-component image of the object is defined as the image of the object contributed only by the aluminum components in M_1 and M_2. Similarly, the PL-component image is the image of the object contributed only by the plastic components in M_1 and M_2. The AL- and PL-component images are sometimes referred, respectively, to as the bone and the soft tissue image. The concept of AL- and PL-component images of an object is essential to understand the dual-energy imaging procedure.

4.4.2 Theory of Dual-Energy Imaging and Its Computational Procedure

4.4.2.1 Transmitted Intensity

In projection radiography within the diagnostic energy range, the transmitted intensity I measured at the detector is given by

$$\frac{I}{I_0} = \int S(E)e^{-[A_1 f_1(E) + A_2 f_2(E)]} \, dE \tag{4.3}$$

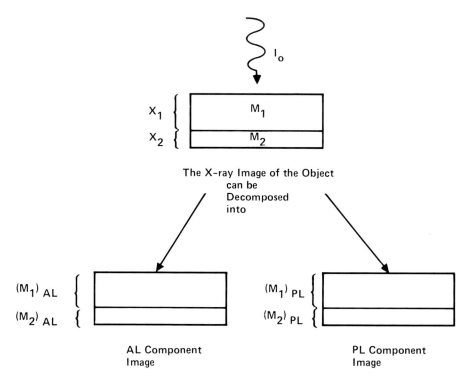

Figure 4.14 Concept of aluminum-component and plastic-component images of an object.

where I_0 = the intensity of the incident beam, measured by a reference detector

$S(E)$ = the incident X-ray spectrum

$f_1(E) \cong 1/E^3$, the energy-dependent part of the photoelectric coefficient at (x,y,z) for $E > k$ electron binding energy

$f_2(E) \cong 1 - 2(E/511) + 5.2(E/511)^2 - 13.3(E/511)^3 + \cdots$

and $E(keV) \ll 511$ is the Compton scattering cross section at (x,y,z), (this is an approximate form of the Klein–Nishina formula for low energy photons). In addition:

$A_i = \int a_i(x,y,z)ds$, $i = 1, 2$, dependent only on the material composition of the object at (x,y,z) along the X-ray paths

$a_1 \cong N_0 Z^4 / A$ is the photoelectric contribution

$a_2 \cong Z\rho N_0 / A$ is the Compton contribution, where Z and A are the atomic number and the atomic weight, respectively, N_0 is Avogadro's number, and ρ is density (g/cm^3)

Assuming that I can be measured, then to obtain A_i, $i = 1, 2$, on more equation is needed.

4.4.2.2 Dual-Energy Model

Let $S_H(E)$ and $S_L(E)$ be the X-ray spectra of two different (high and low) energies, then

$$\ln\left(\frac{I}{I_0}\right)_H = \ln\left\{\int S_H(E)e^{-[A_1 f_1(E)+A_2 f_2(E)]}\, dE\right\} \tag{4.4}$$

and

$$\ln\left(\frac{I}{I_0}\right)_L = \ln\left\{\int S_L(E)e^{-[A_1 f_1(E)+A_2 f_2(E)]}\, dE\right\} \tag{4.5}$$

This is a system of two equations with (theoretically) two unknowns: A_1 and A_2. Since the incident X-ray spectra are difficult to determine, an alternate formulation is needed.

In this formulation, the two basic functions f_1, f_2 (representing the photoelectric and Compton cross sections) are replaced by a set of basis functions representing the total linear attenuation coefficients of aluminum μ_{AL} and of plastic μ_{PL} (other materials can also be used). Each coefficient μ_{AL} and μ_{PL} can be viewed as a linear sum of photoelectric and Compton components:

$$\mu_{AL}(E) = k_1 f_1(E) + k_2 f_2(E) \tag{4.6}$$

$$\mu_{PL}(E) = k_3 f_1(E) + k_4 f_2(E) \tag{4.7}$$

Thus, Eqs. (4.4) and (4.5) can be equivalently written as follows:

$$\ln\left(\frac{I}{I_0}\right)_H = \ln\left\{\int S_H(E)e^{-[t_{PL}\mu_{PL}(E)+t_{AL}\mu_{AL}(E)]}\, dE\right\} \tag{4.8}$$

$$\ln\left(\frac{I}{I_0}\right)_L = \ln\left\{\int S_L(E)e^{-[t_{PL}\mu_{PL}(E)+t_{AL}\mu_{AL}(E)]}\, dE\right\} \tag{4.9}$$

where t_{AL} and t_{PL} are the AL-component and PL-component thickness, respectively.

Equations (4.8) and (4.9) can be solved numerically by approximating both right-hand sides with a quadratic polynomial in t_{PL} and t_{AL}:

$$\ln\left(\frac{I}{I_0}\right)_H = b_0 + b_1 t_{AL} + b_2 t_{PL} + b_3 t_{AL} t_{PL} + b_4 t_{AL}^2 + b_5 t_{PL}^2 \tag{4.10}$$

$$\ln\left(\frac{I}{I_0}\right)_L = c_0 + c_1 t_{AL} + c_2 t_{PL} + c_3 t_{AL} t_{PL} + c_4 t_{AL}^2 + c_5 t_{PL}^2 \tag{4.11}$$

The values for the constant b_i and c_i can be determined using the calibration procedure described in Section 4.4.2.3 and a standard curve-fitting algorithm.

Table 4.6 High Energy X-Ray Transmitted Intensity Value Versus Combination of AL and PL Step Wedges

	PL Step			
AL Step	0	1	2 . . .	17 . . .
0				
1				
.			High energy	
.			X-ray	
.			transmitted	
8			intensities	
.				
.				
.				

4.4.2.3 Calibration Procedure

An aluminum step wedge with steps of ⅛-inch 1100 aluminum ($\rho = 2.70$ g/cm³) and a Lucite step wedge with steps of ¼ inch ($\rho = 1.19$ g/cm³) can be used for calibration. High and low energy digital images of all possible combinations of aluminum and Lucite steps are obtained. With these images, two tables can be generated: one for the high energy spectrum (Table 4.6) and another for the low energy spectrum (Table 4.7).

Table 4.7 Low Energy X-Ray Transmitted Intensity Value Versus Combination of AL and PL Step Wedges

	PL Step			
AL Step	0	1	2 . . .	17 . . .
0				
1				
.			Low energy	
.			X-ray	
.			transmitted	
8			intensities	
.				
.				
.				

Since $(I/I_0)_H$ and $(I/I_0)_L$ can be measured directly from the digital images, and t_{AL} and t_{PL} are known, the coefficients b_i and c_i, $i = 1, \ldots, 5$ in Eqs. (4.10) and (4.11) can be obtained using a standard least-squares-fitting algorithm with the data given in Tables 4.6 and 4.7, respectively.

4.4.2.4 Computational Procedure

After the calibration, with b_i and C_i known, we can decompose the object of interest into its AL and PL components as follows. For each pair of high and low energy images of an object of interest, the corresponding values of $\ln(I/I_0)_H$ and $\ln(I/I_0)_L$ are obtained for each pixel. Equations (4.10) and (4.11) are then solved for t_{PL} and t_{AL} on a pixel-by-pixel basis, using the Newton–Raphson iteration technique with a linear solution as the initial guess. The results are the thicknesses of the plastic-component and aluminum-component images of the object of interest. Figure 4.15 shows some images obtained by using the dual-energy imaging procedure.

4.4.3 The Linear Theory

4.4.3.1 From Nonlinear to Linear Theory

The dual-energy method is a powerful tool for image enhancement in conventional digital radiography. To simplify the procedure, the nonlinear theory can be approximated by the linear theory with the assumption that the X-ray energy is monoenergetic. In this case, Eq. (4.3) can be replaced by

$$I = I_0 e^{-(\mu_1 x_1 + \mu_2 x_2)} \tag{4.12}$$

where μ_1, μ_2 are the linear attenuation coefficients of two materials and x_1, x_2 are the thicknesses.

And Eqs. (4.4) and (4.5) can be replaced by two linear equations with two unknowns t_{AL} and t_{PL}:

$$\ln\left(\frac{I}{I_0}\right)_H = -(\mu_1^H t_{AL} + \mu_2^H t_{PL}) \tag{4.13}$$

$$\ln\left(\frac{I}{I_0}\right)_L = -(\mu_1^L t_{AL} + \mu_2^L t_{PL}) \tag{4.14}$$

For two selected energies H and L, $\mu_1^H, \mu_2^H, \mu_1^L, \mu_2^L$ are known and $\ln(I/I_0)_H$ and $\ln(I/I_0)_L$ can be measured. Equations (4.13) and (4.14) can be solved for the AL-component (t_{AL}) and PL-component (t_{PL}) images.

4.4.3.2 Computational Procedure

AL-Component and PL-Component Images

Diagrammatically, the linear dual-energy imaging procedure is illustrated in Figure 4.16. Let $\ln(I/I_0)_H$ and $\ln(I/I_0)_L$ be the two corresponding pixel values in the high

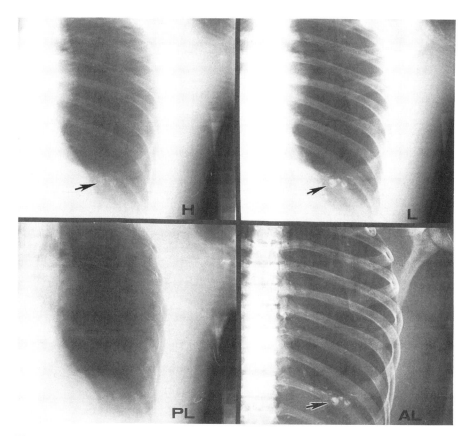

Figure 4.15   Dual-energy images of a Humanoid lung–chest phantom; arrows show calcified nodules: H, 120 kV(p), 16 mA·s (0.5 mm copper filter); L, 60 kV(p), 320 mA·s; PL, soft tissue image with most of the bones eliminated; AL, bone image with most of the soft tissues eliminated. The calcified nodules are clearly seen in the AL image.

Source: Courtesy of Dr. H. Takeuchi.

and low energy images (Fig. 4.16A). Solving Eqs. (4.13) and (4.14) for t_{AL} and t_{PL} will give the corresponding pixel values of the AL-component and PL-component images (Fig. 4.16B).

Simple Subtraction

A simple subtraction between Eq. (4.13) Eq. (4.14) yields

$$\ln\left(\frac{I}{I_0}\right)_H - \ln\left(\frac{I}{I_0}\right)_L = -(\mu_1^H - \mu_1^L)t_{AL} - (\mu_2^H - \mu_2^L)t_{PL} \tag{4.15}$$

To enhance the contrast between the bone (t_{AL}) and the soft tissues (t_{PL}), one needs only select two energies such that

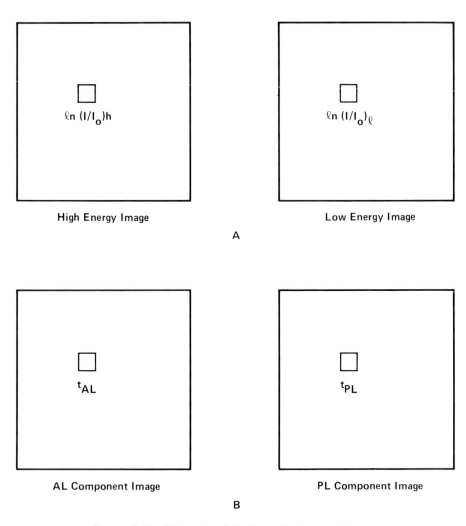

High Energy Image   Low Energy Image

A

AL Component Image   PL Component Image

B

Figure 4.16   Schematic of the linear dual-energy theory.

$$\frac{\mu_1^H - \mu_1^L}{\mu_2^H - \mu_2^L} > \frac{\mu_1}{\mu_2} \tag{4.16}$$

Similarly, if one multiplies Eq. (4.13) by μ_2^L and Eq. (4.14) by μ_2^H, the subtracted image shows only the aluminum component t_{AL}.

A Numerical Example

Perhaps a numerical example is appropriate at this point to reinforce the concept of the linear dual-energy imaging procedure. Consider a hypothetical phantom consisting of two materials M_1 and M_2, with the composition shown in Figure 4.17A. Let the linear attenuation coefficients of these two materials be as follow:

	Low Energy	High Energy
M_1	3	2
M_2	8	4

Then the high and low energy images would look like Figure 4.17B. Consider, for example, the fifth column from the left in the low energy image, where both materials have thickness equal to 2 units. The total attenuation in this column is

$$\ln\left(\frac{I}{I_0}\right)_L = -(\mu_1^L t_{M_1} + \mu_2^L t_{M_1}) = -[(3 \cdot 2) + (8 \cdot 2)] = -22$$

The value is negative because I is always less than or equal to I_0. To obtain an image containing only M_2, the following weighted subtraction is used:

$$3 \ln\left(\frac{I}{I_0}\right)_H - 2 \ln\left(\frac{I}{I_0}\right)_L$$

Consider column 5 of both the low and high energy images in the same example, one obtains

$$(3 \cdot 12) - (2 \cdot 22) = 0\ M_1 + [(2 \cdot 8) - (3 \cdot 4)]M_2$$

or

$$M_2 = -2$$

Similarly, the weighted subtraction $8 \ln(I/I_0)_H - 4 \ln(I/I_0)_L$ will give the M_1 image only. The two resultant images are shown in Figure 4.17C. This method successfully decomposes the object into two images, each of which contains only M_1 or M_2.

4.4.3.3 Method of Producing a High and a Low Energy Image with a Single Exposure

Although the dual-energy imaging procedure is a powerful technique for image enhancement in conventional digital radiography, two images are required to start the procedure. Thus not only must the patient receive two exposures, but movement by the patient during these two exposures will degrade the quality of the resultant images.

To remedy the two-exposure problem, it is possible to insert a physical filter between two X-ray films, two imaging plates, or two image detector systems. A physical filter between the two imaging plates will, in effect, allow the two detectors

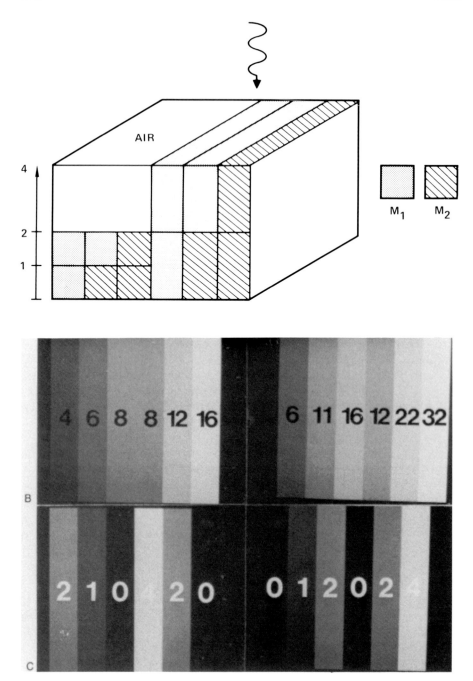

Figure 4.17 Numerical example of the linear dual-energy imaging procedure. (A) Hypothetical phantom consisting of two materials, M_1 and M_2. (B) High and low energy images. (C) M_1-only and M_2-only images; numerals represent thickness.

to produce two images: the low energy image in the front detector and the high energy image in the back detector. This occurs because the energy of the filtered X-ray beam received by the back detector is always higher.

It is also possible to combine the temporal filtering procedure, described in Section 4.2.4, with the dual-energy imaging procedure of Section 4.4.2 to enhance the contrast of the image. This method is called a hybrid dual-energy imaging procedure.

Image Acquisition III: Sectional Imaging

This chapter considers sectional images acquired and presented in digital format: X-ray computed (computerized) tomography (CT), magnetic resonance imaging (MRI), ultrasound (US) imaging, single-photon and positron emission computed tomography (ECT and PET), and digital microscopy. Computed tomography and magnetic resonance imaging, introduced in the early 1970s and 1980s, respectively, are now standard imaging techniques. The ultrasound scanner was originally an analog imaging device, but digital technology has become an integral part of the instrumentation, and US images are now rendered in digital format. ECT and PET use tomographic techniques similar to those of XCT except the energy sources are different. These imaging modalities will be discussed in this chapter. For convenience, nuclear medicine imaging, which is a prerequisite for understanding ECT and PET, is discussed in this chapter along with the imaging modalities just mentioned.

5.1 Image Reconstruction from Projections

5.1.1 The Fourier Projection Theorem

Let $f(x,y)$ be a two-dimensional cross-sectional image of a three-dimensional object. The image reconstruction theorem states that $f(x,y)$ can be reconstructed from cross-sectional one-dimensional projections. In general, 180 different projections in one-degree increments are necessary to produce a satisfactory image, and using more projections always results in a better reconstructed image.

Mathematically, the image reconstruction theorem can be described with the help

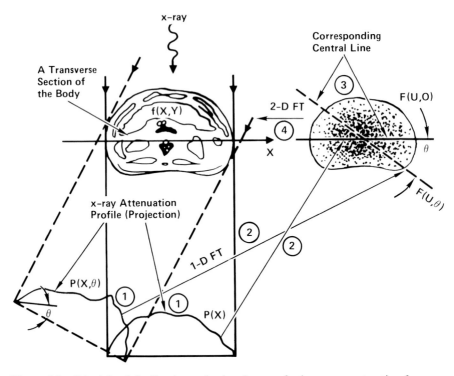

Figure 5.1 Principle of the Fourier projection theorem for image reconstruction from projections. The numerals represent the steps described in the text.

of the Fourier transform (FT) discussed in Chapter 2. Let $f(x,y)$ represent the two-dimensional image to be reconstructed and let $p(x)$ be the one-dimensional projection of $f(x,y)$ onto the horizontal axis, which can be measured experimentally (see Fig. 5.1, the zero-degree projection). Then

$$p(x,o) = \int_{-\infty}^{\infty} f(x,y) \, dy \tag{5.1}$$

The 1-D Fourier transform of $p(x)$ has the form

$$P(u) = \int_{-\infty}^{\infty} \left(\int_{-\infty}^{\infty} f(x,y) dy \right) \exp(-i2\pi ux) \, dx \tag{5.2}$$

$$= \int_{-\infty}^{\infty} \int_{-\infty}^{\infty} f(x,y) \exp[-i2\pi(ux + 0y)] dx \, dy$$

$$= F(u,0)$$

Equations (5.1) and (5.2) imply that the 1-D Fourier transform of a one-dimensional projection of a two-dimensional image is identical to the corresponding central section of the two-dimensional Fourier transform of the object. For example, the two-dimensional image can be a transverse (cross) sectional X-ray image of the body, and the one-dimensional projections can consist of X-ray attenuation profiles (projections) of the same section obtained from a linear X-ray scan at certain angles. If 180 projections at one-degree increments are accumulated and their 1-D FTs performed, each of these 180 Fourier transform projections in one dimension will represent a corresponding central line of the two-dimensional Fourier transform of the X-ray cross-sectional image. The collection of all these transformed projections is the 2-D Fourier transform of $f(x,y)$. A more rigorous mathematical formulation of this Fourier projection theorem, the so-called central slice theorem, is given later (see Section 5.1.3.2).

The steps in the reconstruction of a 2-D image from its 1-D projections are as follows (see Fig. 5.1):

1. Obtain 180 1-D projections of $f(x,y)$.
2. Perform the FT on each 1-D projection.
3. Arrange all these 1-D FTs according to their corresponding angles in the frequency domain: the result is the 2-D FT of $f(x,y)$,
4. Perform the inverse 2-D FT, which gives $f(x,y)$.

The Fourier projection theorem forms the basis of image reconstruction. Other methods that also can be used to reconstruct a 2-D image from its projections are discussed later in this chapter. It is emphasized that the reconstructed image from projections is not always exact; it is only an approximation of the original image. A different reconstruction method will give a slightly different version of the original image. Since all these methods require extensive computation, a computer or special hardware is needed to implement the procedure. The term "computerized (computed) tomography" (CT) is often used to indicate that the image is obtained from its projections using a reconstructed method. If 1-D projections are obtained from X-ray transmission (attenuation) profiles, the procedure is called XCT; the method of obtaining projections from γ-ray emission profiles is called ECT.

5.1.2 The Algebraic Reconstruction Method

The algebraic reconstruction method is often used for the reconstruction of images from an incomplete number of projections (i.e., $< 180°$). A numerical example is given, followed by its mathematical formulation.

5.1.2.1 A Numerical Example

It is easier to understand the concept of this method by first observing an example. Consider $f(x,y)$ to be a 2 × 2 image with the following pixel value:

$$f(x,y) = \begin{array}{|c|c|} \hline 1 & 2 \\ \hline 3 & 4 \\ \hline \end{array}$$

The four projections of this image are as follows:

0° projection	4,6	
45° projection	5 (1 and 4 are ignored for simplicity)	
90° projection	3,7	
135° projection	5 (3 and 2 are ignored for simplicity	

Combining this information, one obtains:

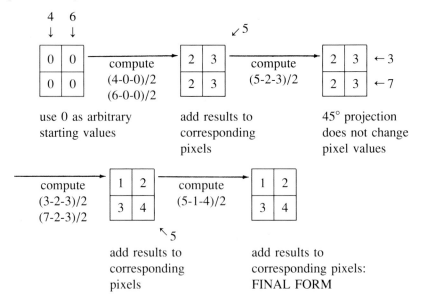

The problem is to reconstruct the 2 × 2 image $f(x,y)$, which is unknown, from these four known projections, which may be obtained from direct measurements. The algebraic reconstruction of the 2 × 2 image from these four known projections proceeds stepwise as follows:

From the last step, it is seen that the result is an exact reconstruction (a pure chance) of the original 2 × 2 image $f(x,y)$. It requires only four projections because $f(x,y)$ is a

2×2 image. This will become apparent when the theory of algebraic reconstruction is discussed in Section 5.1.2.2.

5.1.2.2 Mathematical Formulation

For simplicity, we will use a single subscript to represent a pixel. Thus, with this notation, the principle of algebraic image reconstruction is to approximate the image f_i by a two-dimensional square matrix of N elements based on the known projections p (see Fig. 5.2). The jth beam sum of these projections p_j can be expressed by:

$$p_j = \sum_{i=1}^{N} W_{ij}f_i \qquad\qquad (5.3)$$

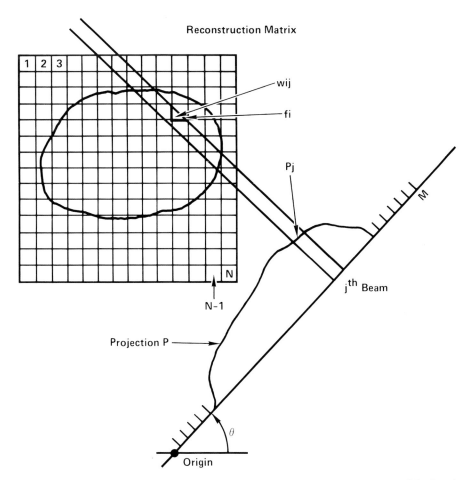

Figure 5.2 Mathematical formulation of the algebraic reconstruction method: f_i is the ith pixel of the object, and W_{ij} is the contribution of the ith pixel to the projection at jth position. One projection of the object at θ is shown.

where W_{ij}, the weighted factor,* is the contribution of pixel i in the image to the jth beam of the projection, and f_i is the pixel value of element i.

Note that W_{ij} are known once the geometry of the system is known, and they are equal to the area of intersection between the ith pixel and the jth beam of the projection, and $W_{ij} = 0$ outside the jth beam. The W_{ij} are precalculated and stored in the computer memory. The reconstruction problem is to obtain f_i for each pixel in the image based on the known values of P_j and W_{ij}.

Equation (5.3) can be solved by inverting the matrix; because of the size of the matrix, however, in practice, this is seldom done. The iteration method, which avoids the problem of matrix inversion, is used more often.

The algebraic reconstruction method, sometimes called the *iteration method,* applies a correction to the initial value of each element during each iteration. The iteration continues until the measured and calculated projection values are within an acceptable threshold.

The correction procedure during the nth iteration can be described by the equation

$$f_i^n = f_i^{n-1} + \sum_{j=1}^{M} \Delta f_{ij}^n \tag{5.4}$$

where f_i^{n-1} and f_i^n are the ith pixel values during and after the $(n-1)$th iteration, and Δf_{ij}^n is the correction value for the ith pixel from jth beam of the projection. Each Δf_{ij}^n is computed as follows.

After the $(n-1)$th iteration, f_i^{n-1} is known, and the jth beam sum of projections P_j^c at a given angle can be calculated by Eq. (5.3). Compute the difference of jth beam, Δp_j, between this calculated projection beam sum P_j^c and the measured p_j. The correction value Δf_{ij}^n can be obtained from Δp_j by either an additive or a multiplicative method according to Eqs. (5.5) and (5.6), respectively.

$$\Delta f_{ij}^n = \frac{W_{ij}\Delta P_j}{\sum_{j=1}^{N} W_{ij}^2} \tag{5.5}$$

$$\Delta f_{ij}^n = \frac{f_i \Delta P_j}{p_j^c} \tag{5.6}$$

The correction process for each iteration continues until all projections have been computed.

5.1.3 The Filtered (Convolution) Back-Projection Method

The selection of the proper filter is the key to obtaining a good reconstruction from filtered (convolution) back-projection. This is the method of choice for almost all XCT scanners.

---

* The two subscripts i and j are not row and column, as commonly used; instead, j represents the jth beam and i the ith pixel in the object.

5.1.3.1 A Numerical Example

Consider the example introduced in Section 5.1.2.1. We now wish to reconstruct the 2×2 matrix $f(x,y)$ from its four known projections using the filtered back-projection method. The procedure is to first convolve each projection with a preselected filter function and then back-project the convolution result to form an image.

For this example, the filter function $(-\frac{1}{2}, 1, -\frac{1}{2})$ will be used. This means that when each projection is convolving with this filter function, the point on the projection under consideration will be multiplied by "1," and both points one pixel away from this point will be multiplied by "$-\frac{1}{2}$." Thus, when the projection [4,6] is convolved with $(-\frac{1}{2}, 1, -\frac{1}{2})$, the result is $(-2, 1, 4, -3)$, since

$$
\begin{array}{r}
-2 \quad 4 \quad -2 \quad \\
+ \quad -3 \quad 6 \quad -3 \\
\hline
-2 \quad 1 \quad 4 \quad -3
\end{array}
$$

Back-projecting this result to the picture, we have:

-2	1	4	-3
-2	1	4	-3

The data points -2, -3 outside the 2×2 reconstructed picture domain are truncated. The result of the following step-by-step illustration of this method, which uses the numerical example described in Section 5.1.2., is an exact reconstruction (again, by pure chance) of the original $f(x,y)$.

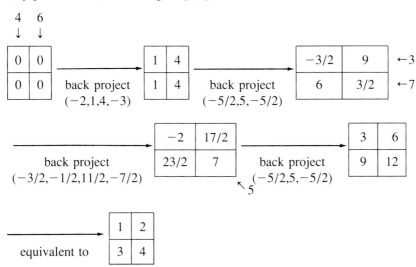

5.1.3.2 Mathematical Formulation

The filtered back-projection method, known as the convolution method, is widely preferred as a reconstruction tool for its speed, accuracy, and versatility. Its mathe-

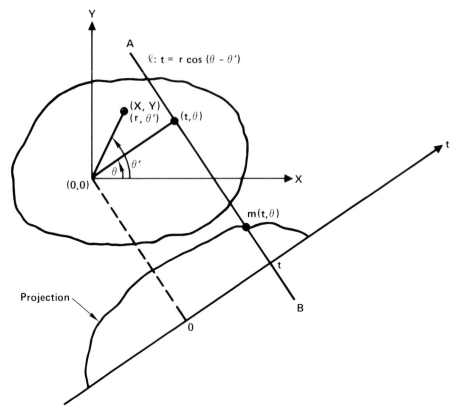

Figure 5.3 Mathematical formulation of the convolution back-projection method; in the projection of the object at angle θ shown, $m(t,\theta)$ is the reading of that projection at a displacement of t.

matical formulation is an extension of the Fourier projection theorem discussed in Section 5.1.1. The following discussion uses the polar coordinate system; the projection is represented by the integral of the product between the image and the delta function. To start, refer to Figure 5.3: the projection through the object with angle θ and a displacement at t from the origin is

$$m(t,\theta) = \int_0^\infty \int_0^\infty f(x,y)\delta[t - (x \cos \theta + y \sin \theta)]dx\, dy \tag{5.7}$$

where δ is the delta function. Since

$$x \cos \theta + y \sin \theta = t \qquad \text{for } (x,y) \text{ on } AB,$$

$$x \cos \theta + y \sin \theta \neq t \qquad \text{for } (x,y) \text{ not on } AB$$

As a result, the integration only accumulates $f(x,y)$ along line AB. Or in polar coordinates Eq. (5.7) can be rewritten as follows:

$$m(t,\theta) = \int_0^{2\pi} \int_0^\infty f(r,\theta')\delta[t - r\cos(\theta - \theta')]r\ dr\ d\theta' \qquad (5.8)$$

where $f(r,\theta')$ is the pixel value of the object at (r,θ'). From the shift property of the delta function, the one-dimensional Fourier transformation of $m(t,\theta)$, $M(\rho,\theta)$, is

$$M(\rho,\theta) = \int_{-\infty}^\infty m(t,\theta)\ \exp(-i2\pi\rho t)dt \qquad (5.9)$$

$$= \int_{-\infty}^\infty \left[\int_0^{2\pi} \int_0^\infty f(r,\theta')\delta[t - r\cos(\theta - \theta')]r\ dr\ d\theta'\right] \exp(-i2\pi\rho t)dt$$

$$= \int_0^{2\pi} \int_0^\infty f(r,\theta')\ \exp[-i2\pi\rho r\cos(\theta - \theta')]r\ dr\ d\theta'$$

Since the two-dimensional Fourier transform of $f(r,\theta)$, $F(\rho,\theta)$ is given by

$$F(\rho,\theta) = \int_0^{2\pi} \int_0^\infty f(r,\theta')\ \exp[-i2\pi\rho r\cos(\theta - \theta')]r\ dr\ d\theta' \qquad (5.10)$$

We can compare Eqs. (5.9) and (5.10) to find that

$$M(\rho,\theta) = F(\rho,\theta) \qquad (5.11)$$

This equation says that the one-dimensional Fourier transform of the projection of an object at angle θ is the central section of the same angle of the two-dimensional Fourier transform of the object. This is the central slice theorem, discussed in Section 5.1.1. The important result of this theorem is that to reconstruct the object completely in the continuous space, an infinite number of projection data are required to fill the whole Fourier space.

Equate the object and its two-dimensional inverse Fourier transform in polar coordinate as follows:

$$f(x,y) = \int_0^{2\pi} \int_0^\infty F(\rho,\theta)\ \exp[i2\pi\rho(x\cos\theta + y\sin\theta)]\rho\ d\rho\ d\theta \qquad (5.12)$$

$$= \int_0^\pi \int_0^\infty F(\rho,\theta)\ \exp[i2\pi\rho(x\cos\theta + y\sin\theta)]\rho d\rho\ d\theta$$

$$+ \int_0^\pi \int_0^\infty F(\rho,\theta + \pi)\ \exp\{i2\pi\rho[x\cos(\theta + \pi)$$

$$+ y\sin(\theta + \pi)]\}\rho\ d\rho\ d\theta$$

Since $F(\rho,\theta + \pi) = F(-\rho,\theta)$, we can write

$$f(x,y) = \int_0^\pi \int_0^\infty F(\rho,\theta)\ \exp[i2\pi\rho(x\cos\theta + y\sin\theta)]\rho\ d\rho\ d\theta$$

$$+ \int_0^\pi \int_0^\infty F(-\rho,\theta)\ \exp[i2\pi(-\rho)(x\cos\theta + y\sin\theta)]\rho\ d\rho\ d\theta$$

Since

$$\int_0^\pi \int_0^\infty F(-\rho,\theta) \exp[i2\pi(-\rho)(x \cos \theta + y \sin \theta)]\rho \ d\rho \ d\theta$$

$$= \int_0^\pi \int_{-\infty}^0 F(\rho,\theta) \exp[i2\pi\rho(x \cos \theta + y \sin \theta)](-\rho)d\rho \ d\theta$$

We can simplify Eq. (5.12) as:

$$f(x,y) = \int_0^\pi \int_{-\infty}^\infty F(\rho,\theta)|\rho| \exp[i2\pi\rho(x \cos \theta + y \sin \theta)]d\rho \ d\theta \tag{5.13}$$

$$= \int_0^\pi \int_{-\infty}^\infty M(\rho,\theta)|\rho| \exp[i2\pi\rho(x \cos \theta + y \sin \theta)]d\rho \ d\theta$$

Define $G(\rho,\theta) = |\rho| M(\rho,\theta)$ and $t = x \cos \theta + y \sin \theta$, then

$$f(x,y) = \int_0^\pi \int_{-\infty}^\infty G(\rho,\theta) \exp(i2\pi\rho t)d\rho \ d\theta \tag{5.14}$$

$$= \int_0^\pi g(t,\theta)d\theta$$

$$= \int_0^\pi g(x \cos \theta + y \sin \theta)d\theta$$

where

$$g(t,\theta) = \int_{-\infty}^\infty G(\rho,\theta) \exp(i2\pi\rho t)d\rho$$

$$= \int_{-\infty}^\infty |\rho| M(\rho,\theta) \exp(i2\pi\rho t)d\rho$$

is the inverse Fourier transform of $G(\rho,\theta)$. The convolution theorem states that the Fourier transform of two multiplicative functions is equal to the convolution of the transform of the function. Thus we have

$$g(t,\theta) = h(t) * m(t,\theta) \tag{5.15a}$$

where $h(t) = \int_{-\infty}^\infty |\rho| \exp(i2\pi\rho t)d\rho$ is the inverse Fourier transform of $|\rho|$, and

$$h(t) * m(t,\theta) = \int_{-\infty}^\infty h(t - \tau)m(\tau,\theta)d\tau \tag{5.15b}$$

is the convolution integral. For $f(x,y)$ such that $M(\rho,\theta) = 0$ for $|\rho| > F$ [i.e., the Fourier transform of projection $m(t,\theta)$ is bounded], we can write the so-called *ramp filter* as follows:

$$h(t) = \int_{-\infty}^\infty |\rho| \exp(i2\pi\rho)d\rho \tag{5.16}$$

$$= \int_{-F}^F |\rho| \exp(i2\rho)d\rho$$

$$= F^2 \left[\frac{\sin(2\pi Ft)}{\pi FT} - \frac{\sin^2(\pi Ft)}{(\pi Ft)^2} \right]$$

Note that $t = x \cos \theta + y \sin \theta$ is equal to the displacement of point (x,y) from the center, when the projection angle is θ. The expression in Eqs. (5.14) and (5.16) means that for any point (x,y) in the object, the reconstruction is the summation of $g(t,\theta)$ for all θ, which is exactly the filtered $[h(t)]$ back-projection $[m(t,\theta)]$. The reconstruction procedure is thus the back-projection of the convolution of the projections and the ramp filter (see Fig. 5.3), that is,

$$f(x,y) = \int_0^\pi h(t) * m(t,\theta) d\theta \tag{5.17}$$

5.2 Transmission X-Ray Computerized Tomography (XCT)

5.2.1 Scanning Mode

A CT scanner consists of a scanning gantry housing an X-ray tube and a detector unit, and a movable bed that can align a specific section of the patient with the gantry. The gantry provides a fixed relative position between the X-ray tube and the detector unit. A scanning mode is the procedure of collecting X-ray attenuation profiles (projections) from a transverse (cross) section of the body. From these projections, the CT scanner's computer program reconstructs the corresponding cross-sectional image of the body.

When the CT scanner was introduced, it utilized a single, pencil-thin X-ray beam as the energy source and took approximately 4.5 minutes to collect the necessary data to perform the picture reconstruction.

During this long 4.5-minute interval, many factors work against the system, including motion from the patient. Patient motion can be categorized into two types: actual physical movement and physiological movement (e.g., heartbeat, respiratory motion, peristalsis). Because of these motions, the reconstructed image will have certain motion artifacts characterized by lines radiating from the center of the movement which can degrade the quality of the image. To overcome this problem, it is necessary to speed up the scanning time. Sections 5.2.1.1 to 5.2.1.5 discuss the scanning modes that represent the evolution of XCT technology.

5.2.1.1 Translation and Rotation Mode Using a Pencil-Thin Collimated X-Ray Beam

The translation and rotation mode is the fundamental CT scanning method. Although it takes 4–5 minutes to perform one cross-sectional scan, the reconstructed image is nonetheless excellent, provided there is no patient motion during the scanning. In this mode (Fig. 5.4), a collimated X-ray beam enters a small area of a body section. Some X-ray photons are absorbed, while others continue to pass through the body and are detected by a detector unit composed of a scintillation

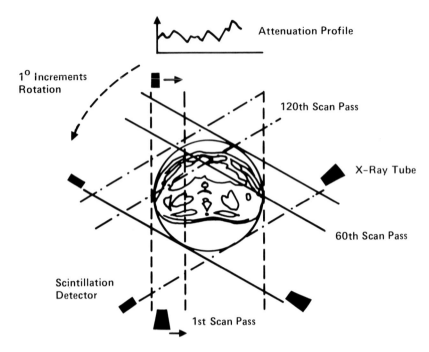

Figure 5.4 Schematic of the translation and rotation scanning mode using a pencil-thin collimated X-ray beam. During each scan-pass, an X-ray attenuation profile is generated. It takes 180 of these profiles at one-degree increments to compile enough data for the computer to reconstruct the cross-sectional image.

crystal and a photomultiplier tube. The amount of absorption depends on the absorption coefficients of the tissues located where the beam passes. A flash of visible light is emitted for each transmitted X-ray photon striking the crystal. The photomultiplier integrates the total light photons in 4 ms intervals. The output from the photomultiplier represents one data point on the profile. As the X-ray beam and the detector translate through the body section as a unit, an X-ray attenuation profile is generated. Then the translation gantry rotates (usually 1°) and another scan-pass is taken.

A completed scan is composed of up to 180 such scan-passes, with the gantry rotating one degree during each pass. Each X-ray attenuation profile is then sampled and fed into the reconstruction program for image reconstruction.

The X-ray energy spectra used in the CT scanner normally are 120 kV(p) and 15 mA, and the maximum X-ray dose to the skin in this case is about 1.8 rads for a complete scan. In XCT, the beam is highly collimated, resulting in a minimal amount of scatter. After a complete scan, the patient's bed is advanced to a certain distance and the next consecutive cross section of the body can be examined. This means that the X-ray energy from the succeeding scan will penetrate a new area. Thus, the radiation dose is not cumulative as long as the distance between two scans is larger than the width of the collimated beam. The dose received by a patient for a series of ten CT scans of the head without overlapping, for example, is approximately the same as that of a single conventional skull X-ray examination.

5.2.1.2 *Translation and Rotation Mode Using a Fan Beam X-Ray Technique*

One obvious approach to speeding up the scanning time is to modify the pencil-thin X-ray beam into small, tightly collimated fan-shaped X-ray beams and to increase the number of scintillator/photomultiplier units in the detector system from 1 to 30. This allows the detector system to collect sufficient data for image reconstruction in much less time. Figure 5.5 shows such a system.

During the scan, the fan-shaped X-ray beams pass through the section under consideration. The transmitted X-rays are then measured by the detectors. Compared to the pencil beam rotation–translation mode, this translation allows one to obtain manyfold additional units of information.

At the end of the first linear traverse, the scanning gantry with the X-ray tube and detector system rotates a certain number of degrees around the patient. Another scan-pass is repeated, and so on, until all necessary data have been collected. The

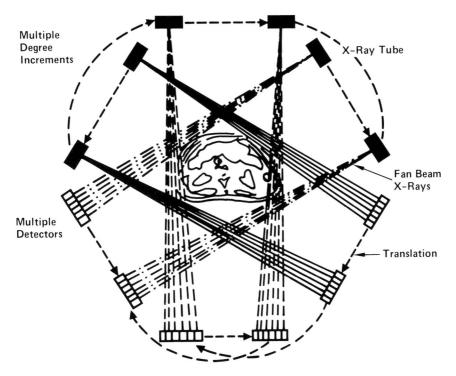

Figure 5.5 Schematic of the translation and rotation scanning mode using a fan beam X-ray technique. The rotation increment is more than one degree, which reduces the scanning time.

scanning time for this type of system ranges from 20 to 30 seconds. The advantage of the 20-second scanning time is that the patient can hold his or her breath, thus minimizing motion artifacts.

The detector system used in this scanning mode is similar to that of the first mode, sodium iodide (NaI), calcium fluoride (CaF), or bismuth germanate (BGO: $Bi_4Ge_3O_{12}$) crystals coupled with photomultiplier tubes.

5.2.1.3 Rotation Mode Using a Large Fan Beam

The translation and rotation scanning mode using fan beam X-rays can be modified to eliminate the translation motion, further reducing the scanning time. Translation is required because the fan beam in this architectural design is not wide enough to cover a complete cross section of the patient. However, if the fan beam is further spread out so that at any angle of the rotation the beam will cover the complete cross section by the detector system without translation, and still collect enough information to permit the reconstruction of the cross-sectional image.

There are two possible configurations in constructing a rotating-only scanning gantry. In the first type (Fig. 5.6), the X-ray tube and the detector system line up at

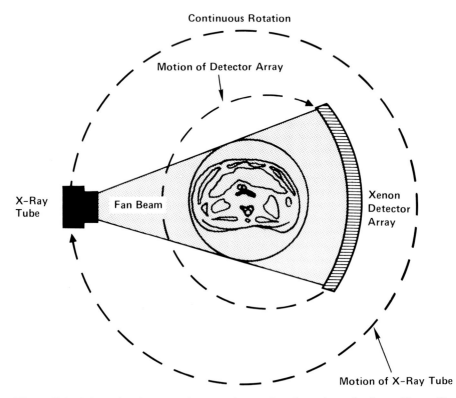

Figure 5.6 Schematic of the rotation scanning mode using a large fan beam X-ray. The detector array (usually pressurized xenon ionization chambers, for compactness) rotates with the X-ray tube as a unit.

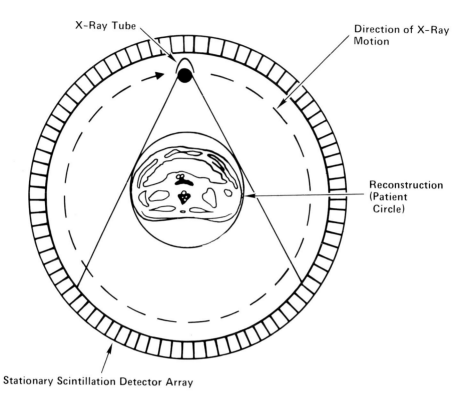

Figure 5.7   Schematic of the rotation scanning mode with a stationary scintillation detector array.

opposite sides of the patient, and both rotate around the cross section of the patient during the 5-second scanning. The detector system used in this configuration is many pressurized ionization chambers (≤ 600) of xenon, or xenon–krypton for two reasons. First, the geometry of this configuration requires a compact array of detectors that can rotate with the X-ray tube as a unit; a scintillator/photomultiplier detector, with its bulky photomultiplier tubes, would constitute a system too large for the gantry. Second, X-ray dose-efficiency calls for each detector element to be shaped differently, which is very difficult to do when a crystal detector is used.

In the second possible configuration for a rotating-only scanning gantry (Fig. 5.7), only the X-ray tube is in motion; the detector array, placed outside the gantry, remains stationary. This configuration maximizes the utilization of X-ray photons because the detector array, which does not have to rotate around the patient, can be placed in the periphery of the gantry. As a result, achieving compactness is not a problem, and the scintillation detectors can be used to optimize the dose efficiency.

However, the difficulty of controlling the gain stability of so many photomultiplier tubes remains a challenge. An alternative is to couple the scintillation crystals with solid state detectors. As many as 1400 detectors can be arranged in the periphery of the gantry. The scanning time of this configuration is about 1–2 seconds.

In the CT industry, devices designed around the translation and rotation mode using a pencil-thin X-ray beam are generally referred to as first-generation scanners; in the second generation the translation and rotation mode uses a small fan beam. The configuration in which both the X-ray tube and the detector system rotate is referred to as the third generation, and architecture in which only the X-ray tube rotates is referred to as the fourth generation. Image quality is about the same for the third and fourth generations.

5.2.1.4 Spiral (Helical) XCT

Two other configurations can further improve the scanning speed: the helical (spiral), discussed here, and the cine (see Section 5.2.1.5). The helical CT is based on the design of the third-generation scanner, whereas the cine CT uses a scanning electron beam X-ray tube.

The four CT configurations described earlier have one common characteristic: the patient's bed remains stationary during the scanning; after a complete scan, the bed advances a certain distance and scanning resumes. The start-and-stop motions retard the scanning operation, however. If the patient's bed could assume a forward motion at constant speed while the scanning gantry rotated continuously, scanning time could be reduced. Such a configuration is not possible, however, because of the high energy cables connected to the gantry and to the transformer, which is external to the gantry. To prevent the cables from becoming tangled, the rotation must be oscillatory. Thus in the spiral or helical CT configuration, the rotation of the gantry and the linear movement of the patient's bed occur simultaneously during the acquisition of projection data.

Figure 5.8 illustrates the principle of spiral CT. There are two possible scanning modes: single helical and cluster helical. In the single helical mode, the bed continuously advances while the gantry rotates for a longer period of time, say 30 seconds. In the cluster helical mode, the simultaneous rotation and translation last only 15 seconds, whereupon both motions stop for 7 seconds before resuming again. The single helical mode is used for patients who can hold their breath for a longer period of time, while the cluster helical mode is for patients who need to take a breath after 15 seconds.

The design of the helical XCT introduced in the late 1980s is based on three technological advances: the slip-ring gantry, improved detector efficiency, and greater X-ray tube cooling capability. The slip-ring gantry contains a set of rings and electrical components that rotate, slide, and make contact to generate both high energy (to supply the X-ray tube and generator) and standard energy (to supply power to other electrical and computer components). For this reason, no electrical cables are necessary to connect the gantry and its components. During the helical scanning, the term "pitch" is used to define the relationship between the X-ray beam collimation and the velocity of the bed movement. Thus, a pitch of 1:1 means that the collimation is 1.0 cm and the bed is moving at 1.0 cm/s. A complete 360° rotation is complete as the bed advances 1.0 cm in one second. During this time, raw data are collected covering 360° and 1.0 cm. For the single helical scan mode, 30

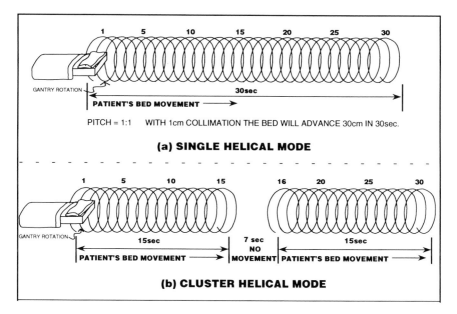

Figure 5.8 Helical (spiral) CT scanning modes.

seconds of raw data are continuously taken while the bed moves 30 cm. After the data collection phase, the raw data are interpolated and/or extrapolated to projections. The projections thus organized are used to reconstruct sectional images. Reconstruction slice thickness can be from 2 mm to 1 cm, depending on the interpolation and extrapolation used.

The advantages of the spiral CT scans are speed of scanning, allowing the user to select slices from continuous data to reconstruct slices with peak contrast medium, retrospective creation of overlapping or thin slices, and volumetric data collection. The disadvantages are helical reconstruction artifacts and potential object boundary unsharpness.

5.2.1.5 Cine XCT

Cine XCT, introduced in 1982, uses a completely different X-ray technology, namely, an electron beam X-ray tube: this scanner is fast enough to capture the motion of the heart. The detector array of the system is based on the fourth-generation stationary detector array (scintillator and photodiode). As shown schematically in Figure 5.9, an electron beam (1) is accelerated through the X-ray tube and bent by the deflection coil (2) toward one of the four target rings (3). Collimators at the exit of the tube restrict the X-ray beam to a 30° fan beam, which forms the energy source of scanning. Since there are four tungsten target rings, each of which has a fairly large area (210°, 90 cm radius) for heat dissipation, the X-ray fan beam can sustain the energy level required for scanning continuously for various scanning modes. In addition, the detector and data collection technologies used in this system allow very

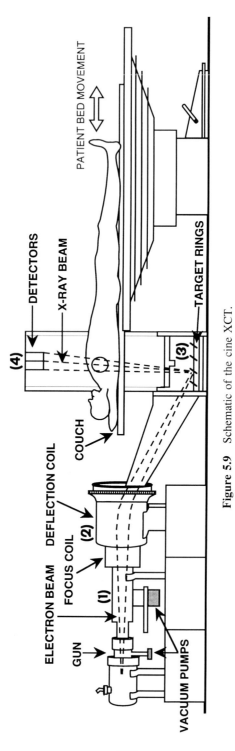

Figure 5.9 Schematic of the cine XCT.

Source: Diagram adapted from a technical brochure of Imatron, Inc.

152

rapid data acquisition. Two detector rings (indicated by 4 in Fig. 5.9) allow data acquisition for two consecutive sections simultaneously. For example, in the slow acquisition mode with a 100 ms scanning time, and an 8 ms interscan delay, cine XCT can provide 9 scans/s, or in the fast acquisition mode with a 20 ms scanning time, 34 scans/s.

The scanning can be done continuously on the same body section (to collect dynamic motion data of the section) or along the axis of the patient (to observe the vascular motion). Because of its fast scanning speed, cine XCT is used for cardiac motion and vascular studies and for emergency room scans.

5.2.2 Operation Principle of an XCT Scanner

Figure 5.10 shows the components of a fourth-generation X-ray CT scanner and their interconnections. Included are a gantry housing the X-ray tube, the detectors, and signal processing/conditioning circuits; a front-end preprocessor unit for data corrections and data reformatting; an image data buffer memory; a controlling computer; a high speed computational processor; a hardware back-projector unit; and a video controller for displaying CT images.

5.2.2.1 Terminology

Before proceeding with the details of operation, it is appropriate to present some definitions and terminology that characterize the operation of a scanner.

1. *Detector circle radius:* the distance from the center of the gantry to the placement of the detectors.
2. *Source circle radius:* the distance from the center of the gantry to the focal spot of the X-ray source.
3. *Scan circle radius:* the distance from the center of the gantry to the edge of the object of interest.
4. *Detector specifications:* the number of detectors used (typically 600–1400) and the detector material composition (e.g., BGO, CaF, Cd_2WO_4).
5. *Scan speed:* the length of time the X-ray tube is turned on during scanning—a factor contributing to the dose received by the patient.
6. *Source fan:* a data file that consists of readings from all detectors for a given source position.
7. *Detector fan:* a data file containing all readings from a single detector, with the X-ray source rotating to all necessary angle positions.
8. *Convolution:* a mathematical operation used in image reconstruction to minimize artifacts.
9. *Back-projector:* a hardware processor that can quickly perform the back-projection (see Eq. 5.17) reconstruction algorithm commonly used in CT.
10. *Slice thickness:* the amount of X-ray collimation with respect to the patient's body axis. This collimation defines the slice thickness, the third dimension of a picture element or pixel. The term "voxel" is sometimes used instead of "pixel."

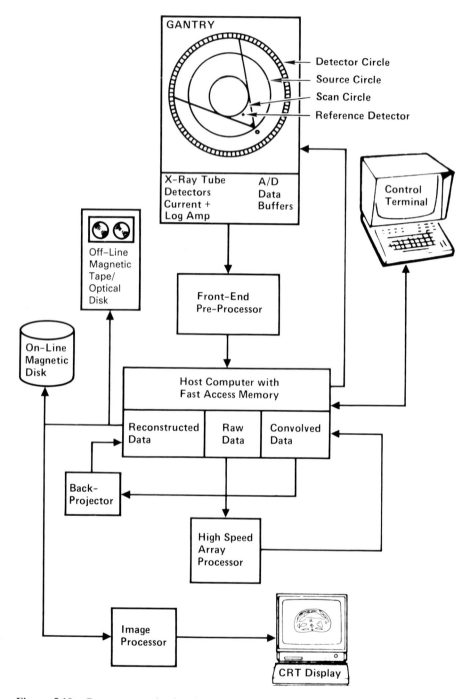

Figure 5.10 Components of a fourth-generation XCT scanner and their interconnections.

11. *CT or Hounsfield number:* a number assigned to a voxel which represents the relative X-ray attenuation coefficient, defined as follows:

$$K \frac{\mu - \mu_w}{\mu_w}$$

where μ is the attenuation coefficient of the material under consideration, μ_w is the attenuation coefficient of water, and K is a constant set by the manufacturer.

12. *Reconstruction matrix size:* the number of voxels in the resulting reconstructed image, typically, 512×512 with 12 bits/voxel.

13. *Reconstruction times:* refers (for a given matrix size) to the average time needed to perform the image reconstruction.

14. *System storage disk size:* the capacity of magnetic disks available in the system to store images. Images stored in these disks can be quickly accessed and displayed. For long-term storage, images are archived onto magnetic tapes or optical disks.

5.2.2.2 Block Diagram of an XCT Scanner

Figure 5.11 is a block diagram giving the data flow of an XCT scanner starting from the detection of transmitted X-rays through the body to the construction of the cross-sectional image. The gantry (refer to Fig. 5.10) housing the X-ray source rotates around the patient. Beam collimators, which determine the beam thickness and the

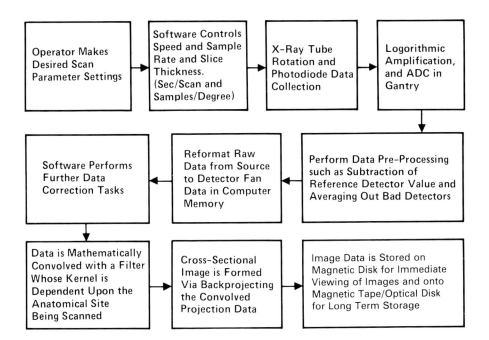

Figure 5.11 Data flow block diagram of an XCT scanner.

angular extent of the fan-shaped X-ray beam, are adjusted to accommodate the operator's selection of scan circle size and slice thickness. The gantry also houses a reference air detector used to calibrate the CT value of air. Located between the X-ray source and the patient, this special detector is in the direct path of the beam and rotates in unison with the source.

Once the transmitted X-ray photons have been detected by the detectors, they are converted to electrical signals. The signals are processed by a series of conditioning circuits. From each detector, the signal is processed by a current amplifier to amplify the small signals from the detectors, as well as to provide electrical impedance matching to the rest of the signal processing system. Next comes a logarithmic amplifier to convert X-ray transmission data (I/I_0) into attenuation (μ) and thickness (x) data:

$$I = I_0 \exp(-\mu x) \quad \text{or} \quad \ln\left(\frac{I_0}{I}\right) = \mu x \quad (5.18)$$

Next, signals are multiplexed from all detectors and fed to analog-to-digital converters. Multiplexing is necessary to take advantage of parallel processing. The signal is then sampled and digitized, typically to 12–16 bits.

Once the signals have been digitized, initial data correction is performed by the front-end preprocessing unit. Some data corrections include subtraction of the air reference detector signal to normalize the attenuation data. Sometimes local averages of detectors are obtained to determine whether any detectors are outside a predetermined standard deviation, since this information can help locate bad detectors. Corrections due to dead time losses (i.e., detection response time losses) by the individual detectors also may be entered.

The front-end preprocessor also provides data reformatting from the source fan to detector fan representation. This data reformatting may be necessary for subsequent optimizing of the computation.

The preprocessed data are stored as reformatted raw data in a fast access memory. At this point, further data processing is performed—for example, detector spacing corrections, to compensate for any deviation in detector center-to-center distances; beam-hardening corrections, to minimize the effects of variations in the X-ray spectrum reaching different points in the object; and corrections due to differences in detector gains. Furthermore, data convolution is performed, the kernel (or filter) of the convolution depending on the anatomical location under consideration (see Section 5.1.3). This convolution is done using a high speed, floating point array processor that can perform mathematical operations on entire arrays of data in a relatively short period of time. The convolution process is necessary to avoid image reconstruction artifacts such as edge overshooting due to ringing phenomenon.

Finally, the image is reconstructed using a hardware back-projector to back-project the detector fan readings. A controlling computer handles the data flow, scheduling, and movement of detector fan data from the fast access memory to the hardware back-projector. The resulting reconstructed image can be archived as well as displayed on a TV monitor. The final display of the resulting image data may include text (e.g., the scan protocol, patient information) overlaid onto the image. For long-term storage of the CT image, the digital images may be archived to magnetic tapes or optical disks.

5.2.2.3 Dual-Energy XCT

Dual energy imaging, described in Section 4.4, can also be used in XCT. In this case, one begins by obtaining all the high and low energy projections of a cross section. Each pair of high and low energy projections of the same angle can be decomposed into two sets of projections (the aluminum component and the plastic component) using the two calibration tables given earlier (Tables 4.6 and 4.7). The cross-sectional images of the aluminum and plastic components, respectively, can be reconstructed from the appropriate set of projections. A proper combination of the aluminum- and plastic-component images will result in images of electron density and effective atomic number, which are true physical properties of the cross section.

The difference between dual-energy scanning in digital radiography and in CT is that the former results in image enhancement that can effectively eliminate the bone and the soft tissues from the final images, whereas the latter gives the true physical properties of the cross section. Figure 5.12 shows examples of images obtained from the dual-energy XCT scanning technique.

5.3 Emission Computerized Tomography

Emission computerized tomography (ECT) has many characteristics in common with transmission X-ray CT. The main difference between these two techniques is the source of radiation used. In ECT the radionuclide, which is administered to patients in the form of radiopharmaceuticals either by injection or by inhalation, is used as a source instead of an external X-ray energy. The basic principle of ECT is based on nuclear medicine scanning, which will be discussed in Section 5.4.1.

It is important to select a dose-efficient detector system for an ECT system for two reasons. First, the quantity measured in ECT is the distribution of radionuclide in the body, which changes with time as a result of flow and biochemical kinetics in the body. Thus, all the necessary measurements must be made in a short period of time. Second, the amount of isotope administered is limited because of the usual dose considerations. Therefore, detector efficiency plays a crucial role in selecting a scintillator for ECT systems.

The basic principle of image reconstruction is the same in ECT and in transmission CT except that the signal in ECT is the attenuation of γ rays during their flight from the emitting nuclei to the detectors. To minimize the contribution from scattered radiation, the ECT uses the characteristics of monoenergetic energy in setting up a counting window to discriminate the lower energy scattered radiation from the high energy primary radiation. There are two major categories in ECT: single-photon emission CT and positron emission CT.

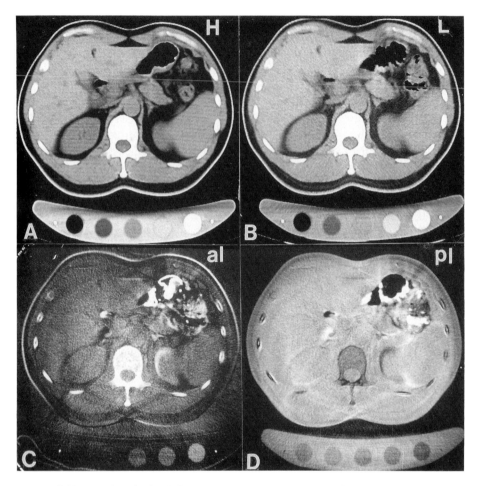

Figure 5.12 Results obtained from the dual energy CT techniques: (A) high energy [140 kV(p), 100 mA·s, 10 mm thickness] scan through the abdominal region, (B) low energy [80 kV(p), 100 mA·s scan through the same area], (C) aluminum component image, and (D) plastic component image. The object beneath each cross section is the bone mineral phantom with five calibration materials: fat equivalent material, water, and K_2HPO_4 (50, 100, and 200 mg/cm^3).

5.3.1 Single-Photon Emission CT (SPECT)

There are many different designs for SPECT, but only rotating gamma camera systems (see Section 5.4.1.2) are commercially available. In a rotating camera system, the gamma camera is rotated around the object and images in a two-dimensional series are reconstructed and stored for processing. The camera is composed of a large scintillation crystal with a diameter of 30–50 cm and a number of photomultiplier tubes (PMTs) attached to the opposite surface of the crystal. When a γ-ray photon interacts with the crystal, the light generated from the photoelectric effect is uniformly distributed among the neighboring PMTs. By measuring the

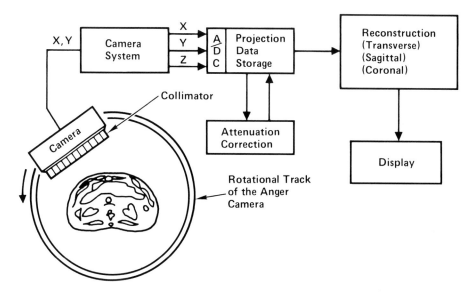

Figure 5.13   Schematic of a single photon emission CT (SPECT).

relative signal of each PMT, the camera can locate the interaction position for each event. The drawback of this system is the difficulty of maintaining uniform speed of rotation of a rather heavy camera. Figure 5.13 shows a flowchart on the operation of a SPECT.

Since typical tomographic study takes 15–20 minutes to complete, it is important to have adequate patient immobilization. To provide the best sensitivity and resolution, it is desirable to have the camera as close to the patient as possible. Since the dimension of body width is greater than thickness, an elliptical orbit of rotation of the camera tends to produce a higher resolution image. Different collimators are used for different applications. In general, the reconstruction algorithm must be modified and the attenuation values corrected for each type of collimator. For example, a single-plane converging collimator will need a fan beam reconstruction algorithm, and a parallel collimator will need a parallel beam algorithm.

Three methods of correcting attenuation values based on the assumption of a constant attenuation value are summarized as follows.

1. *Geometric mean modification.* Each data point in a projection is corrected by the geometric mean of the projection data, which is obtained by taking the square root of the product of two opposite projection data points.
2. *Iterative modification.* This method is similar to the iteration reconstruction method for XCT described earlier. A reconstruction without corrections is first performed, and each pixel in the reconstructed image is compensated by a corrective factor that is the inverse of the average measured attenuation from that point to the boundary pixels. The projections of this modified image are obtained, and the differences between each of the corrected projections and the original measured projections are computed. These difference projections are

reconstructed to obtain an error image. The error image is then added back to the modified image to form the corrected image.

3. *Convolution method.* Each data point in the projection is modified by a factor that depends on the distance from a centerline to the edge of the object. The modified projection data points are filtered with a proper filter function and then back-projected with an exponential weighting factor to obtain the image (see Section 5.1.2).

Currently, SPECT is used mostly for studies of the brain, including brain blood volume (^{99m}Tc-labeled blood cells), regional cerebral blood flow (^{123}I-labeled iodoantipyrine or inhaled Xe^{133}), and physiological condition measurements.

5.3.2 Positron Emission CT (PET)

In PET, a positron instead of a single photon is used as a radionuclide source. The positron emitted from a radionuclide is rapidly slowed down, and annihilated by combination yielding two 511 keV γ-rays oriented at about 180° to each other. The PET system utilizes this unique property of positrons by employing a detector system that requires simultaneous detection of both photons from annihilation, and thus avoids the need for collimators. A pair of detectors is placed at the two opposite sides of the patient, and only events that are detected in coincidence are recorded. Simultaneous detection of two annihilation photons by the detector system thus signals the decay of a positron anywhere along a line connecting the two points of detection (Fig. 5.14). Because of this multiple coincidence logic, PET systems have higher sensitivity than SPECT.

The correction of attenuation is easier in PET than in SPECT because the probability that annihilated photons will reach both detectors simultaneously is a function of the thickness of the body between the two opposite detectors. The correction factor can be obtained by means of a preliminary scan of the body with an external γ-ray source, or a correction table based on a simple geometric shape resembling the attenuation medium can be used. Patient movements, oversimplified geometric shape, and a nonuniform medium will cause errors in attenuation correction.

Thallium-drifted sodium iodide NaI(Tl), bismuth germanate (BGO), and cesium fluoride (CsF) are being used as detector materials. Because of the high energy of the annihilation photon, detector efficiency plays a crucial rule in selecting a scintillator for a PET system. Bismuth germanate is considered to be the most prominent candidate for a PET detector material because of its high detection efficiency, which is due to its high physical density (7.13 g/cm^3) and large atomic number (83), as well as its nonhygroscopicity (which makes for easy packing) and its lack of afterglow.

The ECAT EXACT system (Computer Technology Incorporated) designed for imaging the body, consists of 512 BGO detectors placed in 16 circular array banks with 32 detectors in each bank. During scanning, the system is capable of wobbling to achieve higher resolution via finer sampling. The image spatial resolution for the stationary and wobbled modes are 5–6 mm and 4.5–5 mm, respectively.

A recent PET engineering development is the *whole-body imaging technique*, which produces tomographic images of the entire body with equal spatial resolution

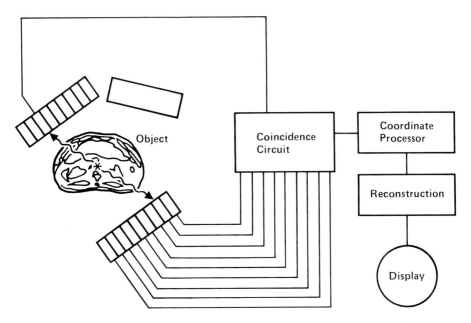

Figure 5.14   Block diagram of a PET system; only two array banks are shown.

in orthogonal image planes. Since the body longitudinal axis is, in general, longer than the other two axes, the patient bed is required to advance during the scanning process to permit the entire body length to be scanned. A complicate data acquisition system in synchrony with the bed motion is necessary to monitor the data collection process. Figure 5.15 illustrates images of the transaxial, coronal, and sagittal orthogonal planes, as well as the anterior posterior projection image of a whole-body PET image with a fluoride ion isotope ($^{18}F^-$).

5.4 Nuclear Medicine and Ultrasound Imaging

5.4.1 Nuclear Medicine

5.4.1.1 Principles of Nuclear Medicine Scanning

Although ECT is sectional imaging, nuclear medicine is not. The topic of nuclear medicine is included here for the convenience of explaining the concept of ECT. The formation of an image in nuclear medicine relies on administering a radiopharmaceutical agent that can be used to differentiate between a normal and an abnormal physiological process. A radiopharmaceutical agent consists of a tracer substance and a radionuclide for highlighting the tracer's position. The tracer typically consists of a molecule that resembles a constituent of the tissue of interest, a colloidal substance that is attacked by reticuloendothelial cells, for example, or a capillary blocking agent. A gamma camera (see Section 5.4.1.2) is then used to obtain an image of the distribution of the radioactivity in an organ.

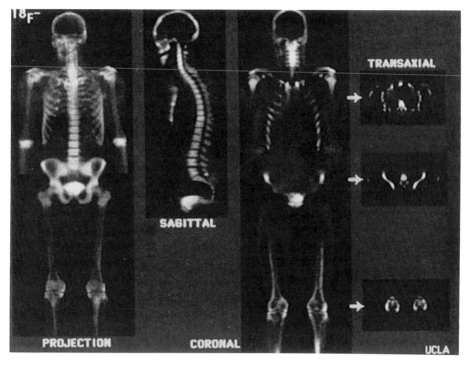

Figure 5.15 Images of the transaxial, coronal, and sagittal orthogonal planes, as well as the anterior–posterior projection image of a whole-body PET image with fluoride ion ($^{-18}$F).

Source: Courtesy of R.A. Hawkins.

The radionuclide is chosen on the basis of its specific activity, half-life, energy spectrum, and ability to bond with the desired tracer molecule. Its activity is important because, in general, one would like to perform scans in the shortest possible time while nevertheless accumulating sufficient nuclear counting decay statistics. As always, the half-life must be reasonably short, to minimize the radiation dose to the patient. The energy spectrum of the isotope is important because if the energy emitted is too low, the radiation will be severely attenuated when passing through the body, hence, nuclear statistics will be poor or scan times unacceptable. If the energy is too high, there may not be enough photoelectric interaction, and absorption in the detector crystal will be low. Typical isotopes used in nuclear medicine have γ-ray emission energies of 100–400 keV.

5.4.1.2 The Gamma Camera and Associated Imaging System

As with most imaging systems, nuclear medicine imagers (e.g., gamma cameras) contain subsystems for data acquisition, data processing, data display, and data archival. A computer is used to control the flow of data and coordinate these subsystems into a functional unit. The operator interactively communicates with the computer via commands from a computer terminal or predefined push buttons on

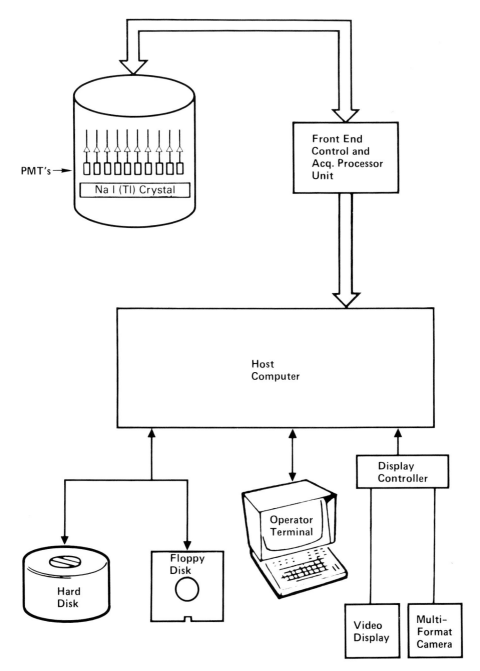

Figure 5.16   Schematic of a scanner used in nuclear medicine: general gamma camera setup.

the system's control terminal. Figure 5.16 shows a schematic of a typical digital nuclear medicine gamma camera.

The data acquisition component consists of a thallium-drifted sodium iodide crystal detector coupled to several photomultiplier tubes. The size of the crystal depends on the desired field of view, which typically ranges from 10 to 21 inches. A radiation incident upon the crystal creates light flashes that are transmitted to the PMTs using a light coupling plate of Lucite or glass; the PMT face may be hexagonal shaped to increase packing efficiency. The signal from each PMT is then sent to its own individual preamplifier, which provides electrical impedance matching for subsequent signal processing stages, as well as a means to balance the response of the camera such that its output is consistent over the entire imaging field of view.

The position encoding of a scintillation event is now described. Individually, a PMT is not able to resolve the exact position of a scintillation event originating in the detector crystal. The signal it produces is proportional to the amount of light it collects. However, the number of resolvable pixels of a gamma camera is much higher than the total number of PMTs used. Light created by a scintillation event is scattered throughout the crystal, and by looking at the relative strengths of the signal from all PMTs whose signal is above a certain threshold value, one can use algebra to determine with reasonable accuracy the positional occurrence of the original event. The amount of light distributed to the various PMTs is a function of the position at which the scintillation occurred. PMTs closer to the scintillation event will produce a stronger signal.

Figure 5.17 illustrates the determination of the position of a scintillation event occurring over the face of the camera. The outputs from all the PMT's are fed into a position-coding matrix circuit that consists of a capacitive network. This network applies an x- and y-direction weighting factor to each PMT according to its positional coordinate. This circuit will extract the orthogonal x and y coordinates relative to the center of the field of view of the location of the scintillation event. The resulting x and y signals are divided in real time by the z (energy) value, using electronic dividing circuits (ratio amplifiers) to remove any energy dependence on the determination of the positional coordinates.

If the camera is tuned correctly, the z signal, which is generated by summing up signals from all contributing PMTs, will be independent of position. The z signal is sent to a pulse height analyzer (PHA), and only z values that correspond to photopeak events are recorded.

The x and y signals are then digitized by using separate analog-to-digital converters and sent to a digital address generating circuit. The z signal is digitized from 8 to 16 bits and is stored in a digital matrix according to its x-y address. Alternatively, the x and y signals can be sent to the x and y deflection circuits of a cathode ray tube (CRT) to control the location of the electron beam spot. The z signal is sent through the PHA circuit and gated to switch on the display of the electron beam spot.

5.4.1.3 Scanning Modes and Image Format

Data may be acquired in three different modes: static, dynamic, and gated. In static mode, the distribution of radioactivity in an organ is relatively stable and a single

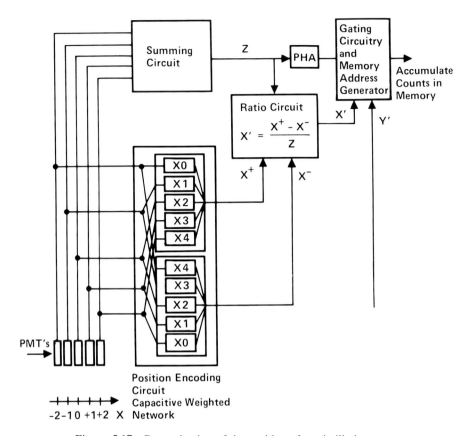

Figure 5.17   Determination of the position of a scintillation event.

image is acquired. The length of the study either is determined manually or can be predefined according to preset counts or a preset time. The digital matrix size can be adjusted to 64 × 64, 128 × 128, 256 × 256, or 512 × 512. Static images are typically digitized to 16 bits, providing a range from 0 to 65,535 counts/pixel.

In dynamic mode, several frames of the radioactive distribution in an organ are acquired, corresponding to different time periods. This model is useful in investigating cardiac performance, renal blood flow, the function of the gall bladder (in cases of suspected blockage) and lungs, cerebral blood flow, and other dynamic flow in studies of other types. In general, images generated in this mode have smaller matrix sizes as well as fewer bits to store the number of counts at a particular pixel location. Each image frame is stored in a separate image memory plane and can be formatted on the video monitor to show many frames on one video screen.

In gated mode, several images are acquired, corresponding to different phases of an organ's movement. For example, the heart cycle can be divided into several phases and a separate image can be acquired for each phase. The signals from the camera are fed into different memory planes according to gated signals generated from an electrocardiograph. Each memory plane acquires counts from different phases of the cycle. The greater the number of phases into which the cardiac cycle is segmented, the better the temporal resolution. For a given scan period, however, the spatial resolution will be lower as a result of lower quantum statistics. Typical matrix sizes are 64×64 or 128×128 by 8 bits, with a maximum of 30 frames per cardiac cycle. In gated mode, useful parameter values such as ejection fraction and stroke volume may be calculated. In addition, the frames of a cardiac cycle may be displayed consecutively and rapidly in cine fashion to evaluate heart wall motion.

5.4.1.4 Data Correction Techniques

The processing of data can be separated into three different categories: primary data corrections, image processing and enhancement, and data analysis. Only primary data corrections are discussed here.

Primary data corrections are concerned mainly with the problem of nonuniform flat field response. There are two major causes of field nonuniformity: variations in point-source sensitivity across the face of the crystal, and spatial distortions due to inaccuracies of the position-coding matrix.

Spatial distortions contribute to the camera's nonuniform response by misplacing events, resulting in local areas in which the recorded counts are too high and other areas in which they are too low. Several methods have been devised to solve this problem. One scheme of correcting nonuniformities involves renormalization of data (Fig. 5.18). A uniform flood source is scanned and the flood image accumulated in the resulting image matrix. The minimum count cell in the image is located, and the ratio of the minimum value to the value stored in each pixel location is used to generate a correction matrix. When the clinical study is performed, a percentage of counts received at each pixel location will be discarded based on the pixel correction factor generated from the flood field image.

A method of deciding which scintillation events will be included in the image involves the use of a random number generator and the application of a rejection technique. If the generated random number (ranging between zero and one) is greater than the correction factor for that pixel, the detected scintillation event is rejected. Otherwise it is accepted and is accumulated in the resulting image. The result is a more cosmetically uniform field.

Other uniformity correction schemes attack the direct causes, not the symptoms. The sliding window and sliding photopeak methods attempt to correct for one of the fundamental causes of nonuniformity, namely, the variations seen in point-source sensitivity. The computer will store an analyzer window setting for each pixel in the image or, alternatively, provide a correction factor that slides the photopeak into the analyzer window. Another correction scheme attacks the second fundamental cause of nonuniformity (spatial distortion) by generating a distortion correction map, which repositions a detected event according to the pixel's positional correction factor. The distortion map is generated by scanning a very regular, well-defined pattern (e.g., a bar phantom) and comparing the relative location of each pixel element to its corresponding point in the real object. In this way, x and y correction factors can be generated for each pixel.

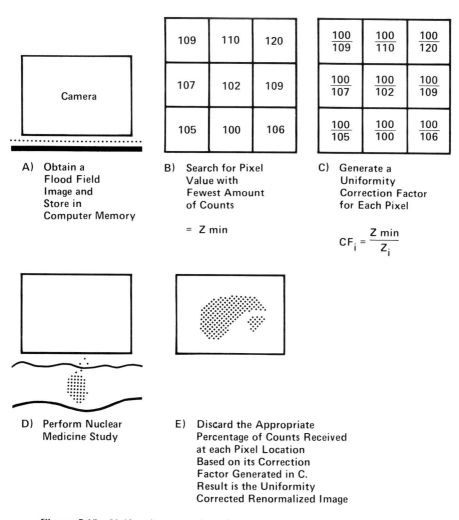

Figure 5.18   Uniformity correction of a gamma camera via renormalization.

Other types of primary data correction include correcting for nonuniform collimator response and subtraction of background noise.

5.4.2 Ultrasound Scanning

Ultrasound imaging has gained widespread application in many areas of medicine including obstetrics, gynecology, pediatrics, ophthalmology, mammography, abdominal imaging, and cardiology, as well as in the imaging of small organs such as the thyroid, prostate, and testicles, and recently in endoscopy. Its wide acceptance is partially due to its noninvasiveness, its use of nonionizing radiation, and its low procedural costs. An ultrasound examination is a widely used first step in attempting to diagnose a presented ailment.

5.4.2.1 Principles of B-Mode Ultrasound Scanning

B-mode ultrasound imaging attempts to reconstruct a cross-sectional view of the patient by way of detecting the amplitudes of acoustical reflections (echoes) that occur at the interface of tissues having different acoustical properties.

Ultrasonic waves are introduced into a patient's body by pressing against the skin with a transducer that generates pulses of high frequency sound waves, which are directed toward the structures of interest. A coupling gel is used to provide efficient transfer of acoustical energy into the body. The acoustical wave propagates through the body tissue, and its radiation pattern will demonstrate high directivity in the near field or Fresnel zone close to the body surface (see Fig. 5.19), and begin to diverge in the far field or Fraunhofer zone. The range of the near and far fields is determined mainly by the wavelength λ of the sonic waves used and the diameter of the transducer. In general, it is preferable to image objects that are within the Fresnel zone, where lateral resolving power is better.

The fate of the acoustical wave is highly dependent on the acoustical properties of the medium in which the wave is propagating. The speed of the wave in media depends on the elasticity and density of the material and affects the degree of refraction (deviation from a straight path) that occurs at a boundary between tissues. The characteristic impedance of the material, which determines the degree of reflec-

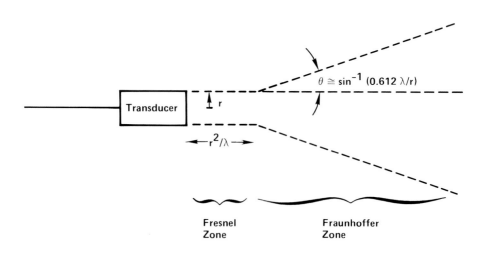

λ: Wavelength of the Sound Wave Used

Figure 5.19 Principle of the ultrasound wave produced by a transducer made of piezoelectric material.

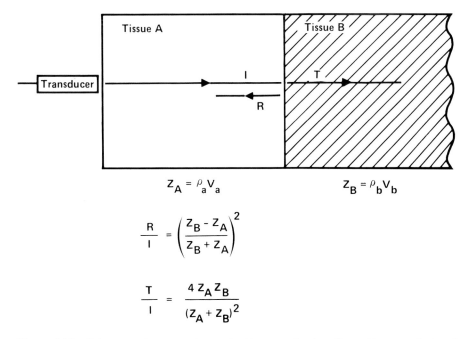

$$Z_A = \rho_a V_a \qquad\qquad Z_B = \rho_b V_b$$

$$\frac{R}{I} = \left(\frac{Z_B - Z_A}{Z_B + Z_A}\right)^2$$

$$\frac{T}{I} = \frac{4\,Z_A\,Z_B}{(Z_A + Z_B)^2}$$

Figure 5.20 Echo strength at normal wave incidence: ρ, density of a medium; *v*, velocity of the ultrasound wave through a medium. See text for definition of other symbols.

tion that occurs when a wave is incident at a boundary, is dependent on the material's density and the speed of sound in the material. The larger the difference between the acoustic impedances (Z_A, Z_B) of two materials forming a boundary, the greater will be the strength of the reflected wave.

Figure 5.20 gives the effects of reflected (R) and transmitted (T) waves on an acoustical boundary. As the reflected and transmitted waves move away from the surface boundary, they, of course, undergo attenuation within their respective propagating media.

Echoes of two different types are normally encountered. *Specular echoes,* which result when the beam encounters a smooth interface whose dimensions are large compared to the wavelength used, send a strong echo signal back to the receiver. *Diffuse echoes,* which occur when the acoustical interface is small or comparable in size to the wavelength used, result in weak echoes that are isotropically scattered and degrade the image.

The rate at which the intensity of the beam changes is dependent on the frequency of the beam and also on inherent material properties of the medium being traversed. The intensity of the beam can be attenuated by partial redirection of the beam via reflection, scatter, or divergence, or by absorption of acoustical energy in the material resulting in the formation of heat. Absorption of the beam is commonly expressed in decibels per centimeter per megahertz (dB/cm/MHz), although the relationship of absorption to frequency is not strictly linear.

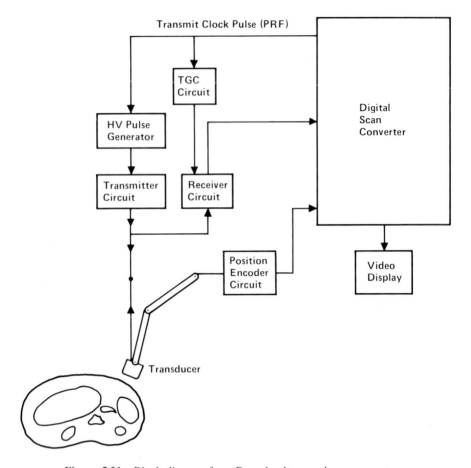

Figure 5.21   Block diagram for a B-mode ultrasound scanner system.

5.4.2.2 System Block Diagram and Operational Procedure

Figure 5.21 shows a general block diagram of a typical B-mode ultrasound scanner. It is composed of a transducer, a high voltage pulse generator, a transmitter circuit, a receiver circuit with time gain compensation (TGC), a mechanical scanning arm with position encoders, a digital scan converter (DSC), and a video display monitor.

The acoustical waves are generated by applying a high voltage pulse to a piezoelectric crystal, resulting in the creation of a longitudinal pressure sonic wave. The rate at which pulses are supplied by the transmitter circuit to the transducer, as determined by a transmit clock, is called the pulse repetition frequency (PRF). Typical PRF values range from 0.5–2.5 kHz. The frequency of the acoustic wave, which is determined by the thickness of the piezoelectric crystal, may range from 1 to 15 MHz. The transducer can serve as acoustical transmitter as well as receiver, since mechanical pressure waves interacting with the crystal will result in the creation of an electrical signal.

Received echo amplitude pulses, which eventually form an ultrasound image, are transferred into electrical signals by the transducer. A radio frequency receiver circuit then amplifies and demodulates the signal. The receiver circuit, a crucial element in an ultrasound scanner, must have a huge dynamic range (30–40 dB) to be able to detect the wide range of reflected signals, which are typically 1–2 V at interfaces near the surface and microvolts at deeper structures. In addition, the receiver must introduce little noise and have a wide amplification bandwidth.

The time gain compensator circuit allows the operator to amplify the echoed signal according to its depth of origin. This feature helps compensate for the higher attenuation of the signal seen from echoes originating from deeper interfaces and results in a more uniform image (i.e., interfaces are not darker closer to the body surface on the image display solely on the basis of being closer to the transducer). The operator is able to obtain the best possible image by controlling the amount of gain at a particular depth.

The output of the receiver is fed into the digital scan converter and used to determine the depth (z dimension) at which the echo occurred. The depth at which the echo originated is calculated by determining the time the echo takes to return to the transducer. The depth of the reflector can be obtained because time and depth are related, and the depth is half the time interval from the transmission of the signal pulse to signal return times the velocity of sound in the traversal medium.

The encoding of the x and y positions of the face of the transducer and the angular orientation of the transducer with respect to the normal of the scanning surface is determined by the scanning arm of the position encoder circuit. The scanning arm is restricted to moving in one linear direction at a time. The arm contains four poten-tiometers whose resistance will correspond to the x and y positions and cosine and sine directions (with angle with respect to the normal of the body surface) of the transducer.

For example, if the transducer is moved in the y direction while keeping x and the angle of rotation fixed, then only the y potentiometer will change its resistance. Position encoders on the arm will generate signals proportional to the position of the transducer and the direction of the ultrasound beam. The x, y, and z data are fed into the digital scan converter to generate addresses that will permit the echo strength signals to be stored in the appropriate memory locations.

The digital scan converter performs A/D conversions of data, data preprocessing, pixel generation, image storage, data postprocessing, and image display. The analog echo signals from the receiver circuit are digitized by an analog-to-digital converter in the DSC, typically to 7–8 bits (128–256 gray levels). Fast A/D converters are normally used because most ultrasound echo signals have a wide bandwidth, and the sampling frequency should be at least twice the highest frequency of interest in the image. Typical A/D sampling rates range from 10 to 20 MHz. The DSC image memory is a random access memory that is normally $512 \times 512 \times 8$ bits for each memory plane.

The data may be preprocessed to enhance the visual display and to match the dynamic range of the subsequent hardware components. Echo signals are typically rescaled, and nonlinear (e.g., logarithmic) circuits often are used to emphasize or de-emphasize certain echo amplitudes.

5.4.2.3 Sampling Modes and Image Display

Three different sampling modes are available on most ultrasound units: the *survey mode,* in which the data stored in memory are continually updated and displayed, the *static mode,* in which only maximum values during a scanning session are stored and displayed, and an *averaging mode,* in which the average of all scans for a particular scan location is stored and displayed.

Once stored in memory, the digital data are subjected to postprocessing operations of several types. These can be categorized according to changing the gray level display of the stored image, temporal smoothing of the data, or spatial operations. Gray scale mean and windowing and nonlinear gray scale transformations are common.

Image display is performed by a video processor and controller unit that can quickly access the image memory and modulate an electron beam to show the image on a video monitor. The digital scan converter allows for echo data to be read continuously from the fast access image memory. This helps to avoid flicker on the display video monitor in real-time imaging. Hard copies of the image are normally obtained using a video multiformat camera or a laser camera.

5.4.2.4 Color Doppler Ultrasound Imaging

Ultrasound scanning using the Doppler principle can detect the movement of blood inside vessels. In particular, it can detect whether the blood is moving away or toward the scanning plane. When several blood vessels are in the scanning plane, it is advantageous to use different colors to represent blood flow direction and speed with respect to the stationary anatomical structures. Thus, colors coupled with the gray scale ultrasound image results in a duplex Doppler ultrasound image. This coupling permits simultaneously imaging of anatomical structures as well as charac-terization of circulatory physiology from known reference planes within the body. The resulting image is called color Doppler or color-flow imaging. For a $512 \times 512 \times 8$ bit ultrasound gray scale image, a color Doppler image will need $512 \times 512 \times 24$ bits, a threefold increase in storage requirement. Figure 5.22 shows a color Doppler US image of a liver scan (see color plate).

5.4.2.5 Cine Loop Ultrasound Imaging

One advantage of ultrasound imaging over other imaging modalities is its noninva-sive nature, which permits the accumulation of ultrasound images continuously through time without adverse effects on the patient. Such images can be played back in a cine loop, which can reveal the dynamic motion of a body organ—for example,

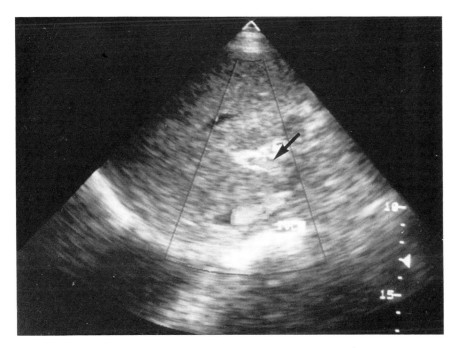

Figure 5.22 Color Doppler ultrasound image of the longitudinal section through the liver indicates that the flow in the inferior vena cava is reversed: blood flow (in red) is directed toward the US scanning plane. Flow in the portal vein (arrow) is hepatopetal. (See color plate.)

Source: Courtesy of E. Grant.

the heartbeat (see also Section 5.2.1.5: Cine XCT). Several seconds of cine loop ultrasound images can produce a very large image file. For example, a 10-second series of color Doppler cine loop ultrasound images will yield $(10 \times 30 \times 0.75) \times 10^6$ bytes $(= 225$ Mbyte$)$ of image information, a very large file to be handled digitally. We will consider how to manage such large data files for storage and for communication in later chapters.

5.5 Magnetic Resonance Imaging

Magnetic resonance imaging (MRI) devices form images of objects through probing the magnetic moments of nuclei, at present usually protons, employing radio frequency (RF) radiation and strong magnetic fields. Information concerning the spatial distribution of nuclear magnetization in the sample is determined from RF signal emission by these stimulated nuclei. The received signal intensity is dependent on five parameters: hydrogen density, spin–lattice relaxation time (T_1), spin–spin relaxation time (T_2), flow velocity (e.g., of arterial blood), and chemical shift.

The purpose of MR imaging is to ascertain spatial (anatomical) information from returned RF signals through filtered back-projection reconstruction or Fourier analysis, ultimately displaying a two-dimensional section of the object for diagnostic evaluation.

There exist distinct advantages for utilizing MRI over other modalities (e.g., XCT) in certain types of examination. The interaction between static magnetic field, RF radiation, and atomic nuclei is free of ionizing radiation; therefore, the imaging procedure is apparently safe. Since, in addition, the scanning mechanism is completely electronic, requiring no moving parts to perform a scan, it is possible to obtain two-dimensional slices of the coronal, sagittal, transaxial planes, and any oblique section. However, the major disadvantage at present is lower spatial resolution compared with XCT.

5.5.1 Basic Physics

Some nuclei (e.g., hydrogen) have a nonzero component of angular momentum arising from their intrinsic spin. The spinning electric charge of the nucleus produces a small magnetic moment μ_N, which will precess about the axis of an applied external magnetic field H, much as a gyroscope does in a gravitational field (Fig. 5.23). The frequency of rotation of the nuclear precession is known as the Larmor frequency

$$\omega = 2\pi\gamma H \tag{5.19}$$

where γ is the gyromagnetic ratio,* a unique value for each nuclear species with nonzero spin, relating Larmor frequency to external magnetic field strength: 42.57 MHz/T for hydrogen [the tesla (T), a unit of magnetic flux density, has the SI units of kilograms per second squared per ampere; $1\ T = 10^4$ gauss]. The precession or resonant frequency of a nucleus is determined solely by the field strength of the external magnetic field. For hydrogen, this external magnetic field also causes an energy splitting of the precessing nuclei into two states (Fig. 5.24), parallel to the external magnetic field (lower energy state) and antiparallel to the external magnetic field (higher energy state). The energy splitting ΔE is proportional to the Larmor frequency

$$\Delta E = \frac{h\omega}{2\pi} = \gamma h H \tag{5.20}$$

where h is Planck's constant. Because these levels have a well-defined energy spacing, transitions from the lower state to the upper state require absorption of photons with frequencies very close to the Larmor precession frequency—a resonance condition, thus the term "nuclear magnetic resonance." For example, in the 0.3 T external magnetic field of a typical clinical MR scanner, the Larmor frequency

---

* In NMR physics literature, the factor 2π is predominantly incorporated into the gyromagnetic ratio γ in the Larmor equation, whereas in MR imaging literature, the factor 2π is not incorporated into the gyromagnetic ratio.

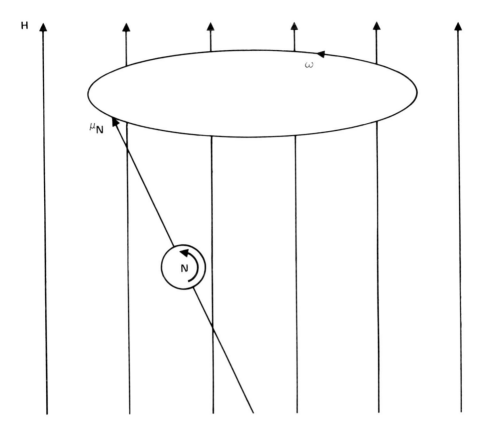

Figure 5.23 Precession and spin. Pictorial representation of a spinning nucleus N with magnetic moment μ_N precessing at the Larmor frequency ω in an external magnetic field H.

for hydrogen is 12.8 MHz, corresponding to an energy separation between parallel and antiparallel states of only 5.3×10^{-8} eV. The population of nuclei in each state at thermal equilibrium is given by Fermi–Boltzmann statistics. Since the two states are separated in energy by a very small amount compared to the mean energy of thermal collisions at room temperature (0.025 eV), only a very minute excess of magnetic moments in the parallel state is realized, 6.8 parts per million (ppm)/T (2 ppm at 0.3 T).

What is observed in the macroscopic domain is the net magnetic behavior of the entire spin ensemble of magnetic moments—the bulk, or macroscopic magnetization vector M. This is zero in the absence of an external magnetic field, since the nuclear magnetic moments are randomly oriented in space. However, in an applied external static magnetic field H_0, there exists a small finite equilibrium magnetization M_0 that aligns parallel to the direction of the field, defining the principal or z axis. As RF energy is absorbed by the ensemble, protons formerly in the lower energy state (parallel to H_0) are promoted to the higher state (antiparallel to H_0),

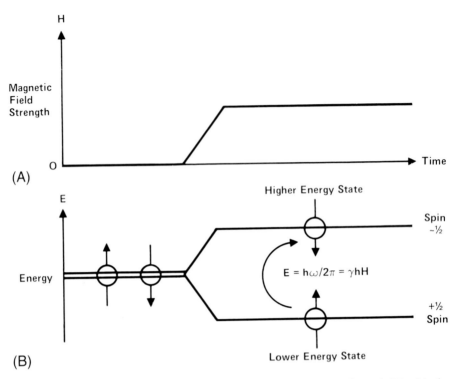

Figure 5.24 Energy splitting. For hydrogen, two energy states are formed (B) with the application of an external magnetic field H (A). The energy separation E is proportional to the magnetic field strength H.

which macroscopically appears as rotation of the magnetization vector away from the z axis (Fig. 5.25). The rotation angle from the z axis is given by:

$$\theta = \gamma H_1 t_w \tag{5.21}$$

where H_1 is the magnitude of the RF magnetic field and t_w is the duration of the applied H_1 pulse. A $\pi/2$ pulse is achieved when θ equals $90°$, M_0 having been tipped into the x–y plane. The torque produced by the interaction of the local magnetization vectors M_0 and H_0 causes the vector to precess about H_0 at the Larmor frequency. To obtain information on the state of the nuclear spins in the object, an RF coil is used to couple to an RF generator first and then to an RF receiver, alternately. Since the RF coil receiver detects only the x–y component of the magnetization vector M_0 (i.e., M_{xy}), a sequence of RF pulses is applied to produce this component for observation.

5.5.2 Pulsing Sequences and Relaxation

The whole process of MRI is based on perturbing the equilibrium magnetization of an object with a series of RF pulses and observing the resulting time-evolving signal

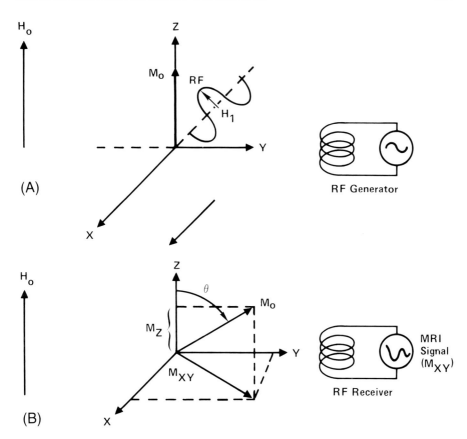

Figure 5.25 RF rotation: application of the RF magnetic field H_1 at the Larmor frequency (A) causes rotation of the equilibrium magnetization (M_0) away from the z axis (B). The component of M_0 in the x–y plane, M_{xy}, is measured by the RF receiver coil; M_z is the longitudinal magnetization.

M_{xy} produced in the RF coil. The observed time-evolving signal is an exponentially damped harmonic oscillation at the Larmor precession frequency, called the free induction decay (FID). The pulsing sequence used depends on the information desired from this time-evolving magnetization signal as it relaxes back to the equilibrium position along the z axis. Several basic pulsing sequences have been derived, including saturation recovery ($\pi/2$ pulse), inversion recovery (a π pulse followed by a $\pi/2$ pulse), and spin–echo sequence ($\pi/2$ pulse followed by one or more π pulses).

The spin–echo sequence (Fig. 5.26) involves tipping the magnetization vector away from its equilibrium position into the x–y plane. The z component of the net magnetization is rotated into the x–y plane by a $\pi/2$ pulse. After a length of time $T_E/2$, a π pulse is applied, causing an echo of the FID to form at the echo time T_E, a sequence parameter determining the temporal appearance of the FID echo. This FID echo is sampled, providing data necessary for image formation. The sequence is

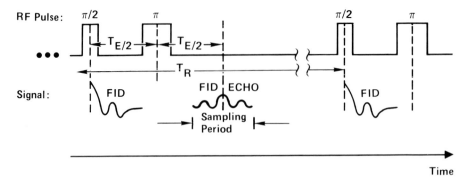

Figure 5.26 Basic spin–echo pulse sequence. See text for symbols.

repeated at intervals of T_R, which is the *repetition time*. The magnitude of the echo depends not only on the sequence parameters T_E and T_R, but also on relaxation characteristics, to be defined in Eqs. (5.22) and (5.23).

Spin–lattice relaxation is represented by an exponential time constant T_1, which characterizes the exchange of energy between excited hydrogen nuclei and their surrounding environment (i.e., lattice). It determines the time required for recovery of the longitudinal magnetization M_z following an RF pulse

$$M_Z = M_0 \left[1 - \exp\left(\frac{-T_R}{T_1} \right) \right]$$ (5.22)

Represented by an exponential time constant T_2, spin–spin relaxation characterizes the exchange of energy between excited and unexcited precessing protons, determining the amplitude of the spin–echo rephasing.

$$M_{xy} = M_z \exp\left(- \frac{T_E}{T_2} \right)$$ (5.23)

Overall, then, the local RF signal intensity (proportional to the magnetization magnitude M_{xy} observed at the spin–echo is given by

$$\text{intensity}_{SE} = \rho_H \left[1 - \exp\left(- \frac{T_R}{T_1} \right) \right] \exp\left(- \frac{T_E}{T_2} \right)$$ (5.24)

where ρ_H is the local relative hydrogen density. Figure 5.27 demonstrates the relationship between relaxation and sequencing times. In addition to T_1, T_2, and ρ_H, flow and chemical shift affect the observed local magnetization, and thus the MR image.

When a substance in the body, say blood, passes through the imaging plane during the pulsing sequence, the protons flowing through the plane experience a magnetic environment different from that of the nonmobile protons in the imaging plane. These factors contribute toward two forms of phenomenological contrast in the final image. At low fluid velocities, there is an actual increase in relative intensity, termed paradoxical enhancement (Fig. 5.28). This phenomenon occurs

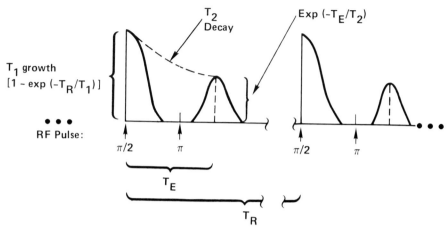

Figure 5.27 Relaxation and sequencing times. The product of $\exp(-T_E/T_2)$, $[1 - \exp(-T_R/T_1)]$ and ρ_H is the relative intensity, Eq. (5.24).

when the nuclei entering the imaging plane during the imaging sequence have not undergone prior excitation. Such particles are in fact fully magnetized, contributing a greater signal than mobile protons in the plane. With increasing velocity, however, the signal falls off, as a result of disruption of the imaging sequence by nuclei quickly traversing the imaging plane. Since at arterial flow velocities, little signal is received compared to mobile protons, the vessels appear much darker than sur-

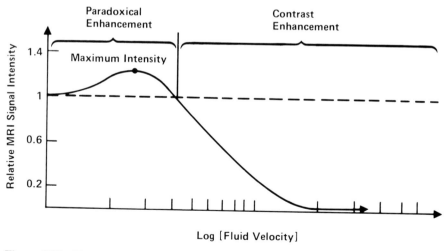

Figure 5.28 Flow velocity and contrast enhancement. For low fluid velocities, paradoxical enhancement occurs, reaching a maximum at $v = $ slice thickness/T_R. Beyond this point, the relative intensity decreases and becomes approximately zero at $v = $ slice thickness/$(T_E/2)$, where the rephasing π pulse no longer orients a magnetization component into the x–y plane.

rounding tissue. In general, flow contrast enhancement is a complex function of velocity, fluid turbulence, and imaging protocol.

Chemical shift occurs when precessing protons experience heterogeneous magnetic environments because of the presence of other species of neighboring nuclei. For instance, protons in the body are predominantly bound up in water (oxygen environment) or lipids (carbon environment); therefore protons in these different environments precess at slightly different frequencies (shift) under the same external magnetic field. Even though these differences only account for 3.5 ppm, they may interfere with desired high frequency spatial information obtained with gradient fields, causing pixel shift artifacts in the final MR image.

5.5.3 Magnetic Resonance Image Production

5.5.3.1 Block Diagram

A simplified block diagram of a typical MR imaging device illustrates the components necessary for the production, detection, and display of the MRI signal (Fig. 5.29). Included are the magnet to produce the H_0 field and RF equipment to produce the H_1 field (transmitter, amplifier, and coil for transmitting mode) and detect the FID (coil for receiving mode, preamplifier, receiver, and signal demodulator); x, y, and z gradient power supplies and coils provide the magnetic field gradients needed for encoding spatial position. Also necessary is the electronics and computer facility to orchestrate the whole imaging process (control interface with computer), digitize the MR image data (A/D converter), reconstruct the image (computer algorithms), and display it (computer, disk storage, image processor, and display system).

5.5.3.2 MR Imaging Fundamentals

Before describing how an MR image is attained, a few fundamental need be explored, namely, achieving spatial resolution, plane selection, free induction decay (FID), and projection gradients. Various techniques are used in sampling the magnetization of the object. These are classified according to the portion of the object sampled at one time: point, line, plane, and volume methods. The present trend is toward use of planar, two-dimensional Fourier transform techniques and the volume method.

Achieving Spatial Resolution in MRI

The basic concept underlying all techniques of achieving spatial resolution is that the resonant frequency of the nuclei is proportional to local magnetic field strength, explicitly stated in the Larmor relation, Eq. (5.19):

$$f = \frac{\omega}{2}\pi = \gamma H$$

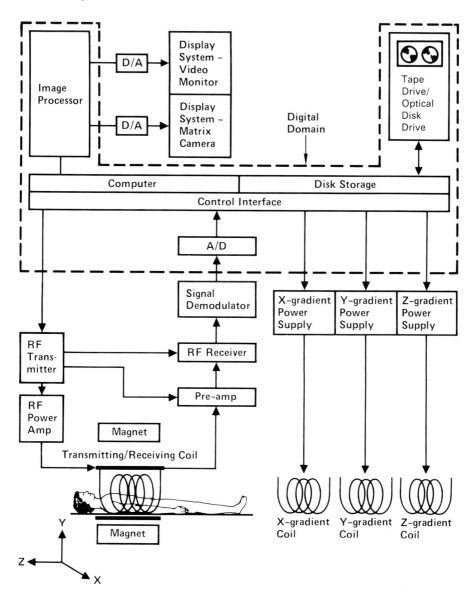

Figure 5.29 Block diagram of a typical MRI system.

To the homogeneous main magnetic field H_0 are added gradient fields:

$$G_x = \delta \left[\frac{H_z(x,y,z)}{\delta x} \right]$$

$$G_y = \delta \left[\frac{H_z(x,y,z)}{\delta y} \right]$$

$$G_z = \delta H_z \left[\frac{(x,y,z)}{\delta z} \right]$$

introducing a positional dependence into the z component of the magnetic field strength at each point: $H_z(x,y,z)$. These gradient fields are generated by three mutually orthogonal gradient coil sets. Relative displacements of resonating nuclei are defined by differences in local resonant frequency produced by the gradients (Fig. 5.30). For example, in one dimension we have

$$H(x) = H_0 + G_x x \tag{5.25}$$

$$\frac{\omega(x)}{2\pi} = \gamma H_0 + \gamma G_x x$$

$$x = \frac{[\omega(x)/2\pi\gamma] - H_0}{G_x}$$

or,

$$x = \frac{[\omega(x) - \omega_0]/2\pi\gamma}{G_x}$$

where $\omega_0/2\pi = \gamma H_0$.

It is apparent that to retrieve the position encoded in the local magnetization Larmor frequency $\omega(x)$, we must have demodulation $\omega(x) - \omega_0$ with respect to the Larmor frequency associated with the static magnetic field ω_0. The demodulation yields $\Delta\omega(x)$, the positionally encoded difference in Larmor frequency due to gradient application:

$$x = \frac{\Delta\omega(x)/2\pi\gamma}{G} \tag{5.26}$$

Thus, the displacement x is determined, providing spatial resolution. In reality, within a subject volume, there exists a continuum of $\Delta\omega$'s from protons precessing in the local gradient field, modulated with the Larmor frequency. It is these local $\Delta\omega$'s that produce through superposition the FID. Typically, gradient fields are on the order of a gauss per centimeter, while the bandwidth of the $\Delta\omega$'s range in the tens of kilohertz.

Plane Selection

With two-dimensional MR imaging techniques, the hydrogen nuclei in the desired image slice are excited through application of a spectrally shaped RF pulse in the presence of a magnetic field gradient perpendicular to the imaging plane.

Both the bandwidth of the RF pulse and the strength of the applied gradient determine the slice thickness (Fig. 5.31). Theoretically, this plane may be produced along any orientation in the imaging volume, provided appropriate gradient fields are applied. The most commonly used orientations correspond to the basic anatomical planes (transaxial, coronal, and sagittal), though some devices can image oblique planes using vectorial combinations of the principal orientations.

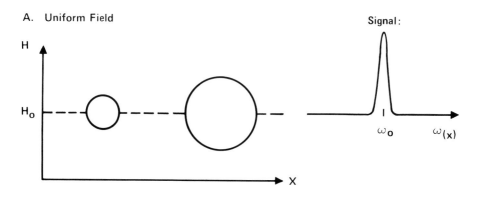

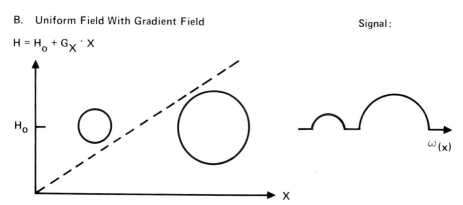

Figure 5.30 Spatial information from gradient application. (A) Two cylindrical volumes of water are placed inside a uniform magnetic field H_0. The MRI signal observed is a superimposed signal from both volumes. (B) With the addition of a linear gradient field, each volume experiences different field strengths, thus separate Larmor frequencies exist for the two volumes. The difference in frequency is proportional to displacement.

Free Induction Decay

The observable in MR imaging, the free induction decay, is observed after application of the plane selecting RF pulse, which rotates the local magnetization vectors in the imaging plane away from the main magnetic field into the $x-y$ plane. There they spontaneously relax and precess, inducing a complex waveform in the receiving coil plane. The portion of the magnetic moment in the plane of the RF coil will induce in the detector an RF voltage which is the FID signal. When the requisite projection gradients are applied after plane selection, the observed FID, a time-varying superposition of all precessing proton frequencies in the plane, will be found to contain all the spectral information necessary for image reconstruction.

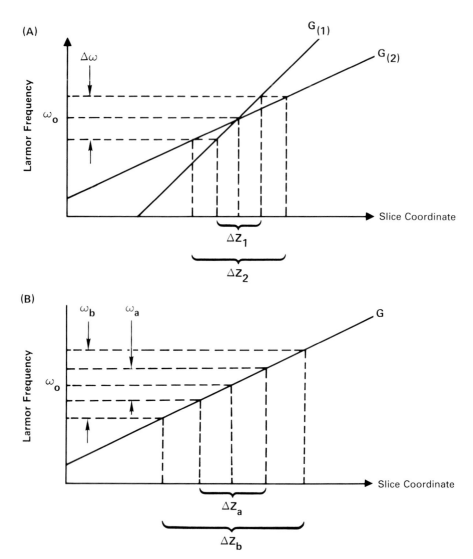

Figure 5.31 Slice thickness as a function of gradient strength and bandwidth. (A) Effect of gradient strength ($G_1 > G_2$) at constant RF bandwidth ($\Delta\omega$). A high field gradient produces a thinner slice thickness ($\Delta z_1 < \Delta z_2$). (B) Effect of RF bandwidth with constant gradient strength. Increased bandwidth ($\Delta\omega_b > \Delta\omega_a$) produces a thicker slice ($\Delta z_b > \Delta z_a$).

Projection Gradients

Previously, a gradient was applied for slice selection through the object. To project the two-dimensional proton spin density onto a line, however, supplemental gradients must be applied antecedent to the sampling of the FID. In the presence of a linear projection gradient, a linear distribution of Larmor frequency across the plane

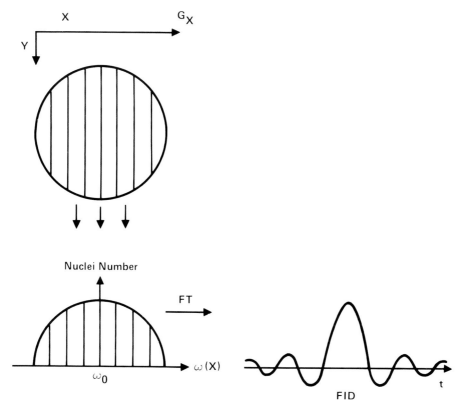

Figure 5.32   Projection through gradient application. Projection onto a line of hydrogen nuclei in a cylindrical water phantom in the selected plane. In the presence of the projection gradient, the nuclei along each vertical line precess at identical Larmor frequencies. Therefore, individual frequency elements in the spectrum correspond to projecting a line of nuclei onto a single point. The superposition of the various Larmor frequencies, due to gradient application, produces the composite FID (i.e., the Fourier transform of the frequency distribution).

is produced. Voxels in each line through the object perpendicular to the projection gradient precess at the same frequency (Fig. 5.32). Therefore, each element of frequency defined by the projection gradient is equivalent to the projection of each line through the plane perpendicular to the projection gradient onto a point along the projection axis. These frequency elements precessing in the axis of the RF receiving coil produce the FID in the time domain, which is the Fourier transform of the precession frequency spectrum.

5.5.3.3 Steps in Producing an MR Image

A spin–echo MR image is produced in the following manner. First, the object is placed inside an RF coil situated in the homogeneous portion of the main magnetic field H_0. Next, a pulsing sequence is applied to the imaging volume (hence spin–echo), which has two effects. The $\pi/2$ pulse applied in the presence of a gradient provides normal selective excitation of a plane through the sample, say the x–y plane; also, the π pulse acts to rephase the local M_{xy} magnetization for the spin–echo.

Next, the FID is observed in the presence of other, yet different linear gradients to provide spatial information/projections by means of recording the demodulated quadrature FID from the RF coil. The demodulated analog signal is sampled with an analog-to-digital converter and stored in a digital data array for processing. This set of data is analogous to one set of projection data in XCT. After the repetition time has elapsed, the pulsing sequence is applied and the FID sampled repeatedly with alternate gradient magnitudes until the desired number of projections has been acquired.

During and after data collection, computed tomographic reconstruction algorithms are performed by computer on the acquired projections (digital data) using filtered back-projection or inverse two-dimensional fast Fourier transform. This yields the final result, a digital image (digital data file) of localized magnetization in the spatial domain whose magnitude follows the spin–echo dependence on relaxation times, hydrogen density, flow, and chemical shift. That the inverse Fourier transform produces an image in the spatial domain is intuitively reasonable, since, as demonstrated earlier, the spatial domain is related via gradient application to the frequency domain, and Fourier transformation of the Larmor precession frequency spectrum produces the FID in the time domain. Therefore, the inverse Fourier transform (IFT) is applied to the collected FID data to reconstruct the spatial distribution of nuclear magnetization in the body section. This procedure can be represented as follows:

$$\text{frequency spectrum} \xrightarrow{\text{FT}} \text{FID} \xrightarrow{\text{IFT}} \text{spatial distribution (image)}$$

This digital image can then be archived on disk storage, or converted to analog form as a video image or hard copy film. Figure 5.33 demonstrates the image information flow.

5.5.3.4 Image Format, Resolution, and Contrast

Image Format

The basic image format of an MR scanner is different from that of other modalities (e.g., XCT). Although both display two-dimensional tomographic slices, MRI, in addition to the transaxial cross sections characteristic of XCT, images the sagittal, coronal, and oblique planes (Fig. 5.34). Research is also being done in obtaining true three-dimensional images both from the FID and through use of postprocessing techniques.

Not only is MRI different from XCT in image plane orientation flexibility, but

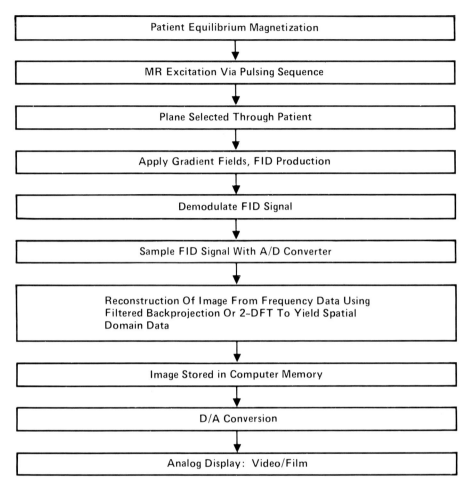

Figure 5.33 Image information flow in an MR imager.

the observable in the MRI scan (the FID) contains information involving many parameters (e.g., T_1, T_2). In XCT, however, the only observable is the linear attenuation coefficient. The challenge of MRI is then attempting to decipher the wealth of information bound up in the FID (T_1, T_2, ρ_H), flow velocity and chemical shift, and how to display all this information adequately. Usually, only the magnetization magnitude is displayed, which is a function of all the above-mentioned parameters, though one may predominate to yield a so-called weighted image. Much work has been performed to obtain true T_1 and T_2 maps for MRI tissue characterization.

Resolution

When discussing resolution, three facets are considered: spatial, density (contrast), and temporal resolution. The density resolution of MRI at the present time is about 8

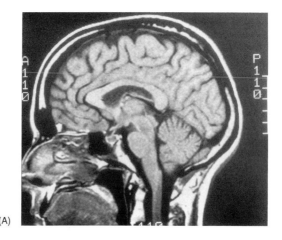

(A)

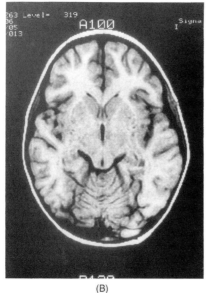

(B)

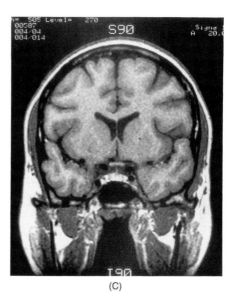

(C)

Figure 5.34 Examples of MR head images: (A) sagittal, (B) transaxial, and (C) coronal.

bits deep, although the A/D converters used to sample the demodulated FID usually sample 2 bytes deep (Fig. 5.35). The spatial resolution of MRI typically varies between 0.3 and 2.0 mm, depending on the coils used to send/receive the RF signal and gradient strength. Because there exists only a 6.8 ppm/T excess of magnetic moments in the lower energy state, the magnetization vector is very small; thus the MR phenomenon is inherently noisy, with low signal-to-noise ratio. This is why the image data are really only about 8 bits deep.

Even though the S/N ratio is lower in MRI than in XCT, MR images rival or

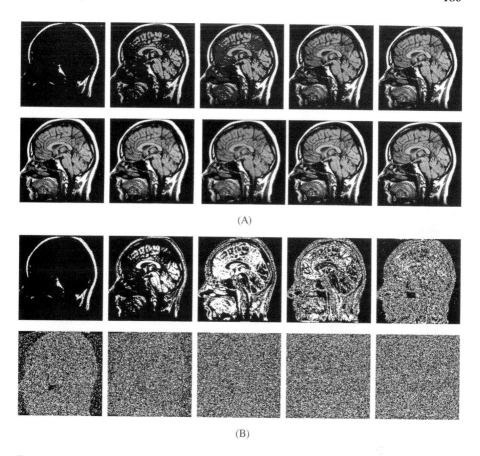

(A)

(B)

Figure 5.35 The original image (second row, last image) was obtained digitally from a GE Signa 5X MR Scanner with 12 bits/pixel. These pictures explore the depth information of the MR image using bit planes. (A) The accumulative bit planes; the top left image displays the most significant bit (1). Moving from left to right, and top to bottom, the next highest bit is added to the previous one: 1 + 2, 1 + 2 + 3, 1 + 2 + 3 + 4, 1 + 2 + 3 + 4 + 5, ... The last image in the second row is the original. No visual differences between the original and rest of the images in the second row are observed. Furthermore, individual bit planes may be observed to determine whether image information is presented at each bit. (B) The individual bit planes. The left-most image in the top row displays the most significant bit (1). Moving from left to right, and top to bottom, the next highest bit is displayed: 2, 3, 4, 5, 6, 7, 8, 9, 10. The bit plane images contain noticeable structural information up to the seventh bit plane. The eighth, ninth and tenth bit planes offer little, if any, structural information.

excel XCT images in some regions of the body partly because of the significantly better tissue contrast realized in MRI. Tissue contrast may be manipulated through choice of pulsing sequence and sequence parameters (e.g., T_R and T_E). The major drawback to MRI is inherently poor temporal resolution. In fact, the three parameters—spatial, contrast, and S/N—are inextricably related, one being augmented only at the expense of one or both of the other two.

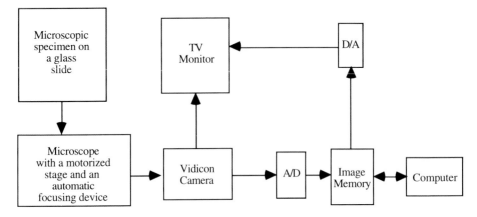

Figure 5.36 Block diagram showing the instrumentation for digital microscopy.

5.6 Microscopic Imaging

5.6.1 Instrumentation

Digital microscopy is used to extract sectional quantitative information from bio-medical microscopic slides. A digital microscopic imaging system consists of the following components:

- a compound microscope with proper illumination for specimen input
- a vidicon (or CCD) camera for scanning microscopic images
- TV monitors for displaying the image
- an analog-to-digital (A/D) converter
- an image memory
- a computer (or image processor) to process the digital image

Figure 5.36 shows the block diagram and the physical setup of the instrumentation.

To do effective quantitative analysis with the microscope, two additional attachments to the microscope are necessary: a motorized stage assembly and an automatic focusing device.

5.6.1.1 Motorized Stage Assembly

A motorized stage assembly promotes rapid screening and locating the exact positions of objects of interest for subsequent detailed analysis. The motorized stage assembly consists of a high precision $x–y$ stage with a specially designed holder for the slide to minimize the vibration due to transmission when the stage is moving. Two stepping motors are used for driving the stage in the x and y directions. A typical motor step is about 2.5 μm, with an accuracy and repeatability to within $±1.25$ μm. The motors can move the stage in either direction with a maximum speed of 650 steps, or 0.165 cm, per second. The two stepping motors can either be controlled manually or automatically by the computer.

5.6.1.2 *Automatic Focusing Device*

The automatic focusing device ensures that the microscope is focusing all the time when the stepping motors are moving the stage from one field to another. It is essential to have the microscope in focus before the vidicon camera starts to scan.

Two common methods for automatic focusing are using a third stepping motor in the z direction, or an air pump. To achieve automatic focusing by means of a third stepping motor, this z-direction motor moves the stage up and down with respect to the objective lens. The z movements are nested in large $+z$ and $-z$ values initially and then gradually to smaller $+z$ and $-z$ values. After each movement, a video scan of the specimen is made through the microscope and some optical parameters are derived from the scan. A focused image is defined as the scan with these optical parameters above certain threshold values. Since nested upward and downward movements of the stage in the z direction are necessary, although the method is automatic, it requires computer processing time to perform the automatic focusing each time the stage moves.

The use of an air pump for automatic focusing is based on the assumption that to have automatic focusing, the specimen lying on the upper surface of a glass slide must be on a perfectly horizontal plane with respect to the objective lens all the time. The glass slide is not of uniform thickness, however, and when it rests on the horizontal stage, the lower surface will form a horizontal plane with respect to the objective, but the upper surface will not, contributing to the imperfect focus of the slide. If an air pump is used to create a vacuum from above, such that the upper surface of the slide is suctioned from above to form a perfectly horizontal plane with respective to the objective, then the slide will be focused all the time. Using an air pump for automatic focusing does not require additional time during operation, but it does require precision machinery.

5.6.2 Resolution

The resolution of a microscope is defined as the minimum distance between two objects in the specimen which can be resolved by the microscope. Three factors control the resolution of a microscope.

1. The angle subtended by the object of interest in the specimen and the objective lens: the larger the angle, the higher the resolution.
2. The medium between the objective lens and the coverslip of the glass slide: the higher the refractive index of the medium, the higher the resolution.
3. The wavelength of light employed: the shorter the wavelength, the higher the resolution.

These three factors can be combined into a single equation (Ernst Abbe, 1840–1905)

$$s = \frac{\lambda}{2(\text{NA})} = \frac{\lambda}{2n \sin i} \tag{5.27}$$

where s is the distance between two objects in the specimen that can be resolved (the smaller the s, the greater the resolution), λ is the wavelength of the light employed, n is the refractive index of the medium, i is the half-angle subtended by the object at the objective lens, and NA is the numerical aperture commonly used for defining the resolution (the larger the NA, the higher the resolution).

Therefore, to obtain a higher resolution for a microscopic image, use as the objective lens an oil immersion lens (large n) with a large angular aperture and select a shorter wavelength of light source for illumination.

5.6.3 Contrast

Contrast is the ability to differentiate various components in the specimen with different intensity levels. Black-and-white contrast is equivalent to the range of the gray scale (the larger the range, the better the contrast). Color contrast is an important parameter in microscopic image processing; in order to bring out the color contrast from the image, various color filters must be used with the adjusted illumination.

It is clear that the spatial and density resolutions of a digital image are limited by the resolution and contrast of a microscope, respectively.

5.6.4 Vidicon Camera and Scanning

When the specimen has been focused under the microscope, a vidicon or a charge-coupled device camera (see Section 3.2.1.1) can be attached to the microscope tube to detect the light emitted from the specimen within the microscopic field of view. The camera scans the specimen point by point from left to right, top to bottom, and forms a light image of the specimen on the photosensitive face of the camera. The brightness $B(x,y)$ of each pixel is converted into an electrical voltage (video signal), which is transmitted to the display monitor. This voltage is used to control the brightness of a corresponding spot on the fluorescent screen of the monitor. These spots reconstruct a video image of the specimen on the TV screen. If the camera is to perform satisfactorily for microscopic imaging, the following specifications should be met:

Gamma (γ) of the camera:	0.65 or less
Dynamic range:	200:1
Resolution:	MTF (modulation transfer function derived by plotting the video amplitude versus the number of line per unit length) should be comparable to that of an ideal Gaussian spot with diameter $\frac{1}{500}$ of the image width
Linearity:	$\pm 0.5\%$ of the pixel value for all pixels

5.6.5 A/D Conversion

There are two methods for digitizing the microscopic image formed by the vidicon camera: The real-time digitizing with a fast A/D converter, usually in the 10 MHz range. It converts the video signal $B(x,y)$ into a digital number $P(x,y)$ and sends it to the (x,y) location of the image memory. A complete TV frame 512 × 512 pixels with 8 bits/pixel) can be digitized in $\frac{1}{30}$ second. Because of the high speed A/D conversion, the signal-to-noise ratio of the real-time digitized image tends to be low. To improve the SNR, it is common to digitize the same frame many times and take the average value for each pixel.

The high resolution digitizer uses an A/D converter with a slower but better signal-to-noise ratio; the digital image thus obtained is of better quality. Since the A/D conversion rate is much slower than the TV scanning rate, the same microscopic field must be scanned many times to produce a complete digital image.

5.6.6 Image Memory

The image memory stores and displays the digitized microscopic image. Once digitized and stored in the memory, the image is continuously refreshed in synchrony with the video scan.

The image memory is not a component of the main computer and should be considered to be a very fast peripheral storage device; the stored image can be accessed by the computer for image processing. The image memory is generally organized into memory planes, and each plane has the storage capacity to refresh a 512 × 512 one-bit gray level image. The most commonly used refresh memory for imaging has 8 or 12 memory planes, which give 256–4096 gray levels. In addition, there should be one extra memory plane for graphic overlay on top of the image memory for interactive image processing.

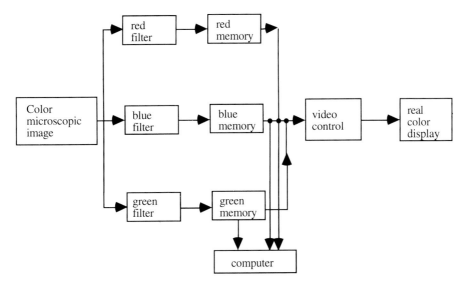

Figure 5.37   Color image processing block diagram. Red, blue, and green filters are used to filter the image before digitization. The three digitized, filtered images are stored in the red, blue, and green memories, respectively. The real color image can be displayed back on the color monitor from these three memories through the composite video control.

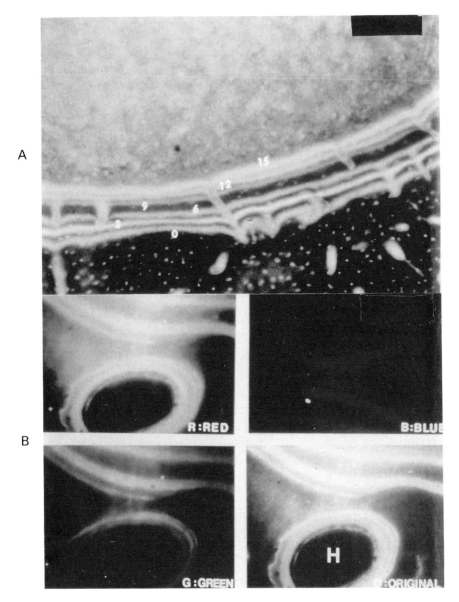

Figure 5.38 (A) Fluorochromic image of a bone cell from the tibia of a rat with five different tetracycline labels shown in orange-red. Each label has its own color characteristics: day 0, oxytetracycline label; day 3, DCAF; day 6, xylenol orange, 90 mg/kg; day 9, hematoporphyrin, 300 mg/kg (did not stain); day 12, doxycycline; day 15, alizarin red 5. The dose is 20 mg/kg. (B) Partial osteonal unit depicting the osteoid and the Haversian canal (H). One tetracycline label is shown in orange-red, the inside ring immediately adjacent to H. The three color images red, blue, and green are also shown (the blue image was accidentally flipped during the photographic process). (See color plate.)

If a real color microscopic image is needed, the color specimen is generally digitized with a red, blue, and green filter, in three separate steps. The three color-filtered images are then stored in the corresponding three image memories, red, blue, and green, each of which with eight planes. Thus, a true color image has 24 bits/pixel. The computer will treat the contents of the three image memories as three individual microscopic images and process them separately. The real color digital microscopic image can be displayed back on a color monitor from these three memories through a color composite video control. Figure 5.37 shows the block diagram of the real color microscopic imaging. In the fluorochromic image of a bone cell with tetracycline labels of Figure 5.38, a partial osteonal unit is shown in the red, blue, green, and the composite color images (see color plate).

5.6.7 Computer

The computer, usually a personal computer with necessary peripherals, serves as a control as well as performing image analysis in the system. The following are the major control function:

movement of the x–y stepping motors
control of the automatic focusing
control of the color filtering
control of the digitization of the microscopic image
image processing

For examples of digitized images of a cell, refer again to the lymphocyte shown in various spatial and density resolutions in Figure 2.2.

CHAPTER

6

Image Compression and Reconstruction

Compressing a radiologic image can save image storage space and transmission time. This chapter describes some compression techniques that are applicable to radiologic images.

6.1 Terminology

The half-dozen definitions that follow are essential to an understanding of image compression/reconstruction.

Original image. The original image is a digital radiologic image $f(x,y)$, where f is a nonnegative integer function, and x and y can be from 0 to 255, 0 to 511, 0 to 1023, and 0 to 2047. The original image is a two-dimensional rectangular array to be compressed into a one-dimensional data file.

Transformed image. The transformed image $F(u,v)$ of the original image $f(x,y)$ is the two-dimensional array after a mathematical transformation. If the transformation is the forward discrete cosine transform, then u, v are nonnegative integers representing the frequencies.

Compressed image file. The compressed image file is a one-dimensional array of encoded information derived from the original or a transformed image by an image compression technique.

Reconstructed image from a compressed image file. The reconstructed image from a compressed image file is a two-dimensional rectangular array $f_c(x,y)$. The technique used for the reconstruction (or decoding) depends on the method of compression. In the case of error-free compression, the reconstructed image is identical to the original image, whereas in irreversible image compression some information will be lost between the original and the reconstructed image. The term "reconstructed image from a compressed image file" should not be confused with the image reconstruction accomplished by means of projections used in computerized tomography as described in Chapter 5.

Difference image. The difference image is the subtracted image between the original and the reconstructed image, $f(x,y) - f_c(x,y)$. In the case of error-free compression, the difference image is the zero image. In the case of irreversible compression, the difference image is the difference between the original image and the reconstructed image. The amount of the difference depends on the compression technique used as well as the compression ratio.

Compression ratio. The compression ratio between the original image and the compressed image file is the ratio between computer storage required to save the original image versus that of the compressed data. Thus, a 4:1 compression on a 512 $\times$ 512 $\times$ 8 = 2,097,152 bit image requires only 524,288 bit storage, 25% of the original image storage required.

6.2 Background

Currently, about 30% of radiologic examinations in the United States have as their output sectional images taken directly in digital format. The major imaging modalities include *computerized tomography, magnetic resonance imaging, ultrasonography, positron emission tomography,* and *single-photon emission computerized tomography,* described in Chapters 4 and 5. These modalities have revolutionized the means of acquiring patient images, providing flexible means of viewing anatomical cross sections and physiological phenomena. The other 70% of examinations on skull, chest, breast, abdomen, and bone are done in conventional projection radiography with the screen–film technique, computed radiography, digital subtraction angiography, and digital fluorography as described in Chapters 3 and 4. *Film digitizers* of different kinds, such as laser scanners, solid state cameras, drum scanners, and video cameras, can be used to convert X-ray films from the screen–film technique into digital format described in Chapter 3. Nuclear medicine images are already in digital format and do not require data conversion.

From this distribution, it is seen that the trend in medical imaging is increasingly digital. The basic motivation is to represent medical images in digital form, supporting image transfer and archiving, and to manipulate visual diagnostic information in useful and novel ways, such as image enhancement and volume rendering. Another push is from the *picture archiving and communication systems* (PACS) community, which envisions a *digital radiology environment* in hospitals for the acquisition, storage, communication, and display of large volumes of images in various modalities (see Chapters 7–11). The amount of digital radiologic images captured per year in the United States alone is at the order of petabytes (i.e., 10^{15} bytes) and is increasing rapidly every year. Image compression provides an impetus for storage and communication of this voluminous amount of digital image data. First, it re-

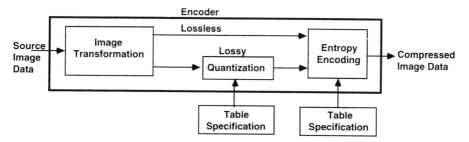

Figure 6.1 The general framework for image data compression. Image transformation can be as simple as the shift of a row, or more complicated, involving mathematical transformation. The decoder is the reverse of the encoder.

duces the bit size required to store and represent images, while maintaining relevant diagnostic information. Second, it enables fast transmission over a network of large medical images for display at workstations, where diagnostic, review, and teaching purposes can be served.

Technically, all image data compression schemes can be broadly categorized into two types. One is *reversible* or "lossless" *compression,* shown in Figure 6.1. A reversible scheme achieves modest compression ratios of the order of 2 to 3, but will allow exact recovery of the original image from the compressed version. An *irreversible scheme* will not allow exact recovery after compression but can achieve much higher compression ratios (e.g., ranging from 10 to 50 or more). Generally speaking, more compression is obtained at the expense of more image degradation; that is, image quality declines as the compression ratio increases. Another type of compression used in medical imaging is *clinical image compression,* which stores a few medically relevant images, as determined by the physicians, out of a series of real-time images, thus reducing the total number of images in an examination file. The stored images may or may not be further compressed by the reversible scheme. In an ultrasound examination, for example, the radiologist may collect data for several seconds, at 30 images per second, but keep only 4 to 8 frames for recording, and discarding the rest.

Image degradation from irreversible compression may or may not be visually apparent. The term "visually lossless" has been used to characterize lossy schemes that result in no visible loss under normal radiologic viewing conditions. An image reconstructed from a compression algorithm that is visually lossless under certain viewing conditions (e.g., a 19 in. video monitor with 1024 × 1024 pixels at a viewing distance of 4 ft could result in visible degradations under more stringent conditions, e.g., printed on a 14 in. × 17 in. film.

A related term used by the American College of Radiology and the National Electrical Manufacturers Association (ACR-NEMA) is *information preserving.* The ACR-NEMA standard report defines a compression scheme as "information preserving" if the resulting image retains all the significant information of the original image. Both "visually lossless" and "information preserving" are subjective terms, and extreme caution must be taken in their interpretation.

Currently, lossy algorithms are not being used by radiologists in primary diagnoses because physicians and radiologists are concerned with the legal consequences of an incorrect diagnosis based on a lossy compressed image. Indeed, lossy compression has raised legal questions for manufacturers and users alike, and the U.S. Food and Drug Administration (FDA) has instituted new regulatory policies. However, large-scale clinical tests are under way by several research laboratories to develop reasonable policies and acceptable standards for the use of lossy processing on medical images. This topic is discussed in Section 6.8.

6.3 Error-Free Compression

This section presents three error-free image compression techniques. The first technique is based on some inherent properties of the image under consideration; the second and third are standard data compression methods.

6.3.1 Clipping and Bit Truncation

The technique of clipping and bit truncation is applied to cross-sectional images obtained from picture reconstruction from projections like MR, CT, PET, and SPECT. The image is first compressed through a clipping procedure (Fig. 6.2). In this case, only the information within the rectangle that includes the outer boundary of the cross section is retained. The size and relative location of the rectangle with respect to the original image are saved in the image descriptors for image reconstruction.

The value of each pixel within the rectangle can be further compressed through a bit truncation procedure. For example, picture reconstruction from X-ray CT projec-

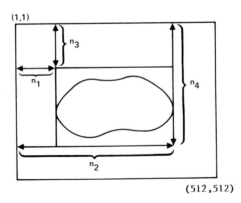

Figure 6.2   A simple boundary search algorithm yields n_1, n_2, n_3, and n_4, the four parameters required to compress a 512 $\times$ 512 CT image to a smaller rectangular area with dimensions of $(n_2 - n_1) \times (n_4 - n_3)$. These parameters also give the relative location of the rectangle with respect to the original image. Each pixel in this rectangular area can be compressed further by means of a bit truncation procedure.

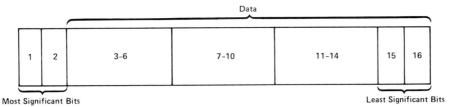

Figure 6.3   After the CT image has been reconstructed from projections, each pixel occupies 16 bits. In one type of CT scanner, bit 1 and bit 2 (the most significant bits) are generally equal to zero; bit 15 and bit 16 (the least significant bits in the data) are mostly the reconstruction noise. To achieve compression, these four bits are dropped during the transfer from image memory to a storage device.

tions maintains computational accuracy by requiring each pixel to have 16 bits. At the end of the reconstruction, about 12-bit information giving 4096 gray levels is significant. Therefore, each pixel can be compressed from 16 bits to 12 bits before it is transferred to a storage device.

Figure 6.3 shows an example of a CT pixel compressed from 16 bits to 12 bits. Figure 6.4 depicts the format of the compressed CT image file on a sequential storage device (e.g., a magnetic tape). Using both clipping and bit truncation, a 2:1 compression ration can be achieved.

6.3.2 Run-Length Coding

Run-length coding, which is based on the repeatability of adjacent pixel values, can be used to compress an image rowwise or columnwise. A run-length code consists of three sequential numbers: the mark, the length, and the gray level. The compression procedure starts with obtaining a histogram of the image. The mark is chosen as the gray level in the image that has the lowest frequency of occurrence. If more than one gray level has the same lowest frequency of occurrence, the higher gray level will be chosen as the mark. The image is then searched line by line, and sets of three sequential numbers are encoded.

For example, assume that the lowest frequency of occurrence gray level in a 512 $\times$ 512 $\times$ 8 image is 128. During the search, suppose the search program encounters

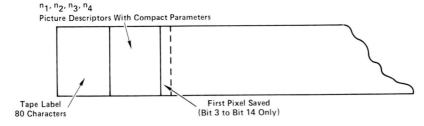

Figure 6.4   An example of the format of a compressed CT image file on magnetic tape.

25 pixels, all having a value of 10, the run-length code for these numbers would then be:

128	25	10
Mark	Length	Gray level

If the length is the same as the mark, the three-number set should be split into two sets. Thus the set 128 128 34 would be split into the sets 128 4 34 and 128 124 34 (the lengths 4 and 124 are arbitrary but should be predetermined before the encoding).

There are two special cases in the run-length code:

1. Since each run-length code set requires three numbers, there is no advantage to compressing adjacent pixels with value repeating less than four times. In this case each of these pixel values is used as the code.

2. The code can consist of two sequential numbers only:

   128   128:   next pixel value is 128

   128   0:   end of the coding

To decode run-length coding, the procedure checks the coded data sequentially. If a mark is found, the following two codes must be the length and the gray level, except for the two special cases. In the first case, if a mark is not found, the code itself is the gray level. In the second case, a 128 following a 128 means that the next pixel value is 128, and a 0 following a 128 means the end of the coding.

Figure 6.5 provides an example: the run-length codes of two horizontal lines from a CT head scan (Fig. 6.5C, E) yield compression ratios for these lines of about 9:1 and 1.5:1, respectively.

A modified run-length coding called run-zero coding is sometimes more practical to use. In this case, the original image is first shifted one pixel to the right and a shifted image is formed. A subtracted image between the original and the shifted image is obtained, which is to be coded. A run-length code on the subtracted image requires only the mark and the length because the third code is not necessary: either it is zero or it is not required because of the two special cases described earlier. The run-zero coding requires that the first pixel value be saved for the decoding procedure.

6.3.3 Huffman Coding

Huffman coding, which is based on the probability (or the frequency) of occurrence of the gray levels in the image, can be used to compress the original image. The encoding procedure is best described with an example.

1. *Original image.* Consider a 10 × 10 image with eight gray levels (C, F, G, B, E, D, H, A), as shown in Fig. 6.6A.
2. *Histogram.* Obtain the histogram of the original image (Fig. 6.6B).

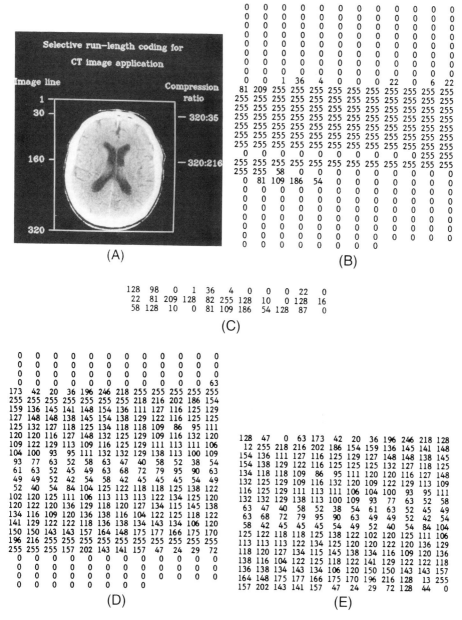

Figure 6.5 (A) Head CT scan (320 × 320 matrix); for convenience of explanation, only the 8 most significant bits per pixel are used during the compression. (B) Pixel values in horizontal line 30 of the scan: total bytes, 320. (C) Run-length coding for line 30: code mark, 128; total bytes required, 35; compression ratio, 320/35 (9.1:1). (D) Pixel values in horizontal line 160: total bytes, 320. (E) Run-length coding for line 160: code mark, 128; total bytes required, 216; compression ratio 320/216 (1.5:1). The compression ratios in (C) and (E) are quite different because of the backgrounds outside the CT image.

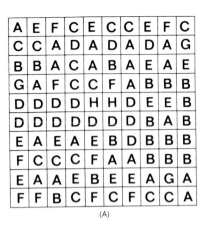

(A)

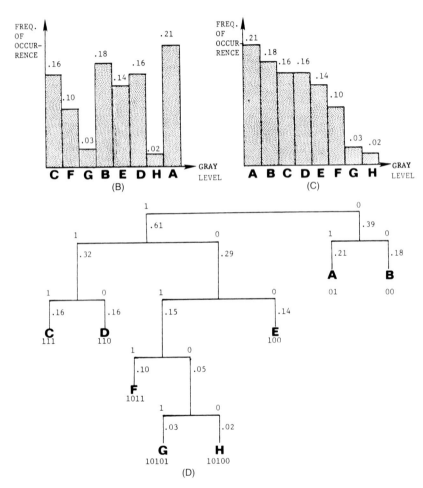

Figure 6.6 The procedure for generating Huffman coding: (A) original 10 × 10 image with eight gray levels (C, F, G, B, E, D, H, A), (B) histogram of the original image, (C) the rearranged histogram, and (D) the Huffman tree and its corresponding codes.

3. *Rearrangement of the histogram.* Rearrange the histogram according to the probability (or frequency) of occurrence of the gray levels and form a new histogram (Fig. 6.6C).

4. *The Huffman tree.* A Huffman tree with two nodes at each level is built as follows. To start, take the two gray levels with the lowest probability of occurrence, in this case G and H, to form the first level; always put the gray level with a higher probability value to the left. Add the total probabilities of these two nodes (0.03 + 0.02 = 0.05). Take the next gray level in the rearranged histogram (F) and form a higher level branch with G and H; put F at the left because of its higher probability value (0.1). Continue until the branch reaches a probability of 0.29. At this point no gray levels in the rearranged histogram have a higher probability value than 0.29. Take the next two available gray levels in the rearranged histogram (C and D) and form a new branch. Always follow the rule that the higher probability gray level is placed on the left. Join this new branch with the previously established branches, which gives a probability of 0.61. Return to the rearranged histogram and repeat the procedure until all the gray levels have been used. This completes the first step of forming a Huffman tree.

Next, designate a "1" to the left and a "0" to the right node throughout all branches of the tree. The last step is to assign bits to each gray level according to its location in the tree. For example, gray level H would be assigned "10100" because it is at the fifth level with the trace of the probabilities as

$$1 \longrightarrow 0 \longrightarrow 1 \longrightarrow 0 \longrightarrow 0 \longrightarrow \text{"H"}$$
$$0.61 \quad 0.29 \quad 0.15 \quad 0.05 \quad 0.02$$

The complete Huffman tree is shown in Figure 6.6D.

5. *The Huffman code.* The Huffman code for these eight gray levels are:

A: 01	2 bits	
B: 00	2 bits	
C: 111	3 bits	
D: 110	3 bits	
E: 100	3 bits	
F: 1011	4 bits	
G: 10101	5 bits	
H: 10100	5 bits	

Therefore, the first row of the original image (Fig. 6.6A) can be encoded as follows:

01	100	1011	111	100	111	111	100	1011	111
A	E	F	C	E	C	C	E	F	C

6. *Compression ratio.* To compute the compression ratio, assume that each pixel in the original image requires 3 bits to preserve the information ($2^3 = 8$ gray

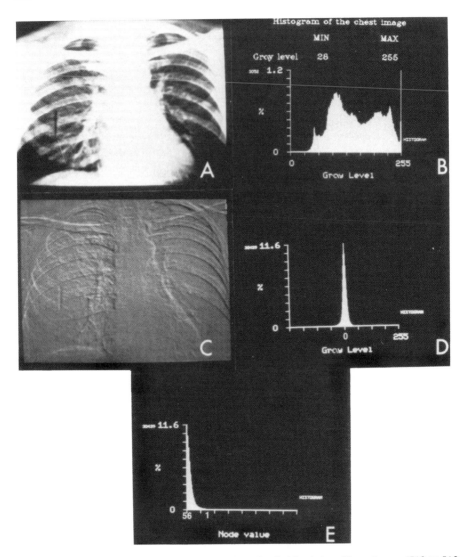

Figure 6.7 An example of the Huffman coding of a digitized chest X-ray image ($512 \times 512 \times 8$). Shifting the image one pixel down and one pixel to the right, produces a subtracted image, from which the Huffman coding is obtained. Huffman coding of the subtracted image (i.e., the original image minus the shifted image) yields a higher compression ratio than that of the original image. The first row and the first column of the original image are needed during the decoding process.

(A) The original digitized chest image. (B) histogram of the original image. (C) The subtracted image. (D) Histogram of the subtracted image. (E) The rearranged histogram. (F) The Huffman tree with codes. The histogram of the subtracted image has 56 gray levels: see (E). Branch node 57 (see last row in Table 6.1) consists of the left node 2 (gray level 26) and right node 1 (gray level 66), each of which has frequency of occurrence equal to 1; the total frequency of occurrence of node 57 is 2. The compression ratio of the subtracted image is about 2.1:1.

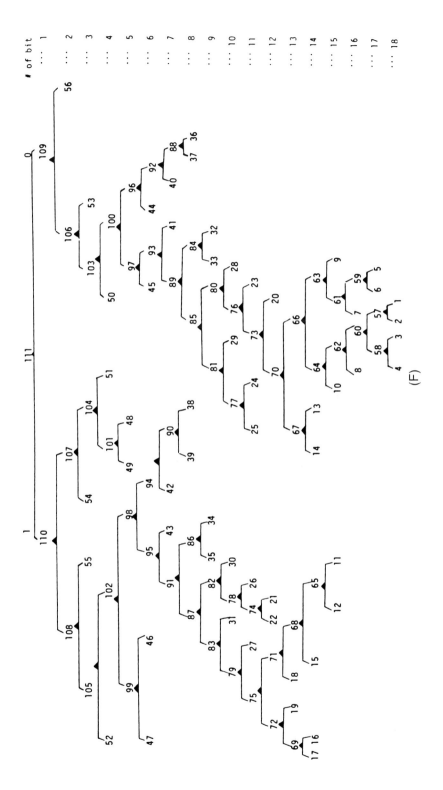

(F)

207

Table 6.1.   The Huffman Tree of the Chest Image: Compression Ratio, 2.1 : 1

	Branch		Gray Level		Histogram*		
Node	Left (1)	Right (0)	Left	Right	Left	Right	Sum
111	110	109			157947	104197	262144
110	108	107			85399	72548	157947
109	106	56†		0†	55417	48780	104197
108	105	55		1	46639	38760	85399
107	54	104	−1		38546	34002	72548
106	103	53		−2	29787	25630	55417
105	52	102	2		25493	21146	46639
104	101	51		3	18400	15602	34002
103	50	100	−3		15473	14314	29787
102	99	98			11176	9970	21146
101	49	48	−4	4	9244	9156	18400
100	97	96			7334	6980	14314
99	47	46	−5	5	5618	5558	11176
98	95	94			5173	4797	9970
97	45	93	−6		3692	3642	7334
96	44	92	6		3607	3373	6980
95	91	43		7	2645	2528	5173
94	42	90	−7		2416	2381	4797
93	89	41		8	1937	1705	3642
92	40	88	−8		1699	1674	3373
91	87	86			1434	1211	2645
90	39	38	−9	9	1198	1183	2381
89	85	84			1031	906	1937
88	37	36	−10	10	847	827	1674
87	83	82			769	665	1434
86	35	34	11	−11	613	598	1211
85	81	80			558	473	1031
84	33	32	12	−12	473	433	906
83	79	31		−13	404	365	769
82	78	30		13	337	328	665
81	77	29		14	297	261	558
80	76	28		−14	249	224	473
79	75	27		−15	214	190	404
78	74	26		15	175	162	337
77	25	24	16	−16	150	147	297
76	73	23		−17	131	118	249
75	72	71			110	104	214
74	22	21	17	18	98	77	175
73	70	20		−19	74	57	131
72	69	19		−18	56	54	110
71	18	68	19		53	51	104
70	67	66			42	32	74
69	17	16	−20	20	29	27	56
68	15	65	21		26	25	51
67	14	13	−22	−21	22	20	42
66	64	63			19	13	32
65	12	11	22	24	13	12	25

Table 6.1.   *(Continued)*

Node	Branch Left (1)	Branch Right (0)	Gray Level Left	Gray Level Right	Histogram* Left	Histogram* Right	Sum
64	10	62	−24		10	9	19
63	61	9		23	7	6	13
62	8	60	25		5	4	9
61	7	59	−23		4	3	7
60	58	57			2	2	4
59	6	5	−25	−36	2	1	3
58	4	3	−28	−26	1	1	2
57	2	1	26	66	1	1	2

* The count of each terminal node is the frequency of occurrences of the corresponding gray level in the subtracted image. The count of each branch node is the total count of all the nodes initiated from this node. Thus, the count in the left column is always greater than or equal to the right column by convention, and the count in each row is always greater than or equal to that of the row below. The total count for the last node "111" is 262144 = 512 × 512, which is the size of the image.

† Each terminal node (1–56) corresponds to a gray level in the subtracted image: minus signs are possible because of the subtraction.

levels). The average number of bits required to compress this image using this Huffman code can be computed by:

$$\text{average number of bits} = \sum_{i=1}^{8} P_i[\text{bit required for gray level "}i\text{"}]$$

$$= 0.21 \times 2 + 0.18 \times 2 + 0.16 \times 3 + 0.16 \times 3$$

$$+ 0.14 \times 3 + 0.1 \times 4 + 0.03 \times 5 + 0.02 \times 5$$

$$= 2.81$$

where i is any of A, B, . . . , H and P_i is the probability of occurrence of gray level "i."

The compression ratio, in this case, 3:2.81 = 1.1:1, is not a very good result. In general, Huffman coding will give low compression ratios for flat histogram images and higher compression ratios for sharp histograms.

In practice, Huffman coding should also be applied to the subtracted image obtained from the original and the shifted image as described in Section 6.3.2. To reconstruct the image, the compressed image file is searched sequentially, bit by bit, to match the Huffman code, and then decoded accordingly.

Figure 6.7 presents an example of error-free image compression using the Huffman coding on a shifted-then-subtracted digitized chest X-ray image (512 × 512 × 8). The associated Huffman tree is listed in Table 6.1.

To obtain higher error-free compression ratios, the run-length method can be used first, followed by the Huffman coding.

6.4 Two-Dimensional Irreversible Image Compression

6.4.1 Introduction

Irreversible compression is most often done in the transform domain and is called transform coding. The procedure of transform coding is to first transform the original image into the transform domain with a two-dimensional transformation—for example, Fourier, Hadamard, cosine, Karhunen–Loeve, or wavelet. The transform coefficients are then quantized and encoded (see Fig. 6.1). The result is a highly compressed data file.

The image can be compressed in blocks or in its entirety. In block compression, before the image transformation, the entire image can be subdivided into equal size blocks (e.g., 8 × 8), whereupon the transformation is applied to each block. A statistical quantitation method is then used to encode the 8 × 8 transform coefficients of each block. The advantages of the block compression technique are that all blocks can be compressed in parallel, and it is easier to perform the computation for a small block transformation than for an entire image. A disadvantage is that a blocky artifact, which is not desirable for radiologic applications, may appear in the reconstructed image. Further image processing on the reconstructed image is sometimes necessary to smooth out such an artifact.

The full-frame compression technique, on the other hand, transforms the entire image into the transform domain. Quantitation is applied to *all* the transform coefficients of the entire transformed image. The full-frame technique is computationally tedious, expensive, and time-consuming. Since, however, it does not produce a blocky artifact, it is more suitable for radiologic applications.

6.4.2 Block Compression Technique

The most popular block compression technique using forward two-dimensional discrete cosine transform is the JPEG (Joint Photographic Experts Group) standard. Sections 6.4.2.1–6.4.2.4 summarize this method, which consists of four steps: two-dimensional forward discrete cosine transform (DCT), bit allocation table and quantitation, DCT coding, and entropy coding.

6.4.2.1 Two-Dimensional Discrete Cosine Transform

Discrete cosine transformation (see Section 2.4.5) has been proven to be an effective method for image compression because the energy in the transform domain is concentrated in a small region. As a result, the DCT method can yield larger compression ratios and maintain the image quality. The forward discrete cosine transform of the original image $f(j, k)$ is given by

$$F(u,v)$$

$$= \left(\frac{2}{N}\right)^2 C(u)\, C(v) \left[\sum_{k=0}^{N-1} \sum_{j=0}^{N-1} f(j,k) \cos \frac{u(j + 0.5)}{N} \cos \frac{v(k + 0.5)}{N} \right] \quad (6.1)$$

The inverse discrete cosine transform of $F(u,v)$ is the original image $f(j,k)$:

$$f(j,k) = \sum_{v=0}^{N-1} \sum_{u=0}^{N-1} F(u,v)C(u)C(v) \cos \frac{u(j + 0.5)}{N} \cos \frac{v(k + 0.5)}{N} \qquad (6.2)$$

where
$$\begin{aligned} C(O) &= (0.5)^{|1/2|} &&\text{for} \quad u,v \neq 0 \\ &= 1 &&\text{for} \quad u,v = 0 \end{aligned}$$

and $N \times N$ is the size of the image.

Thus, for the block transform, $N \times N = 8 \times 8$, whereas for the full-frame compression of a 2048 × 2048 image, $N = 2048$.

6.4.2.2 Bit Allocation Table and Quantization

The two-dimensional DCT of an 8 × 8 block yields 64 DCT coefficients. The energy of these coefficients is concentrated among the lower frequency components. To achieve a higher compression ratio, these coefficients are quantized with no greater precision than is necessary to achieve the desired image quality. In doing so, the original values of the coefficients are compromised, hence some information lost. Quantization of the DCT coefficient $F(u,v)$ can be obtained by

$$F_q(u,v) = \text{NINT}\left(\frac{F(u,v)}{Q(u,v)} \right) \qquad (6.3)$$

where $Q(u,v)$ is the quantizer step size, and NINT is the nearest integer function.

One method of determining the quantizer step size is by manipulating a bit allocation table $B(u,v)$ which is defined by

$$\begin{aligned} B(u,v) &= \log_2[|F(u,v)|] + K &&\text{if} \quad |F(u,v)| \geq 1 \\ &= K &&\text{otherwise} \end{aligned} \qquad (6.4)$$

where $|F(u,v)|$ is the absolute value of the cosine transform coefficient, and K is a real number that determines the compression ratio. Notice that each pixel in the transformed image $F(u,v)$ corresponds to one value of the table $B(u,v)$. Each value in this table represents the number of computer memory bits for saving the corresponding pixel value in the transformed image. The value in the bit allocation table can be adjusted to increase or decrease the amount of compression by assigning a certain value to K. Thus, for example, if a pixel located at (p,q) and $F(p,q) = 3822$, then $B(p,q) = 11.905 + K$. If one selects $K = +0.095$, then $B(p,q) = 12$ (i.e., 12 bits are allocated to save the value 3822). On the other hand, if one selects $K = -.905$, then $B(p,q) = 11$ [i.e., $F(p,q)$ is compressed to 11 bits].

Based on Eq. (6.4), Eq. (6.3) can be rewritten as follows:

$$F_q(u,v) = \text{NINT}\left[(2^{|B(m,n)-1|} - 1) \frac{F(u,v)}{|F(m,n)|} \right] \qquad (6.5)$$

where $F(u,v)$ is the coefficient of the transformed image, $F_q(u,v)$ is the corresponding quantized value, (m,n) is the location of the maximum value of $|F(u,v)|$ for $0 \leq$

$u,v \le N - 1$, and $B(m,n)$ is the corresponding number of bits in the bit allocation table assigned to save $|F(m,n)|$. It is seen in this formula that $F(u,v)$ has been normalized with respect to $(2^{|B(mn)-1|} - 1)/|F(m,n)|$.

The quantized value $F_q(u,v)$ is an approximate value of $F(u,v)$ because of the value K described in Eq. (6.4). This procedure introduces an approximation to the compressed image file.

6.4.2.3 DCT Coding and Entropy Coding

For block quantization with an 8×8 matrix, the $F(0,0)$ is the DC coefficient and is normally the maximum value of $|F(u,v)|$. Starting from $F(0,0)$, the other 63 coefficients can be coded in a zigzag sequence shown in Figure 6.8. This zigzag sequence will facilitate entropy coding by placing low frequency components which normally have larger coefficients before high frequency components.

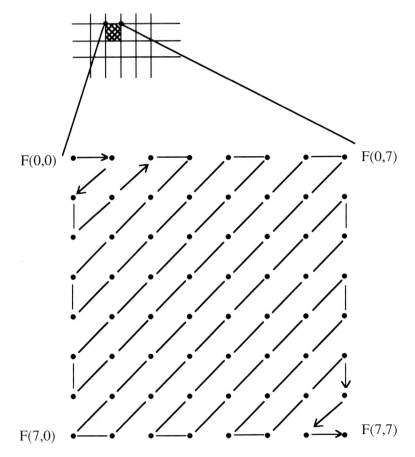

Figure 6.8   The zigzag sequence of an 8×8 matrix used in block quantitation.

The last step in block compression is entropy coding, which provides additional lossless compression by using a reversible technique—for example, run-length coding or Huffman coding, as described in Sections 6.3.2 and 6.3.3.

6.4.2.4 Decoding and Inverse Transform

The block-compressed image file is a sequential file containing the following information: entropy coding, zigzag sequence, bit allocation table, and the quantization. This information can be used in reverse order to reconstruct the compressed image. The compressed image file is decoded by using the bit allocation table as a guide to form a two-dimensional array $F_A(u,v)$, which is the approximate transformed image. The value of $F_A(u,v)$ is computed by

$$F_A(u,v) = \frac{|F(m,n)|\, F_q(u,v)}{2^{|B(m,n)-1|} - 1} \tag{6.6}$$

Equation (6.6) is almost the inverse of Eq. (6.5), and $F_A(u,v)$ is the approximation of $F(u,v)$. Inverse cosine transform (Eq. (6.2) is then applied on $F_A(u,v)$, which gives $f_A(x,y)$, the reconstructed image. Since $F_A(u,v)$ is an approximation of $F(u,v)$, some differences exist between the original image $f(x,y)$ and the reconstructed image $f_A(x,y)$. The compression ratio is dependent on the amount of quantization and the efficiency of the entropy coding. Figure 6.9 shows some block compression results with a compression ratio of 20:1 using the JPEG standard.

6.4.3 Full-Frame Compression

6.4.3.1 The Full-Frame Bit Allocation Algorithm

The full-frame bit allocation (FFBA) compression technique in the cosine transform domain is developed primarily for radiologic images. It is different from the JPEG block method in that the transform is done on the entire image. Image compression using blocks of the image gives blocky artifacts that might affect diagnostic accuracy.

Basically, the FFBA is similar to the block compression technique, as indicated by the following steps. The transformed image of the entire image is first obtained by using the cosine transformation (Eq. 6.1). A bit allocation table (Eq. 6.4) designating the number of bits for each pixel in this transformed image is then generated, the value of each pixel is quantized based on a predetermined rule (Eq. 6.5), and the bit allocation table is used to encode the quantized image, forming a one-dimensional sequentially compressed image file. The one-dimensional image file is further compressed by means of lossless entropy coding. The compression ratio between the original image and the compressed image file depends on the information in the bit allocation table, the amount of quantization on the transformed image, and the entropy coding. The compressed image file and the bit allocation table are saved and used to reconstruct the image. Figure 6.10 shows the data flow of the full-frame bit allocation technique.

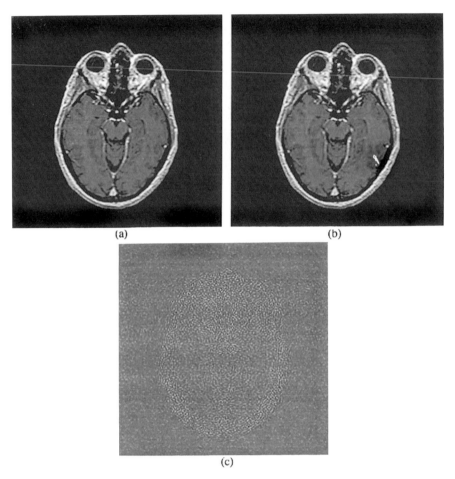

(a)   (b)

(c)

Figure 6.9 An MR image compressed at a compression ratio of 20:1, in accordance with the JPEG standard: (a) the original image, (b) the decompressed image, and (c) the difference image.

Source: Courtesy of Jun Wang.

During image reconstruction, the bit allocation table is used to decode the one-dimensional compressed image file back to a two-dimensional array. An inverse cosine transform is performed on the two-dimensional array to form the reconstructed image. The reconstructed image does not exactly equal the original image because approximation is introduced in the bit allocation table generation and in the quantization procedure.

Despite this similarity, however, the implementation of the FFBA is quite different from the block compression method for several reasons. First, it is computationally tedious and time-consuming to carry out the 2-D DCT when the image size is large. Second, the bit allocation table given in Eq. (6.4) is large when the image size is large, and therefore it becomes an overhead in the compressed file. In the case of block compression, one 8×8 bit allocation table is sufficient for all blocks.

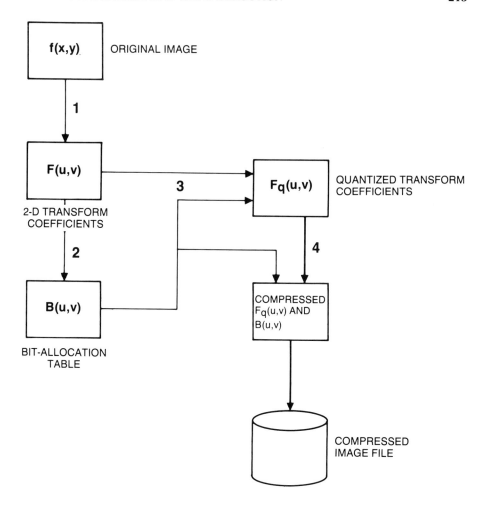

OPERATIONS:

1. FORWARD DISCRETE COSINE TRANSFORM

2. BIT-ALLOCATION PROCESS

3. QUANTIZATION

4. BIT-ALLOCATION ENCODING

Figure 6.10 Data flow of the full-frame bit allocation technique.

Third, zigzag sequencing provides an efficient arrangement for the entropy coding in a small block of data. In the FFBA, zigzag sequencing is not a good method for rearranging the DCT coefficients because of the large matrix size. The implementation of the FFBA is best accomplished by considering a fast DCT method and a compact full-frame bit allocation table, as described in Sections 6.4.3.2 and 6.4.3.3.

6.4.3.2 Fast Discrete Cosine Transform Algorithms

Narasimha–Peterson Algorithm

The discrete cosine transformation given in Eq. (6.1) is time-consuming when N is large, which is the case in the FFBA technique. Many elegant and computationally efficient methods have been developed during the past years, however, by Chen, Narasimha and Peterson, Makhoul, and others. The following algorithms were derived by Narasimha and Peterson. Consider a real sequence $x(n)$; $n = 0, \ldots, N - 1$. The DCT of $x(n)$ can be computed by means of the following steps:

1. Form a new sequence:

$$r(n) = x(2n); \qquad\qquad n = 0,1, \ldots, N/2 - 1 \qquad\qquad (6.7)$$

$$ = x(2N - 2n - 1); \qquad n = N/2, \ldots, N - 1$$

   This reordering consists of all the even elements of $x(n)$ followed by the odd elements in reverse order.
2. Compute $R(k)$, the Fourier transform of $r(n)$.
3. Compute $F(k) = 2c(k) \, \mathrm{Re}[\exp(-i\pi k/2N) \, R(k)]$; $k = 0, 1, \ldots, N - 1$, where $c(0) = 1/\sqrt{2}$ and $c(k) = 1$ for $k = 0, 1, \ldots, N - 1$.

The DCT of $x(n)$ is then given by $F(k)$. If N is a power of 2, the Fourier transform may be computed using the FFT. Further efficiency may be achieved because the FFT of a real sequence can be computed by doing an $N/2$-point complex FFT. Alternatively, one can simultaneously compute the FFT of two real N-point sequences $r(n)$ and $s(n)$, by doing a single N-point complex FFT. This can be done by forming the complex sequence $z(n) = r(n) + i \, s(n)$, and computing $Z(k)$. The Fourier coefficients can then be extracted [using $Z(N) = Z(0)$] from:

$$R(k) = \frac{1}{2} \, \mathrm{Re}[Z(k) + Z(N - k)] + \frac{i}{2} \, \mathrm{Im}[Z(k) - Z(N - k)] \qquad (6.8)$$

$$S(k) = \frac{1}{2} \, \mathrm{Im}[Z(k) + Z(N - k)] - \frac{i}{2} \, \mathrm{Re}[Z(k) - Z(N - k)]$$

The Narashimha–Peterson algorithm allows us to compute an N-point DCT for the cost of some reordering, an $N/2$-point complex FFT, and some phase corrections. Or, one can compute two N-point DCTs with reordering, an N-point complex FFT, Fourier coefficient extraction, and phase corrections. Figure 6.11 shows the cosine transforms of a chest radiograph (CH), a renoarteriogram (RE), the SMPTE phantom (PH) shown in Figure 6.12, and a CT image.

Computational Precision Required

The similarities between the DCT and the FFT imply that we can extrapolate the computational precision required in DCT from that of FFT. The effect of numerical errors and finite word lengths in the computation of the FFT has been analyzed for both fixed and floating point arithmetic. Results are extensively reviewed in Oppenheim. Mostly, these highly theoretical analyses have concentrated on analyzing

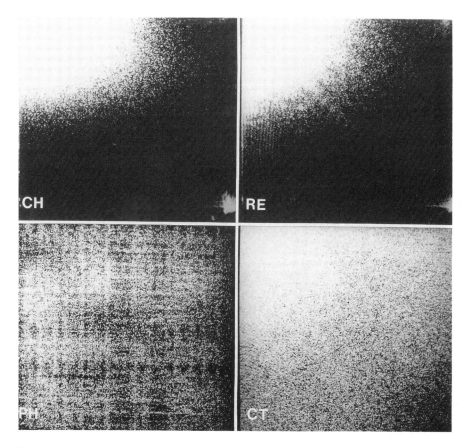

Figure 6.11 The cosine transforms of a chest radiograph (CH: shown later in Fig. 6.17), a renoarteriogram (RE: Fig. 3.17(1)), a CT scan (CT: Fig. 6.20), and an SMPTE phantom (PH: Fig. 6.12). The origin is located at the upper left-hand corner of each image. It is seen that the frequency distributions of the cosine transforms of the chest radiograph and the renoarteriogram are quite similar; they concentrate in the upper left-hand corner, representing the lower frequency components. The frequency distribution of the cosine transform of the CT is spread more toward the higher frequency region, whereas in the case of the SMPTE phantom, the frequency distribution of the cosine transform is all over the transform domain.

noise sources, calculating the effect on the signal-to-noise ratio in the transform coefficients. A white noise image input is often assumed.

For full-frame radiologic image compression, the salient questions involve the dynamical range that can be expected in the transform coefficients and the precision to which they must be calculated. "Sufficient precision" is defined as transform followed by inversion without any gray level errors in the reconstructed image. Irreversible compression due to quantization will be accompanied by some errors; however, these arise from bit allocation rather than loss of precision in the transform.

Assume that the initial image has been digitized to b bits resolution, on a fixed gray level scale ranging from 0 to the maximum $|x(n)|$.

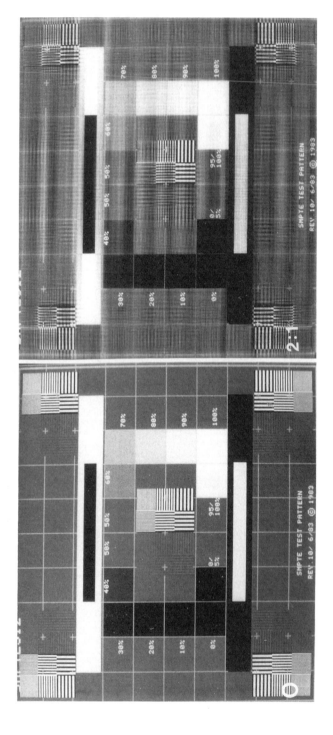

Figure 6.12 The digital SMPTE phantom (Society of Motion Picture and Television Engineers), and the reconstructed image with compression ratio of 2:1. Observe the vertical and horizontal edge artifacts in the reconstructed image.

Oppenheim and Schafer provided a main sequence value estimation of the signal-to-noise ratio in digital computation of the *FFT X(k)* of *x(n)*:

$$X(k) = \frac{1}{N} \sum_{n=0}^{N-1} x(n) \exp \left(\frac{-i2\pi \, nk}{N} \right) \qquad k = 0, 1, \ldots, n-1 \qquad (6.9)$$

as

$$(\text{SNR})^2 = \frac{E[|N(k)|^2]}{E[|X(k)|^2]} = N2^{-2b} = 2^s 2^{-2b} \qquad (6.10)$$

where *s* is the number of stages in FFT computation and *N(k)* is the noise level of *X(k)*.

For a 2-D 1K-point FFT full frame, if one assumes white computational noise, *s* = 20. If the image is digitized to 8 bits, then the SNR should be kept below 2^{-9}. Equation (6.10) becomes

$$|2^{-9}|^2 = 2^{20}2^{-2b} \qquad \text{or} \qquad b = 19 \qquad (6.11)$$

Thus, to maintain computation accuracy for a 1K × 1K FFBA, the minimum number of bits required in the computation is 19.

6.4.3.3 Bit Allocation Table and Quantization

Storage of the bit allocation table is an overhead in the compression algorithm because it must be included in the compressed file. For block compression, this table is small (maximum 8 × 8) and does not require elaborate schemes for its storage. In full-frame compression, this table becomes very large, and it is desirable to reduce its size by invoking some rules. One rule is to assume radial symmetry in the transform domain from which the table is reduced to a one-dimensional bit allocation table with only *N* entries for an *N* × *N* image. This rule suffers from making undesirable compromises in the quantization of high frequency components. As a result, the FFBA becomes extremely sensitive to any artificially sharp edges (e.g., from patient labels, orientation markers, sharp-edged prosthetic devices, edges of the X-ray collimator). In particular, this rule cannot be applied to linear pair phantoms. Refer again to Figure 6.12, which shows the digital SMPTE phantom and the reconstructed image with a compression ratio of 2:1.

Another rule is to combine the bit allocation table and the quantization into one step, which can treat all frequencies as equally important. The quantized coefficient $F_q(u,v)$ can be obtained from the DCT coefficients $F(u,v)$ by:

$$F_q(u,v) = \text{NINT}[2^p F(u,v)] \qquad (6.12)$$

where NINT is the nearest integer function and *p* is a constant that determines the compression ratio. Equation (6.12) in effect rounds off $F(u,v)$ to the *p*th linear place. The selection of *p* depends on the spectral properties of the transform image itself to ensure that large magnitude components are concentrated in a small, low frequency region of the transform domain.

In general, p determines the compression ratio, and sometimes a change in p can drastically affect the compression ratio. Equation (6.12) can be modified to alleviate this problem.

$$F_q(u,v) = \text{NINT}[2^{p'}F(u,v)] \tag{6.13}$$

where

$$
\begin{aligned}
p' &= p + 1 & u < k & \quad \text{and} & y < k, k = 0, 1, \ldots, N - 1 \\
&= p & u \geq k & \quad \text{or} & v \geq k
\end{aligned}
$$

and k is a second parameter in determining the compression ratio. It is seen from Eq. (6.13) that components with both u and v less than k are kept to one extra bit of precision. For a given p, a larger value of k means more coefficients kept to one extra bit of precision.

The bit allocation table can be divided into a number of rectangular zones. These zones are fixed for a given class of images (e.g., size of image, CT, MR, CR). Within each zone, the coefficient with the largest absolute value determines how many bits are allocated for each coefficient in that zone. The quantized coefficients in this zone are packed into a one-dimensional file in a predetermined order. The compact bit allocation table now is many sets (usually thousands) of (u,v) coordinates instead of a large two-dimensional table representing the boundaries of each zone. The sets of coordinates are stored along with the one-dimensional file forming the compressed image file. Too few zones results in either inefficient bit packing or loss of information; too many zones results in lower compression ratio.

Image reconstruction from compressed data is accomplished by reversing the procedure described earlier and diagrammed in Figure 6.10, using the compact bit allocation table. The compressed image file is unpacked for each zone to recover the $F_q(u,v)$. The quantized $F_q(u,v)$ is rescaled with

$$F_A(u,v) = 2^{-p'}F_q(u,v) \tag{6.14}$$

An inverse DCT is then applied on $F_A(u,v)$, giving $f_A(j,k)$, which is the reconstructed image.

6.4.3.4 Hardware Module

The FFBA algorithm described in Sections 6.4.3.1–6.4.3.3 can be implemented in a hardware module for fast image compression and reconstruction. A module developed at UCLA is shown in Figure 6.13. The processor board consists of four DSP 56001 (digital signal processing) chips for parallel computing. The one-dimensional FFT can be computed on four image lines utilizing one DSP each (see Section 2.4.3). This module can compress a 1K × 1K image in about one second.

6.4.3.5 Variations of the Full-Frame Compression Technique

As discussed earlier, the full-frame compression technique is very sensitive to anatomical or artificial sharp edges, especially when the bit allocation table is condensed based on radial symmetry. Under these conditions, the high frequency

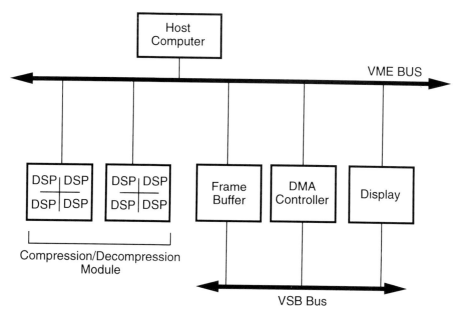

Figure 6.13   A hardware compression module (UCLA). Four Motorola DSP 56001 chips are mounted on a VME card to achieve 40 million instructions per second (mips) for processing the compression algorithm. Also on the board are the glue logic and static RAMs associated with each DSP. The driver chips separate individual processing regions for each DSP to run independently. Two boards are used for compression and decompression.

components of the transform coefficients are compromised, resulting in edge artifacts. Figures 6.14 and 6.15 show two examples. Figure 6.14A is a digitized chest radiograph with the patient's identification label; the reconstructed image (Fig. 6.14B) has a compression ratio of 9:1. Figure 6.15A is a CT head image; its reconstructed image (Fig. 6.15B) has a compression ratio 12:1. The first case shows vertical and horizontal edge artifacts adjacent to the artificially induced identification label, whereas the second case shows ringing artifacts due to an anatomical feature in the edge of the skull. These artifacts can be minimized with composite compression. Considering the CT head scan as an example, the composite compression technique consists of the following steps as shown in Figure 6.16:

1. The original image is subdivided into two regions, the brain and the skull. This can be done by means of a standard automatic segmentation image processing technique.
2. A brain tissue image is formed by filling the region outside the brain tissue with the average CT value of the brain tissue.
3. The FFBA method is applied to the brain tissue image to form a compressed data file.
4. A skull image is formed by filling zeros inside and outside the skull.
5. The skull image is compressed with a conventional error-free method (e.g., run-length coding), and a second compressed data file is formed.

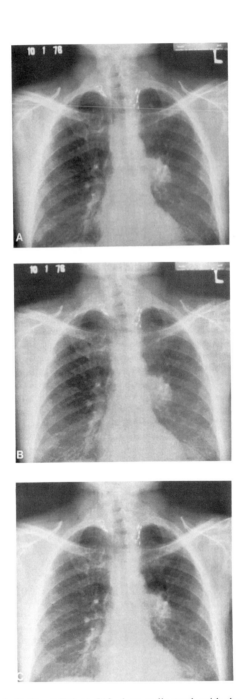

Figure 6.14 (A) A digitized 512 × 512 chest radiograph with the patient's identification label. (B) The reconstructed image from (A) with a compression ratio of 9:1. Observe the vertical and horizontal edge artifacts near the label. (C) The reconstructed image from (A) with composite compression, after removal of the patient's identification label; compression ratio is also 9:1.

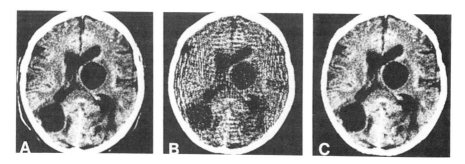

Figure 6.15 Application of the FFBA technique to a CT image of the head. (A) Original image. (B) Reconstructed image from a 12:1 compression image file obtained without the use of composite compression. Observe the ringing artifacts in the brain. (C) Reconstructed image from a 12:1 compressed image file obtained with the use of composite compression.

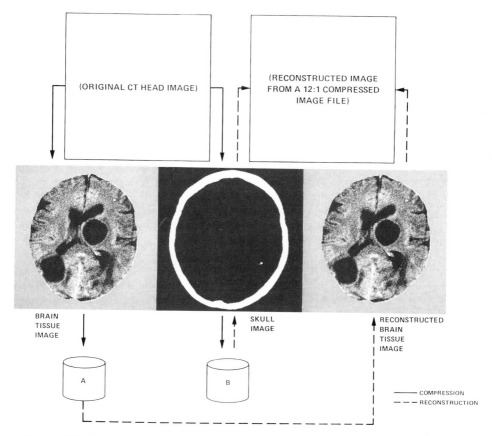

Figure 6.16 Example of composite compression. The CT head image is segmented into a brain image and a skull image. The full-frame bit allocation algorithm is used to compress the brain image, and run-length coding is used for the skull image. The composite reconstructed image is obtained by assembling the brain and the skull reconstructed images.

The skull image and the brain tissue image are reconstructed separately from their corresponding compressed data files by using the proper decoding method. A single substitution algorithm can be used to assemble the two reconstructed images into one reconstructed CT image. Figures 6.14C and 6.15C show the reconstructed chest radiograph and the CT head image using the composite compression technique with compression ratios identical to those of Figures 6.14B and 6.15B. Both the horizontal and vertical line artifacts and the ringing artifacts disappear.

6.5 Measurement of the Difference Between the Original and Reconstructed Images

It is natural to raise the question, How much can an image be compressed to yield compressed data that preserve sufficient information for a given clinical application? This section discusses some parameters and methods used to measure the trade-off between image quality and compression ratio.

6.5.1 Quantitative Parameters

6.5.1.1 Normalized Mean Square Error

The normalized mean square error (NMSE) between the original $f(x,y)$ and the reconstructed $f_A(x,y)$ image can be used as a quantitative measure of the closeness of the reconstructed image to the original image. The formula for the normalized mean square error is given by

$$\text{NMSE} = \frac{\displaystyle\sum_{x=0}^{N-1}\sum_{y=0}^{N-1}[f(x,y) - f_A(x,y)]^2}{\displaystyle\sum_{x=0}^{N-1}\sum_{y=0}^{N-1}f(x,y)^2} \tag{6.15}$$

or

$$\text{NMSE} = \frac{\displaystyle\sum_{u=0}^{N-1}\sum_{v=0}^{N-1}[(F(u,v) - F_A(u,v)]^2}{\displaystyle\sum_{u=0}^{N-1}\sum_{v=0}^{N-1}F(u,v)^2} \tag{6.16}$$

because the cosine transform is a unitary transformation.

NMSE is a global measurement of the quality of the reconstructed image; it does not provide information on the local measurement. It is obvious that NMSE is a function of the compression ratio. A high compression ratio will yield a high NMSE value.

6.5.1.2 Peak Signal-to-Noise Ratio

Another quantitative measure is the peak signal-to-noise ratio (PSNR) based on the root mean square error of the reconstructed image, which is very similar to the NMSE:

$$\text{PSNR} = \frac{20 \log(f(x,y)_{\text{max}})}{\dfrac{\left\{ \sum\limits_{x=0}^{N-1} \sum\limits_{y=0}^{N-1} [f(x,y) - f_A(x,y)]^2 \right\}^{1/2}}{N \times N}} \tag{6.17}$$

where $f(x,y)_{\text{max}}$ is the maximum value of the entire image, $N \times N$ is the total number of pixels in the image, and the denominator (under the heavy rule) is the root mean square difference of the reconstructed image.

6.5.2 Qualitative Measurement: Difference Image and Its Histogram

The difference image between the original and reconstructed images gives a qualitative measurement that compares the quality of the reconstructed image with that of the original. The corresponding histogram of the difference image provides a global qualitative measurement of the difference between the original and reconstructed images. A very narrow histogram means a small difference, whereas a broad histogram means a very large difference.

6.5.3 Acceptable Compression Ratio

Consider the following experiment. Compress a $512 \times 512 \times 8$ bit digitized chest X-ray film using the FFBA with compression ratios 4:1, 7:1, 12:1, 19:1, and 32:1. The original digitized image and the five reconstructed images are shown in Figure 6.17. All six images are displayed simultaneously in random order on a multi-viewing station with six identical video monitors. Observers are to evaluate these images qualitatively. Only the original image is identified, and the observers are requested to write down the comparative order of the five reconstructed images based on the quality of each image.

Table 6.2 shows one of the tabulated results, which demonstrates that most observers can order only three images correctly. To understand the reason for this, consider Figure 6.18, which shows the difference images between the original and reconstructed images. It is difficult to detect any residual anatomical structures from these images for compression ratios lower than 12:1; hence the observers have difficulty putting the 4:1, 7:1, and 12:1 images in a proper order.

Figure 6.19 shows the histograms of the original and all the difference images. The range of the 4:1 compression ratio histogram is very narrow, and as the compression ration becomes higher, the range of corresponding histogram becomes

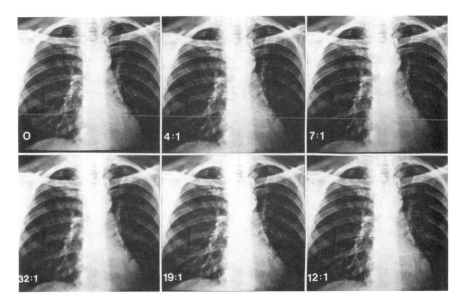

Figure 6.17 Reconstructed images: upper left, chest radiograph digitized to $512 \times 512 \times 8$; clockwise, five reconstructed images with compression ratios of 4:1, 7:1, 12:1, 19:1, and 32:1. (The FFBA method was used.)

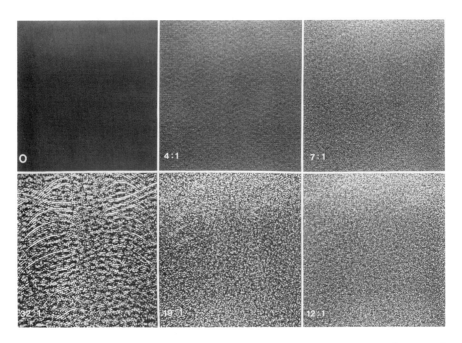

Figure 6.18 Difference images: the difference created by image compression is seen to be evenly distributed throughout the whole image; the higher the compression ratio, the larger the difference. To afford better visualization of the difference images, each pixel value in the difference image has been magnified by a factor of 10 and added to a constant 127 before the display. Clockwise from upper left, difference images between the original (Fig. 6.17) and the 1:1, 4:1, 7:1, 12:1, 19:1, and 32:1 reconstructed images.

226

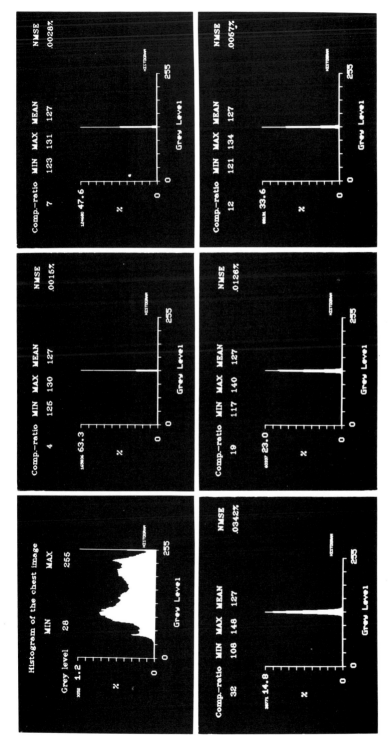

Figure 6.19 Histograms of the original image and the difference images, showing minimum, maximum, mean, and standard deviation of each histogram on the top; the normalized mean square error (NMSE) between the original image and the reconstructed image is also depicted. Clockwise from upper left: histograms of the original image (Fig. 6.17, O), and the corresponding 4:1, 7:1, 12:1, 19:1, and 32:1 difference images (Fig. 6.18). It is seen that the range of the 4:1 compression ratio histogram is very narrow, and as the compression ratio becomes higher, the range of the corresponding histogram becomes broader.

Table 6.2   Evaluation of Quality of Reconstruction
Images with Compression Ratios 4:1,
8:1, 12:1, 16:1, and 32:1 on a Chest
Radiograph (See Figs. 6.17, 6.18 and 6.19)

Performance	Number of People	Percentage
Non-Radiologists with Some Image Processing Background: Total Samples, 25		
Score*		
5	1	4%
4	0	0%
3	1	4%
2	4	16%
1	7	28%
0	12	48%
Identify 4:1 correctly	2	8%
Identify 32:1 correctly	9	36%
Radiologists: Total Samples, 12		
Score*		
5	0	0%
4	0	0%
3	5	41.0%
2	5	41.7%
1	2	16.7%
0	0	0%
Identify 4:1 correctly	2	16.7%
Identify 32:1 correctly	11	91.7%

*   A score of 5 means that the observer identifies the order of all five
reconstructed images correctly based on the quality of the displayed images.
A score of 3 means the observer identifies the order of any three of the five
reconstructed images.

broader. Figure 6.19 also displays the normalized mean square errors between the
original image and the reconstructed images (upper right-hand corner, under
NMSE): for compression ratios 4:1, 7:1, 12:1, 19:1, and 32:1, they are 0.0015%,
0.0028%, 0.0057%, 0.0126%, and 0.0342%, respectively. Clearly the NMSEs of all
these difference images are very small.

The body CT image shown in Figure 6.20 offers another example. Reconstructed
images with compression ratios less than and equal to 8:1 do not exhibit deteriora-
tion in image quality. The experiment described illustrates that for this particular
image, reconstructed images from compression ratios less than 10:1 are indis-
tinguishable from the original image; that is, there are no residual anatomical structures appearing in the difference image. In other words, a compression ration 10:1 or

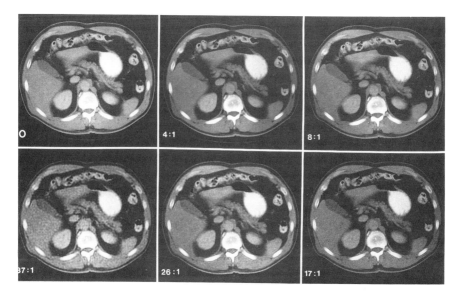

Figure 6.20 Body CT scan (upper left), followed, clockwise, by reconstructed images with compression ratios of 4:1, 8:1, 17:1, 26:1, and 37:1. (The FFBA method was used.)

less is acceptable for this image. It is obvious that the acceptable compression ratio is not universal and is a function of many variables, such as type and quality of the image to be compressed, the digitizer used, the size of the digitized image, and the display method. This functional relationship can be studied with the experiment described in Section 6.5.4.1.

6.5.4. Quality of the Reconstructed Image

6.5.4.1 The Experiment

This section describes an experiment to study the quality of reconstructed images based on the FFBA technique with the radial symmetrical bit allocation table based on Lo (1985). The first requirement is a collection of good quality X-ray films from conventional radiographic procedures, including AP chest, lateral chest, abdominal, mask, contrast and subtracted neuroangiograms, hand and skeletal films, and pulmonary arteriorgrams. Each film is digitized to a 2048 × 2048 matrix with a high resolution laser film scanner. Each 2048 × 2048 image is averaged to a 1024 × 1024 image and a 512 × 512 image. After each of these matrices has been subjected to image compression, it is possible to study acceptable compression ratios under each condition.

Table 6.3 describes the images used in one of these experiments, which included, in addition to the aforementioned images, 10 computed tomographic images (CT). Column 5 in the table shows the number of digitized film images and CT images

Table 6.3 Images Used for Image Compression Study

Image Source	Number of Cases	Acquisition Method	Image Size	Number of Images	Number of Reconstructed Images	Number of Difference Images	Total
Extremities	2	Drum scan	$1024 \times 1024 \times 8$	2	2	2	6
Pulmonary arteriogram	1	Laser scan	$2048 \times 2048 \times 8$	1	5	5	11
		2×2 average	$2048 \times 2048 \times 10$	1	5	5	11
			$1024 \times 1024 \times 8$	1	5	5	11
			$1024 \times 1024 \times 10$	1	5	5	11
		4×4 average	$512 \times 512 \times 8$	1	5	5	11
			$512 \times 512 \times 10$	1	5	5	11
Chest radiograph (PA view)	5	Laser scan	$2048 \times 2048 \times 8$	5	25	25	55
		2×2 average	$1024 \times 1024 \times 8$	5	25	25	55
		4×4 average	$512 \times 512 \times 8$	5	25	25	55
Chest radiograph (Lateral view)	5	Laser scan	$2048 \times 2048 \times 8$	5	25	25	55
		2×2 average	$1024 \times 1024 \times 8$	5	25	25	55
		4×4 average	$512 \times 512 \times 8$	5	25	25	55
Gastrointestinal radiograph	5	Laser scan	$2048 \times 2048 \times 8$	5	25	25	55
		2×2 average	$1024 \times 1024 \times 8$	5	25	25	55
		4×4 average	$512 \times 512 \times 8$	5	25	25	55
Neuroangiogram (1 mask, 2 contrast, and 2 subtraction images)	5	Laser scan	$2048 \times 2048 \times 8$	5	25	25	55
		2×2 average	$1024 \times 1024 \times 8$	5	25	25	55
		4×4 average	$512 \times 512 \times 8$	5	25	25	55
CT (Body)	5	Digital	$512 \times 512 \times 12$	5	25	25	55
CT (Head)	5	Digital	$512 \times 512 \times 12$	5	25	25	55
Total	33			78	382	382	842

selected for this experiment. The following parameters were used to interpret the results: compression ratio, difference image, and normalized mean square error.

Figures 6.21–6.26 depict the results of the compression study using the FFBA on the pulmonary arteriogram. Figures 6.21, 6.23, and 6.25 show the pulmonary arteriogram digitized to 512×512, 1024×1024, and 2048×2048, and the respective reconstructed images from different compression ratios. Figures 6.22, 6.24, and 6.26 are their corresponding difference images. Qualitative comparison of these images demonstrates that it is possible to compress these images to very high compression ratios (512 image: 11:1, 1024 image: 20:1; 2048 image: 40:1), and that in the difference images for compression ratios lower than 16:1 (512), 26:1 (1024), and 40:1 (2048), no residual anatomical structures are seen from these figures. For these reasons, one can compress the images to high compression ratios without sacrificing the diagnostic value of the images.

Figure 6.27 shows the relationship between the normalized mean square error and the compression ratio of the pulmonary arteriogram; the point with the *shortest radial distance* from the origin on each curve (arrows) can be used as a measure of the acceptable compression ratio of each image size. In the case of the 512×512 image, the point is at the compression ratio of about 8:1, which corresponds to the NMSE of about 0.010%. And in the cases of 1024 and 2048, the points correspond to compression ratios of 15:1 and 20:1 respectively. Thus, these parameters can be used as a means of measuring the acceptable compression ratio, and they appear to be quite consistent.

In general, images from conventional projection radiography (e.g., chest or gastrointestinal X-rays; angiograms) give higher acceptable compression ratios than images from pulmonary arteriograms.

Since a higher compression ratio corresponds to greater loss of information, one must determine an optimal compression ratio for a given image for a particular clinical application. Results from this experiment show that a normalized mean square error of 0.02% can be used as an acceptable threshold for most of the images described in Table 6.3. Reconstructed images with a NMSE larger than 0.02% tend to have visible artifacts, and their corresponding difference images also show some visible residue anatomical structures. Table 6.4 lists acceptable compression ratios using the full-frame bit allocation compression technique based on a NMSE of 0.02% and the observation of the difference images. Figures 6.28, 6.29, 6.30, 6.31, 6.32, and 6.33 show the relationship between the NMSE and the compression ratio of AP chest radiographs, lateral view chests, neuroangiograms, gastrointestinal radiographs, CT body images, and CT head images, respectively.

6.5.4.2 Some Observations

1. Results from experiments conducted according to the protocol of Section 6.5.4.1 show that digitized X-ray film with a larger matrix always yields a higher acceptable compression ratio. This is true for all categories of projection radiography. One explanation is that when a projection radiograph is digitized into a

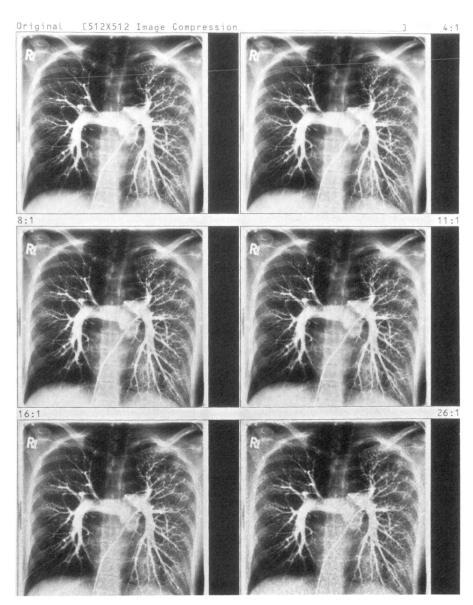

Figure 6.21 Original (upper left) and reconstructed images from compressed data on a pulmonary arteriogram. An X-ray film digitized with a laser scanner to dimensions of 2048 × 2048 × 8 was subsampled to 512 × 512 × 8. The images reconstructed from compressed image data have compression ratios of 4:1, 8:1, 11:1, 16:1, and 26:1.

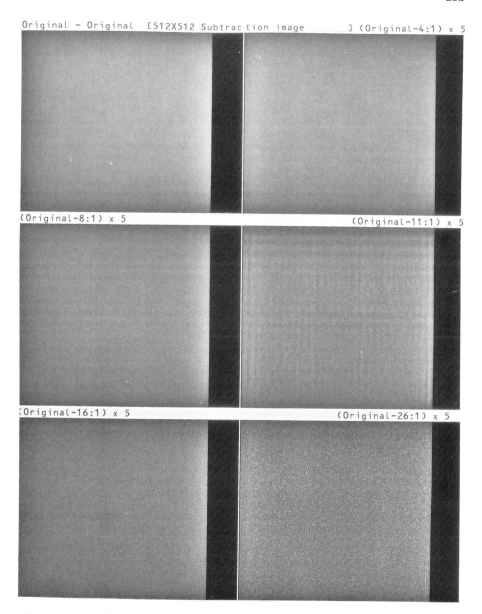

Figure 6.22   Difference images: upper left, the difference between the original and itself, followed clockwise by images that are the difference between the original and each reconstructed image shown in Figure 6.21. The difference created by image compression is evenly distributed throughout the whole image; the higher the compression ratio, the larger the difference. To afford a better visualization of the difference images, each pixel value in the difference image was multiplied by 5 and added to a constant 127 before the display. The acceptable compression ratio is 11:1; at higher ratios, anatomic structural patterns start to appear in the difference image.

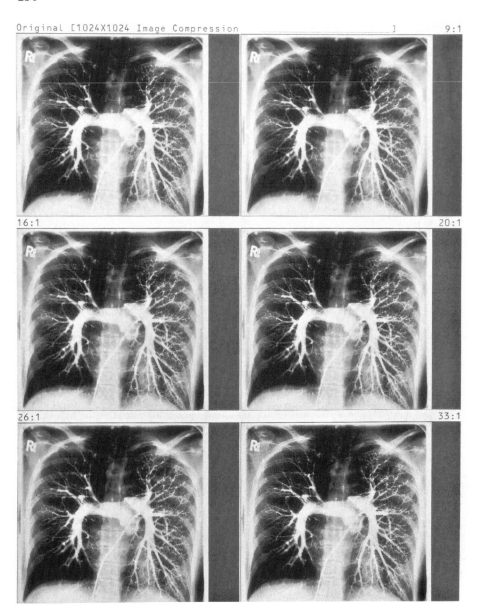

Figure 6.23 Original and reconstructed images from compressed data on the pulmonary arteriogram of Figure 6.21, digitized with a laser scanner and subsampled to 1024 × 1024 × 8 bits. The reconstructed images are from data with compression ratios of 9:1, 16:1, 20:1, 26:1, and 33:1.

Figure 6.24 Difference images from the pulmonary arteriogram subsampled to 1024 × 1024 × 8 bits as in Figure 6.23. The differences are obtained between the original and itself at compression ratios of 9:1, 16:1, 20:1, 26:1, and 33:1, respectively. The acceptable compression ratio is 20:1.

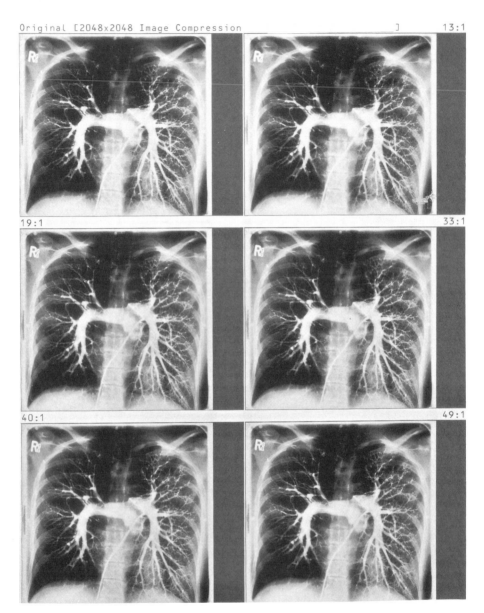

Original [2048x2048 Image Compression   ]   13:1

19:1   33:1

40:1   49:1

Figure 6.25 Original and reconstructed images from compressed data on the pulmonary arteriogram of Figure 6.21 digitized to 2048 × 2048 × 8 bits. The reconstructed images are from data with compression ratios of 13:1, 19:1, 33:1, 40:1, and 49:1.

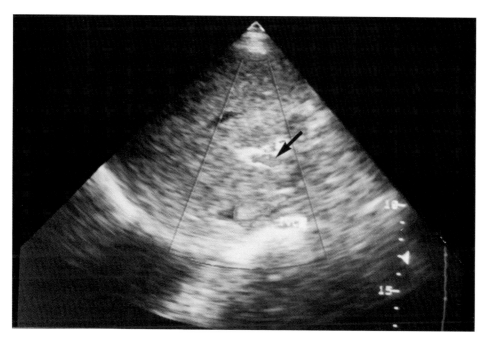

Figure 5.22 Color Doppler ultrasound image of the longitudinal section through the liver indicates that the flow in the inferior vena cava is reversed: blood flow (in red) is directed toward the US scanning plane. Flow in the portal vein (arrow) is hepatopetal.

Source: Courtesy of E. Grant.

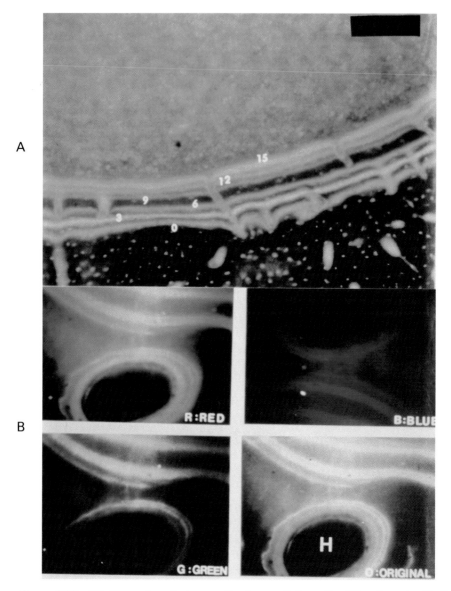

Figure 5.38 (A) Fluorochromic image of a bone cell from the tibia of a rat with five different tetracycline labels shown in orange-red. Each label has its own color characteristics: day 0, oxytetracycline label; day 3, DCAF; day 6, xylenol orange, 90 mg/kg; day 9, hematoporphyrin, 300 mg/kg (did not stain); day 12, doxycycline; day 15, alizarin red 5. The dose is 20 mg/kg. (B) Partial osteonal unit depicting the osteoid and the Haversian canal (H). One tetracycline label is shown in orange-red, the inside ring immediately adjacent to H. The three color images red, blue, and green are also shown (the blue image was accidentally flipped during the photographic process).

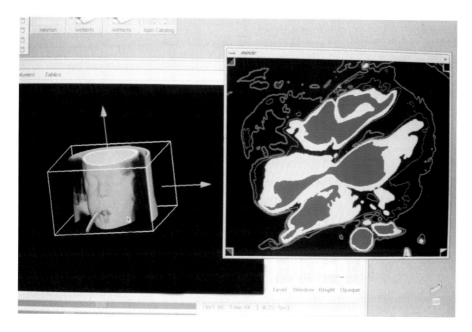

Figure 9.4 High end analysis workstation (Reality Station, ONYX) at UCSF showing 3-D rendering of a CT examination of a child's head and simulated blood flow (blue) in the four chambers of her heart.

Source: (Courtesy of SiliconGraphics Computer Systems, Mountian View, CA, S. Wong and E. Grant).

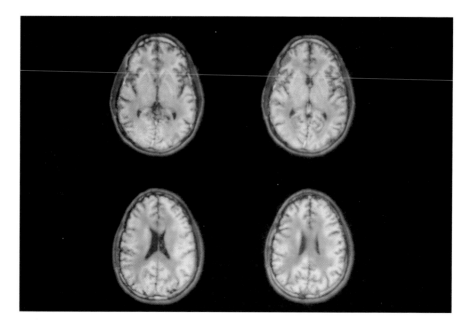

Figure 11.8 Mapping of brain function to anatomy. The four gray level images are from the MR, the color images are from PET of the same patient: red shows high metabolic rates; registration of these two images required sophisticated mathematics and computer programming.

Source: Courtesy of D. Valentino, 1991.

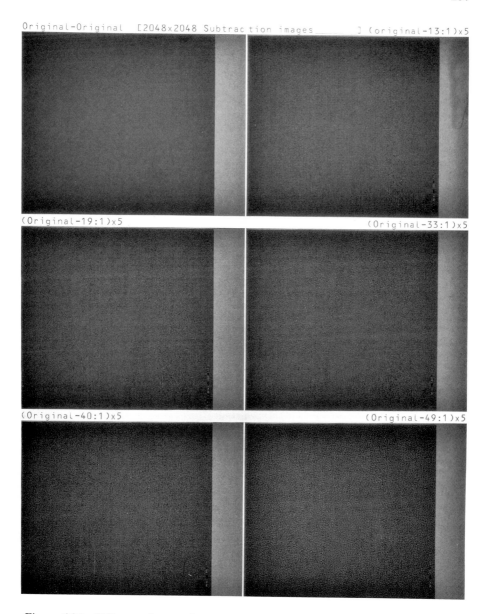

Figure 6.26 Difference images from the digitized pulmonary arteriogram with 2048 × 2048 × 8 bits (Fig. 6.25). The differences are obtained between the original and itself at compression ratios of 13:1, 19:1, 33:1, 40:1, and 49:1, respectively. The acceptable compression ratio is 33:1.

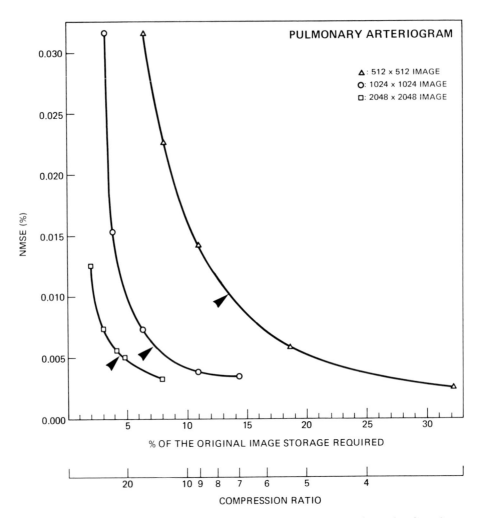

Figure 6.27 Normalized mean square error (NMSE) versus compression ratio of a pulmonary arteriogram digitized to 2048, 1024, and 512.

Table 6.4 Acceptable Compression Ratio Radiologic Images of Various Types*

Image Size	CT (H)	CT (B)	Chest (AP)	Extremities	Chest (L)	GI	Angio
			Acceptable Compression Ratio				
2048			25:1		20:1	25:1	25:1
1024			20:1	15:1	15:1	20:1	20:1
512	10:1	10:1	10:1	6:1	6:1	10:1	10:1

*H, head; B, body; AP, anterior–posterior view; L, lateral view; GI, gastrointestinal; Angio, neuroangiogram.

larger matrix, the correlation between pixels is higher. A higher correlation image gives a higher compression ratio.

2. An image with many edges (e.g., a pulmonary arteriogram) and/or with high contrast regions (e.g., barium inside the stomach and gastrointestinal tract) always gives a lower acceptable compression ratio compared to that of a similar radiograph without the contrast medium.

3. The acceptable compression ratio of all AP chest X-rays is quite predictable as seen in Figure 6.28 where all five 1K images cluster together. This is probably due to three reasons:

   (a) A chest X-ray has relatively few sharp edges.

   (b) The background area outside the chest wall is small.

   (c) The image is relatively symmetrical with respect to the medial line of the image.

4. The acceptable compression ratio for lateral chest X-rays is comparatively lower than that of the AP chest image (comparing Figs. 6.29 and 6.28). This effect probably is attributable to three characteristics of the lateral view:

   (a) The background outside the chest wall in the image is relatively larger compared to that in the AP view.

   (b) The boundary between the image and the background is relatively sharp compared to the AP view.

   (c) The image has a relatively larger area in the neck region, the optical density of which contrasts quite markedly to the adjacent background area.

5. In the case of barium contrast study in the gastrointestinal region (Fig. 6.31), case d has the highest acceptable compression ratio. This is because the image itself is low contrast compared to the others. Cases a, c, and e are all high contrast, having large regions filled with contrast medium, and as a group they have a relatively lower acceptable compression ratio. A high contrast image and/or an image with large contrast regions always gives a lower compression ratio.

6. In the case of neuroangiograms (Fig. 6.30), the five images are mask, contrast-enhanced images, and subtracted images. The mask and contrast images, which can be grouped together, have a relative higher acceptable compression ratio than the subtracted images. This is due to the existence of many edges and fine details in the subtracted images compared to the mask and the contrast images.

   In general, in digital subtraction angiography the area outside the circular field of the image intensifier and the area inside the four edges of the X-ray field in conventional radiography do not create problems in image compression. However, the background area between the skull and the circular field of the image intensifier in neuroangiogram, which shows up as an overexposed (black) area, will lower the acceptable image compression ratio. The reason is similar to that given in item 5 with respect to a high contrast area inside an image.

7. The patient's identification label in each radiograph will also lower the acceptable image compression ratio. This label, which is quite large and has four sharp edges, will give horizontal and vertical edge artifacts on the reconstructed images even at a very low compression ratio. It is advantageous to perform some

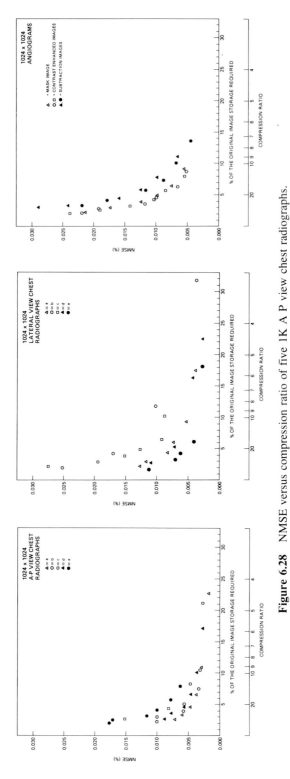

Figure 6.28 NMSE versus compression ratio of five 1K A P view chest radiographs.

Figure 6.29 NMSE versus compression ratio of five 1K lateral view chest radiographs.

Figure 6.30 NMSE versus compression ratio of five 1K neuroangiograms.

240

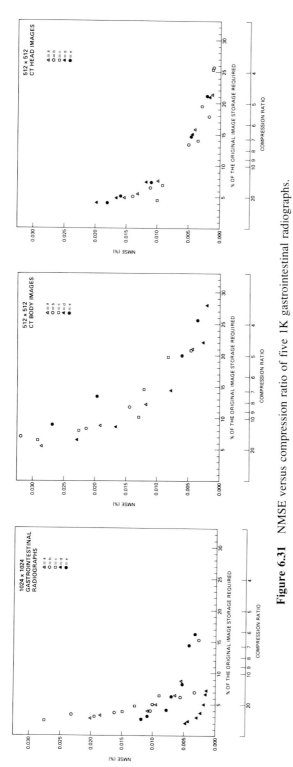

Figure 6.31 NMSE versus compression ratio of five 1K gastrointestinal radiographs.

Figure 6.32 NMSE versus compression ratio of five CT body images.

Figure 6.33 NMSE versus compression ratio of five CT head images.

Table 6.5   Relationship between Image Compression Ratio, Matrix
Size, Number of Bits Per Pixel, and Quality of the Digitizer

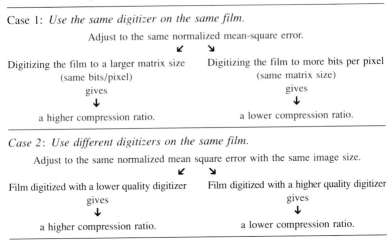

Case 1: *Use the same digitizer on the same film.*

Adjust to the same normalized mean-square error.

Digitizing the film to a larger matrix size (same bits/pixel)	Digitizing the film to more bits per pixel (same matrix size)
gives	gives
↓	↓
a higher compression ratio.	a lower compression ratio.

Case 2: *Use different digitizers on the same film.*

Adjust to the same normalized mean square error with the same image size.

Film digitized with a lower quality digitizer	Film digitized with a higher quality digitizer
gives	gives
↓	↓
a higher compression ratio.	a lower compression ratio.

image preprocessing before the image is compressed. Preprocessing includes deleting labels, and filling up the area with pixel values similar to the background in the original image (see Figure 6.14).

8. For body CT images, scans in the lower abdominal region always give a lower acceptable compression ratio than scans in the chest and the upper abdominal region. This is because the small intestine, in the lower abdominal region, contains air, which results in high contrast compared to the organs. In Figure 6.32, the CT body scan images a, c, and d have a higher acceptable compression ratio compared to the lower abdominal scans b and e.

9. CT head images can be preprocessed and separated into a skull image and a brain tissue image (see Fig. 6.16). Error-free compression can be used to compress the skull image, and the full-frame bit allocation technique can be applied for the brain tissue image.

Table 6.5 summarizes the relationship between image compression ratio and the matrix size and number bits per pixel, and the quality of the digitizer.

6.5.5 Receiver Operating Characteristic Analysis

Another method of measuring the difference between the quality of the original image and the reconstructed image is receiver operating characteristic (ROC) analysis, based on the work of Swets and Pickett. This method was developed for comparing image quality between two modalities. To begin, a set of good quality images of a certain category (e.g., AP chest radiographs) is selected by a panel of experts. The selection process includes considerations of types of disease, method of determination of the "truth" of the disease, number of images, distribution between normal and abnormal images, and subtlety of the disease appearing on images. The images in the set are then compressed to a predetermined compression ratio and reconstructed; the result is two sets of images, the original and the reconstructed.

Observers with expertise in diagnosing the subject diseases participate as observers to review all the images. For each image, an individual observer is asked to give an ROC confidence rating on a scale of 1–5 representing his or her impression of the likelihood of the presence of the disease. A confidence value of 1 indicates that the disease is definitely not present, and a confidence value of 5 indicates that the disease is present. Confidence values 2 and 4 indicate that the disease process probably is not present and probably is present, respectively. A confidence value of 3 indicates that the presence of the disease process is equivocal or indeterminate. Every image is read by every observer. The ratings of all images by a single observer are graded based on the "truth." The two plots that result show true positive (TP) versus false positive (FP). The first plot is an ROC curve representing the observer's performance of diagnosing the selected disease from the original images; the curve in the second plot indicates performance on the reconstructed images. The area Az under the ROC curve is an index of quantitative measure of the observer's performance on this image. Thus, if the Az (original) and the Az (reconstructed) of the two ROC curves are very close to each other, we can say that diagnoses of this disease based on the reconstructed image with the predetermined compression ratio will be as good as those made (by this observer) from the original image. In other words, this compression ratio is acceptable for this image type with the given disease.

In doing the ROC analysis, the statistical "power" of the study is important: the higher the power, the more confidence can be placed in the result. The statistical power is determined by the number of images used and the number of observers. A meaningful ROC analysis often requires many images (100 or more) and five or six observers to determine one type of image with several diseases. Although performing an ROC analysis is tedious, time-consuming, and expensive, this method for determination of the quality of the reconstructed image is accepted by the radiology community.

Sections 6.5.5.1 and 6.5.5.2 show results of two ROC analyses: hand radiographs with subperiosteal resorption and thoracic images with various types of intrathoracic pathology. The compression method used was the FFBA with zone bit allocation table implemented in a hardware module described in Section 6.4.3.4.

6.5.5.1 Thoracic Imaging with Lung Modules and Interstitial Lung Disease

In a study based on work by Aberle et al. (1993) 122 posteroanterior chest radiographs were obtained on patients in an ambulatory patient setting: 30 cases of interstitial lung disease, 45 images containing combinations of lung nodules ($N = 37$) or mediastinal masses ($N = 39$), and 47 normal images containing none of these

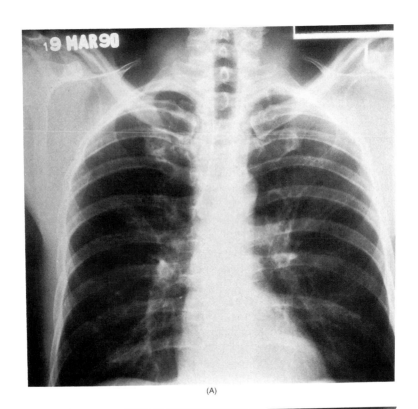

(A)

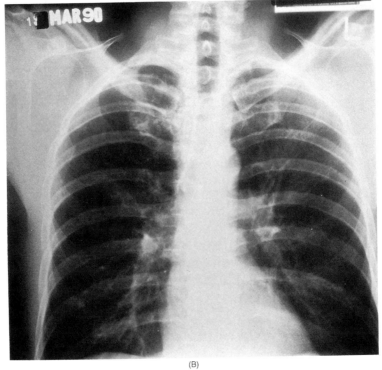

(B)

244

(C)

Figure 6.34 Example of using the full-frame image compression hardware in thoracic imaging. (A) Digitized 2048 × 2048 × 12 bit AP chest image printed back on a film. (B) Reconstructed image with a compression ratio of 20:1. (C) The difference image between the original and the reconstructed image (Aberle et al.).

Source: Aberle et al. (1993).

pathologies. The images were digitized (nominal 2K × 2K × 12 bit resolution), printed in a hard copy format (14 in. × 14 in.), and compressed at an approximate compression ratio of 20:1. Figure 6.34 shows three images: original, reconstructed, and subtracted.

Observer performance tests were conducted in which five radiologists used ROC analysis on digitized uncompressed and compressed hard copy images. Tables 6.6 and 6.7 show the ROC area (Az) for interstitial disease and lung nodules, respectively: there are no significant differences between the two display conditions for the detectability of either thoracic abnormality. Thus irreversible image compression at ratios of 20:1 may be acceptable for use in digital thoracic imaging.

Table 6.6   Reader Specific Areas Under the ROC Curves (Az)
for Interstitial Disease*

Observer	Az ($\pm$SD)		P Value	95% Confidence Intervals for Area Differences
	Digitized Image	Compressed Image		
A	.967 ($\pm$ 0.24)	.988 ($\pm$ .011)	.16	$-$.063, .021
B	.956 ($\pm$ .028)	.889 ($\pm$ .055)	.12	$-$.013, .147
C	.947 ($\pm$ .047)	.957 ($\pm$ .031)	.42	$-$.092, .072
D	.978 ($\pm$ .017)	.989 ($\pm$ .011)	.27	$-$.041, .019
E	.884 ($\pm$ .065)	.902 ($\pm$ .059)	.38	$-$.041, .019
Mean score	.946 ($\pm$ .036)	.945 ($\pm$ .033)	.43	$-$.151, .115

Source: Aberle et al. (1993).

6.5.5.2 *Hand Radiographs with Subperiosteal Resorption*

A study based on work by Sayre et al. (1992) entailed the analysis of 71 hand radiographs, of which 45 were normal and 26 had subperiosteal resorption. The images were digitized to 2K $\times$ 2K $\times$ 12 bit resolution and printed on film (14 in. $\times$ 17 in.). The digitized images were compressed to 20:1 and printed on film of the same size. Figure 6.35 shows original, reconstructed, and subtracted images. An ROC analysis with five observers was performed. Figure 6.36 shows the ROC curves of the original and the reconstructed images from the five observers: statistics demonstrate that there is no significant difference between results obtained using original and reconstructed images with 20:1 compression ratio for the diagnosis of subperiosteal resorption from hand radiographs.

6.6   Three-Dimensional Image Compression

6.6.1   Background

So far, we have discussed only two-dimensional image compression, however, acquisition of three- and four-dimensional medical images is becoming more common in CT, MR, US, and DSA. The third dimension can be in the spatial domain (e.g., sectional images) or in the time domain (e.g., in an angiographic study). Such processes significantly increase the volume of data gathered per study. To compress 3-D data efficiently, one must consider decorrelation images. Some work done on 3-D compression reported by Sun and Goldberg (1988), Lee (1993), and Koo (1992) considered the correlation between adjacent sections. Chan, Lou, and Huang (1989) reported a full-frame DCT method for DSA, CT, and MR. They found that by grouping four to eight slices as a 3-D volume, compression was twice as efficient as it was with 2-D full-frame DCT for DSA. The 3-D method of compressing CT images was also more efficient than 2-D. However, 3-D compression did not achieve very high efficiency in the case of MR images. In Sections 6.6.2 and 6.6.3

Table 6.7 Reader Specific Areas Under the ROC Curves (Az)
for Lung Nodules

	Az ($\pm$SD)		P	95% Confidence Intervals for
Observer	Digitized Image	Compressed Image	Value	Area Differences[i]
A	.871 ($\pm$ .053)	.902 ($\pm$ .039)	.23	$-.131, .069$
B	.848 ($\pm$ .073)	.900 ($\pm$ .047)	.20	$-.185, .081$
C	.839 ($\pm$ .061)	.846 ($\pm$ .051)	.45	$-.141, .128$
D	.915 ($\pm$ .066)	.886 ($\pm$ .072)	.25	$-.113, .172$
E	.856 ($\pm$ .050)	.876 ($\pm$ .053)	.32	$-.121, .081$
Mean score	.866 ($\pm$ .061)	.882 ($\pm$ .052)	.30	

Source: Aberle et al. (1993).

we discuss the wavelet transform in 3-D image compression based on Wang's work (1995).

The wavelet transform has drawn significant attention since the publication of the papers by Daubechies (1988) and Mallat (1989). Wavelet theory and its applications have been developed substantially in the past few years. Wavelet transform data supply both spatial and frequency information, whereas conventionally in the Fourier transform there is only frequency information. Because of this characteristic, wavelet image compression has lately shown promising results.

6.6.2 Wavelet Theory and Multiresolution Analysis

6.6.2.1 Wavelet Theory

A transform is an operation that transforms a function from one domain to another. The basis is a set of functions that is used for the transformation. In the Fourier transform, the basis functions are a series of sine and cosine functions, and the resulting domain is the frequency domain.

In a one-dimensional wavelet transform, there exists a mother wavelet function $\psi(x)$. The basis functions are formed by dilation and translation of the mother wavelet

$$\psi_{a,b}(x) = \frac{1}{\sqrt{a}}\, \psi\left(\frac{x-b}{a}\right) \tag{6.18}$$

where a and b are the dilation and translation factors, respectively. The continuous wavelet transform of a function $f(x)$ can be expressed as follows:

$$F_{w}(a,b) = \frac{1}{\sqrt{a}} \int_{-\infty}^{\infty} f(x)\psi^*\left(\frac{x-b}{a}\right) dx \tag{6.19}$$

where * is the complex conjugate operator.

The basis functions given in Eq. (6.18) are redundant when a and b are continu-

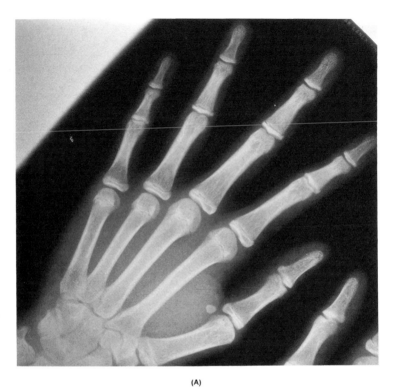

(A)

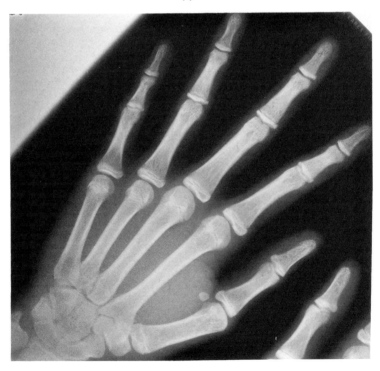

(B)

248

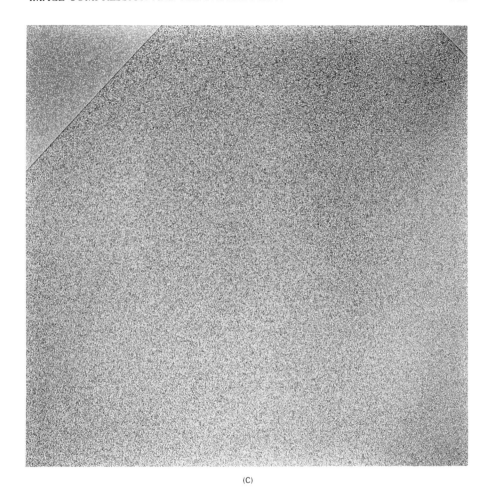

(C)

Figure 6.35 Example of using full-frame image compression hardware in hand radiographs with evidence of subperiosteal resorption (arrows). (a) Digitized 2048 × 2048 × 12 bit hand image printed on a film. (b) Reconstructed image with a compression ratio of 20:1. (c) The subtracted image.

Source: Sayre et al. (1992).

ous. It is possible, however, to discretize a and b to form an orthonormal basis. One way of discretizing a and b is to let $a = 2^m$ and $b = 2^m n$, so that Eq. (6.18) becomes

$$\psi_{m,n}(x) = 2^{-m/2}\psi(2^{-m}x - n) \tag{6.20}$$

where m and n are integers. The wavelet transform then becomes

$$F_w(m,n) = 2^{-m/2}\int_{-\infty}^{\infty} f(x)\psi(2^{-m}x - n)dx \tag{6.21}$$

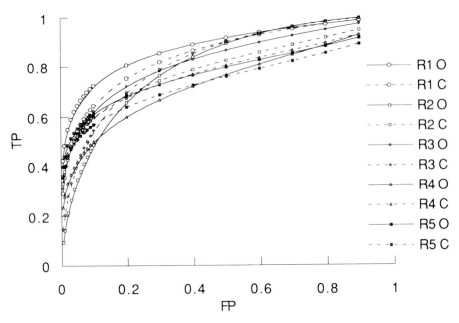

Figure 6.36 Comparison of five observer ROC curves obtained from a hand image compression study: *TP*, true positive; *FP*, false-positive; *O*, original image; *C*, reconstructed image.

Since m and n are integers, Eq. (6.21) is called a wavelet series. It is seen from this representation that the transform contains both spatial and frequency information.

6.6.2.2 Multiresolution Analysis

Multiresolution analysis decomposes a signal into a series of smooth signals and their associated detailed signals at different resolution levels. At each level, the smooth signal and its detailed signal can be used to reconstruct the smooth signal in the next higher resolution level. The multiresolution decomposed signal lies between the spatial and frequency domains. The 3-D wavelet method discussed here is based on Mallat's definition of multiresolution theory using a pyramid algorithm.

We use a one-dimensional case to explain the concept of multiresolution analysis. Consider the discrete signal f_m at level m, which be decomposed into the $m + 1$ level by convoluting it with h (low pass) and g (high pass) filters to form a smooth signal f_{m+1} and a detailed signal f'_{m+1}, as shown in Figure 6.37. This can be implemented in following equations using the pyramidal algorithm:

$$f_{m+1}(n) = \sum_k h(2n - k)f_m(k) \tag{6.22}$$

$$f'_{m+1}(n) = \sum_k g(2n - k)f_m(k)$$

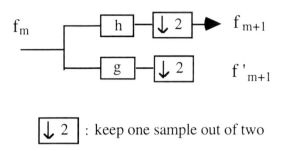

Figure 6.37 Decomposition of a signal f_m into a smooth resolution f_{m+1} and a detailed signal f'_{m+1}.

where f_{m+1} is the smooth signal and f'_{m+1} is the detailed signal at the resolution level $m + 1$.

The total number of discrete points in f_m is equal to that of the sum of f_{m+1} and f'_{m+1}. The same process can be further applied to f_{m+1}, creating the detailed and smooth signal at the next lower resolution level, until the desired level is reached.

Figure 6.38 depicts the components resulting from three levels of decomposition of the signal f_1. The horizontal axis indicates the total number of discrete points of the original signal, and the vertical axis is the level of the decomposition. At the resolution level $m = 3$, the final signal is composed of the detailed signals of the other resolution levels f'_1, f'_2, and f'_3 plus one smooth signal f_3. Signals at each level can be compressed by quantization and encoding methods described in earlier sections. Accumulation on all these compressed signals at different levels can be used to reconstruct the original signal.

The primary advantage of the wavelet transform compared with the Fourier transform is that the wavelet transform is localized in both the spatial and frequency domains, therefore the transformation of a given signal will contain both spatial and frequency information of that signal. On the other hand, the Fourier transform basis extends infinitely, with the result that any local information in space is spread out over the whole frequency domain.

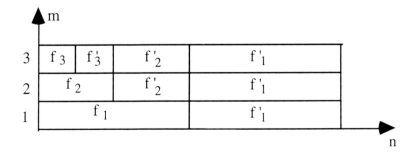

Figure 6.38 Three-level wavelet decomposition of a signal.

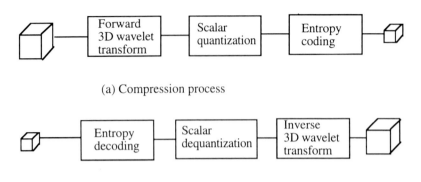

(a) Compression process

(b) Decompression process

Figure 6.39   Block diagrams of the compression and decompression of a 3-D wavelet.

6.6.3 Three-Dimensional Image Compression with Wavelet Transform

6.6.3.1 The Block Diagrams

Figure 6.39 shows the block diagrams of three-dimensional wavelet compression and decompression. In the compression process, a 3-D wavelet transform is first applied to the 3-D image data, resulting in a 3-D multiresolution representation of the image. Then the wavelet coefficients are quantized using scalar quantization. Finally, run-length and Huffman coding are used to impose entropy coding on the quantized data.

Decompression is the inverse of the compression process. The compressed data are first entropy-decoded. Second, a dequantization procedure is applied to the decoded data. Finally, an inverse 3-D wavelet transform is applied, resulting in the reconstructed 3-D image data.

6.6.3.2 Three-Dimensional Wavelet Transform

For the three-dimensional case, a wavelet ψ and a scaling function ϕ are chosen such that the three-dimensional scaling and wavelet functions are separable. That is, the scaling function has the form

$$\Phi(x,y,z) = \phi(x)\phi(y)\phi(z) \tag{6.23}$$

and the wavelet functions are written as follows:

$$\Psi^1(x,y,z) = \phi(x)\phi(y)\psi(z) \qquad \Psi^2(x,y,z) = \phi(x)\psi(y)\phi(z) \qquad \Psi^3(x,y,z) = \psi(x)\phi(y)\phi(z) \tag{6.24}$$

$$\Psi^4(x,y,z) = \phi(x)\psi(y)\psi(z) \qquad \Psi^5(x,y,z) = \psi(x)\phi(y)\psi(z) \qquad \Psi^6(x,y,z) = \psi(x)\psi(y)\phi(z)$$

$$\Psi^7(x,y,z) = \psi(x)\psi(y)\psi(z).$$

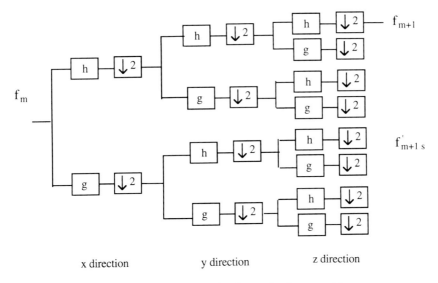

Figure 6.40   Three-dimensional wavelet decomposition.

Three-dimensional wavelet transforms can be computed by extension of the one-dimensional pyramidal algorithm. One level of the decomposition process from f_m to f_{m+1} is shown in Figure 6.40. We first convolute each line in the x direction separately with filters h and g, followed by subsampling every other pixel. The resulting signals are convoluted with h and g in the y direction, again followed with subsampling. Finally the same procedure is applied to the z direction.

The resulting signal has eight components. Since h is a low pass filter, only one component contains low frequency information, f_{m+1}. The rest of the components convolute at least once with the high pass filter g, and therefore contain the detailed signals f'_{m+1} in different directions. The same process is repeated for the low frequency signal f_{m+1} until the desired level is reached.

Figure 6.41 shows two levels of 3-D wavelet transform on a volume data set. The

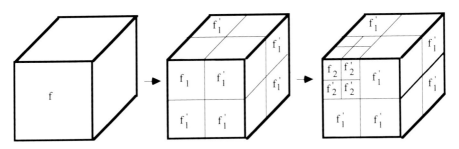

Figure 6.41   The result of a 3-D wavelet transform on a volume data set.

first level decomposes the data into eight components: f_1 is the low resolution portion of the image data, and the remaining blocks are high resolution components. As Figure 6.41 indicates, f_1 can be further decomposed into eight smaller volumes labeled f_2 and f_2'. The detailed images on level 1 contain higher frequency components than those of level 2 f_2'.

With properly chosen wavelets, the low resolution component in the m level is $1/(2^3)^m$ of the original image size after the transformation, but it contains about 90% of the total energy in the m level, where m is the level of the decomposition and the high resolution components are separated into different resolution levels. For these reasons, the wavelet transform yields a better presentation of the original image for compression purposes. Different levels of representation can be coded differently to achieve a desired compression ratio.

6.6.3.3 Quantization

The second step of compression is quantization. The purpose of quantization is to map a large number of input values into a smaller set of output values by reducing the precision of the data. This is the step in which information may be lost. Wavelet-transformed data are floating point values and consist of two types: low resolution image components, which contain most of the energy, and high resolution image components, which contain the information from sharp edges.

Since the low resolution components have most of the energy, we want to maintain the integrity of such data. To minimize data loss in this portion, we map each floating point value to its nearest integer neighbor (NINT). In the high resolution components of the wavelet coefficients, there are many coefficients of small magnitude that correspond to the flat areas in the original image. These coefficients contain very little energy, and we can eliminate them without creating significant distortions in the reconstructed image. A threshold number T_m is chosen, such that any coefficients less than T_m will be set to zero. Above T_m, a range of floating point values are mapped into a single integer. If the quantization number is Q_m, quantized high frequency coefficients can be written as follows:

$$a_q(i,j,k) = \text{NINT}\left[\frac{a(i,j,k) - T_m}{Q_m}\right] \qquad a(i,j,k) > T_m \qquad (6.25)$$

$$a_q(i,j,k) = 0 \qquad\qquad\qquad -T_m \leq a(i,j,k) \leq T_m$$

$$a_q(i,j,k) = \text{NINT}\left[\frac{a(i,j,k) + T_m}{Q_m}\right] \qquad a(i,j,k) < -T_m$$

where $a(i,j,k)$ is the wavelet coefficient, $a_q(i,j,k)$ is the quantized wavelet coefficient, and m is the number of the level in the wavelet transform; T_m and Q_m are functions of the wavelet transform level. The function T_m can be set as a constant, and $Q_m = Q2^{m-1}$, where Q is a constant.

6.6.3.4 Entropy Coding

In the third step, the quantized data are subjected to run-length coding followed by Huffman coding. Run-length coding is effective when there are pixels with the same gray level in a sequence. Since thresholding of the high resolution components results a large number of zeros, run-length coding can be expected to significantly reduce the size of data. Applying Huffman coding after run-length coding can further improve the compression ratio.

6.6.3.5 Some Results

This section presents some compression results using a 3-D MR data set from a GE 5x Signa Scanner with 124 images with 256 × 256 × 12 bits per image. A 2-D wavelet compression is also applied to the same data set, and the results are compared with the 3-D compression results. The 2-D compression algorithm is similar to that of the 3-D compression algorithm except that a two-dimensional wavelet transform is applied to each slice.

Figure 6.42 compares the compression ratios for the 3-D and 2-D algorithms; the horizontal axis is the peak signal-to-noise ratio (PSNR) defined in Section 6.5.1.2, and the vertical axis represents the compression ratio.

At the same PSNR, compression ratios of the 3-D method are about 40–90% higher than that of the 2-D method. From Figure 6.43 a slice of MR volume image data compressed with 3-D wavelet method, we can see that at the compression ratio

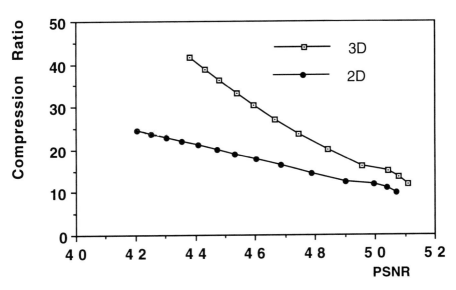

Figure 6.42   Data for 3-D wavelet compression plotted versus data for 2-D wavelet compression.

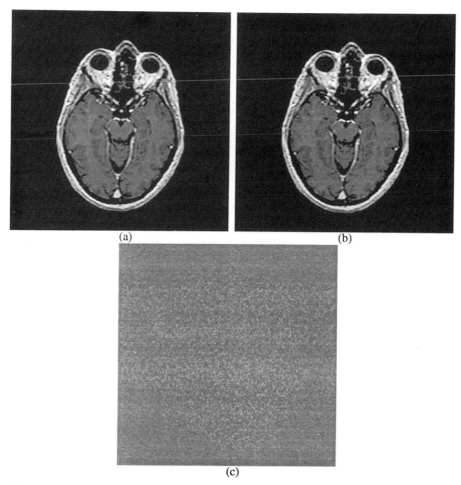

(a)   (b)

(c)

Figure 6.43 Slice of 3-D MR volume data compressed at a compression ratio of 20:1 with the 3-D wavelet compression method: compare with Figure 6.9. (a) Original image. (b) Decompressed image. (c) Difference image.

Source: Courtesy of Jun Wang [1995].

of 20:1, the quality of the decompressed image is nearly the same as that of the original image.

6.7 Color Image Compression

6.7.1 Examples of Color Images in Radiology

Color images are very important in microscopy but very seldom used in radiology because traditionally, radiology uses an X-ray source, which produces monochromatic images. Color, when used, is mostly for enhancement purposes. In this case, a certain gray level or a range of gray levels is converted to colors, to enhance visual appearance. Examples are found in nuclear medicine, PET, and most recently, in Doppler ultrasound (US) (see Fig. 5.22). In Section 5.4.2, we noted that a 10-second Doppler US study can produce an image file as large as 225 Mbyte because of the pseudocolor images. We now discuss a method of compressing US color Doppler images.

6.7.2 The Color Spaces

Traditionally, a color $512 \times 512 \times 24$ bit image is decomposed into a red, a green, and a blue image in the RGB color space, each with $512 \times 512 \times 8$ bits (see Section 5.6). Each image is treated independently as an individual image. For display, the display system combines the images on a color monitor through a color composite video control. This scheme is referred to as the color space, and the three-color decomposition is determined by drawing a triangle on a special color chart developed by the Commission Internationale de L'Eclairage (CIE) with each of the base colors as an end point. The CIE color chart is characterized by isolating the luminance (or brightness) from the chrominance (or hue). Based on this characteristic as a guideline, the National Television System Committee (NTSC) defined a new color space YIQ, representing the luminance, in-phase chrominance, and quadrature chrominance coordinates, respectively. In digital imaging a color space called YCbCr is used, where Cr and Cb represent two chrominance components. The conversion between the standard RGB space to YCbCr is given by

$$
\begin{bmatrix} Y \\ Cb \\ Cr \end{bmatrix} = \begin{bmatrix} 0.2990 & 0.587 & 0.114 \\ -0.1687 & -0.3313 & 0.5 \\ 0.5 & -0.4187 & -0.0813 \end{bmatrix} \begin{bmatrix} R \\ G \\ B \end{bmatrix} \tag{6.26}
$$

where R, G, and B pixel values are between 0 and 255.

There are two advantages of using the YCbCr system. First, it distributes most of the image information into the luminance component (Y), with less going to chrominance (Cb and Cr). As a result, the YCbCr elements are less correlated and, therefore, can be compressed separately without loss in efficiency. Second, through field experience, the variations in the Cb and Cr planes are known to be less than that in the Y plane. Therefore, Cb and Cr can be subsampled in both the horizontal and the vertical direction without loss much of the chrominance. The immediate compression from converting the RGB to YCbCr is 2:1. This can be computed as follows:

Original RGB color image size:	$512 \times 512 \times 24$ bits		
YCbCr image size:	$(512 \times 512 \times 8) +$	2	$\times (0.25 \times 512 \times 512 \times 8 \text{ bits})$
	(Y)	(Cb and Cr)	subsampling

That is, after the conversion, each YCbCr pixel is represented by 12 bits: eight bits for the luminance (Y), and eight bits for each of the chrominances (Cb and Cr) for every other pixel and every other line. The Y, Cb, and Cr image can be compressed further as three individual images by using error-free compression. JPEG, the Joint Photographic Experts Group, uses this technique for color image compression.

6.7.3 Compression of Color Ultrasound Images

Normal US Doppler studies generate an average of 13 ± 6 Mbyte per image file. There are cases that can go up to 80–100 Mbyte. To compare a color Doppler image (see Fig. 5.22), the color RGB image is first transformed to the YCbCr space with Eq. (6.26). But instead of subsampling the Cb and Cr images as described earlier, all three images are subject to a run-length coding independently. Two factors favor this approach. First, a US image possesses information within a sector. Outside the sector, it contains only background information. Background information can yield a very high compression ratio. Second, the Cb and Cr images contain little information except at the flow regions, which are very small compared with the entire anatomical structures in the image. Thus, run-length coding of Cb and Cr can give a very high compression ratio, eliminating the need for subsampling. On average, two-dimensional, error-free run-length coding can give a 3:5:1 compression ratio, and it can be as high as 6:1. Even higher compression ratios can result if the third dimension (time) of a temporal US study is considered.

6.8 Legal and Regulatory Issues

In this section, we discuss the legal and regulatory issues of radiologic image compression. Reversible or lossless compression does not cause any legal complications, but provides modest reduction in image size, with a compression ratio of 2:1. Therefore intense research effort has been focused on lossy compression schemes of low bit rate that discard image data of no diagnostic significance but retain medically relevant information in an examination. The results of many studies indicate that a digital chest image conceivably can be compressed to 10:1 or higher with acceptable diagnostic quality.

In recent years there has been a marked increase in the number of medical image communication and storage devices that use data compression as a means of reducing storage space and transmission time. This increase is prompted by the immediate need to store large volumes of accumulating digital images and the shift toward the digital radiology environment, especially the widespread use of picture archiving and communications (PACS) and teleradiology applications (to be discussed in Chapters 8 to 11). To a certain extent, this trend is also influenced by the formation of industrial data interchange and communication standards, such as those of the ACR-NEMA (American College of Radiology/National Electrical Manufacturers Association) and DICOM (Digital Imaging and Communication in Medicine) groups.

Product comparison in the literature also shows the increased availability of medical devices that implement lossy compression. A summary of premarket notifications reviewed by the U.S. Center for Devices and Radiological Health (CDRH) of the Food and Drug Administration (FDA) in 1992 indicated that most PACS devices submitted for marketing clearance are all-new products or significant modifications of existing products. Of the 19 products reviewed, 15 implement some form of compression and 6 incorporate lossy compression; some even have a compression ratio as high as 80:1.

The availability of lossy compression has raised new regulatory and legal questions for manufacturers, users, and the FDA. Regulatory policy, however, is concerned less with patents and copyright matters, as in commercial software systems, and more with the safety and the quality of medical devices that incorporate compression hardware and software, including the following considerations: indication for use and labeling, existence of a suitable measure of compression that properly characterizes the degree of information, and the effects of compression on image postprocessing. The legal questions frequently asked involve the possibility of standards for image compression and product liability guidelines. All these pertinent questions and issues raised are interrelated. To transfer lossy compression technology into the marketplace, the researchers, as well as the developers, must properly understand the technical implications and challenges derived from these issues.

6.8.1 Use of Irreversible Compression

Should lossy coding techniques be restricted to uses other than primary diagnosis? Lossy techniques are being used for teaching files, reviewing reports, general archives with known diagnosis, and presenting research conclusions. Radiologists are concerned, however, that the use of lossy compression at the primary diagnosis might cause loss of fine details or subtle information of original images and result in incorrect diagnosis or interpretation, with the accompanying possibility of malpractice suits. Since primary diagnosis is an important activity that has a significant impact on health care service, excluding the use of lossy coding from its practice hinders the move toward a digital radiology environment. Thus, another regulatory issue to be undertaken is the rendering of an informed decision as to whether lossy compression can be used for specific primary diagnoses that do not require high resolution. Also worthy of study is the issue of tailoring the degree of lossy compression for different kinds of radiological application.

6.8.2 Measure of Image Compression

Although there exist many methods of evaluating image quality, such as subjective ratings, paired comparisons, free response ROC, sensitivity and specificity, and signal-to-noise ratio, classical ROC analyses as described in Section 6.5.5 are still the radiologist's most credible and acceptable way of measuring image quality. A great deal of work has been done to determine ROC curves for different specific radiological tasks using images reconstructed under various degrees of lossy compression. It would be almost impossible, however, to attempt this work as the basis of regulation. This is because there is a wide variety of diagnostic radiological tasks, and the acceptable degree of compression is task dependent.

The FDA has chosen to place such decisions in the hands of the user. The agency, however, has taken steps to ensure that the user has the information needed to make the decision by requiring that the lossy compression statement as well as the approximate compression ratio be attached to lossy images. The manufacturers also are required to provide in their operator's manuals a discussion on the effects of lossy compression on image quality. Data from laboratory tests are required in a premarket notification only when the medical device uses new technologies and asserts new claims, however. The PACS guidance document from the FDA (1993) allows the manufacturers to report the normalized mean square error (NMSE) of their communication and storage devices using lossy coding techniques. This measure was chosen because it has often been used by the manufacturers themselves and there is some objective basis for comparisons. However, as discussed in Section 6.5, NMSE does not provide any local information regarding type of loss (e.g., spatial location or spatial frequency). The development of a better, and general, method for characterizing compression losses is urgently needed and should be a *high priority research topic* in medical imaging.

6.8.3 Image Postprocessing

The effect of lossy compression on image postprocessing software has received little attention. Postprocessing image software includes filtering (e.g., smoothing, edge enhancement, morphological operations), mensuration algorithms (e.g., surface and volume determinations), and image feature extraction (e.g., identification of lung nodules and breast cancer microcalcifications). The postprocessing of lossy images is seldom used because the physician would not need to apply these techniques. On the other hand, for storing large volumes of image data for transmitting images to a referring physician at a remote location, such as in a PACS image database, and for performing certain kinds of examination, such as cine-type examinations, postprocessing is desirable. The basic position of the FDA on lossy image postprocessing is to have the developers demonstrate that the software will function with the chosen level of compression and submit test data to support their claims.

6.8.4 Legal Standards for Compression

Presently no legal standards exist for radiologic image compression. The absence of such standards means that there is no objective clinical reference for a court to use in judging a malpractice case that involves the use of a medical device incorporating lossy algorithms. To be acceptable, a compression algorithm requires thorough clinical validation tests, carried out on a large number of images and involving many clinicians, to ensure that diagnostic accuracy is not jeopardized by lossy compression. This approach could conceivably comprise a "reasonable" standard before the courts. Such a task would be difficult, though not impossible, to carry out for measuring the image quality of the wide variety of modalities available. Currently, when a misdiagnosis is the subject of a legal trial, radiologists testifying for the plaintiff and for the defense will argue image quality before the jury, and the judge will give instructions regarding reasonableness as related to issue of the duty owed by the defendant to the plaintiff as well as image quality. We then let the jury to decide whether there was a breach of duty to provide reasonable image quality. One obvious question is: Should courts dictate compression schemes? Our position is that it is the clinical and engineering professionals who should dictate clarity in legal compression standards, not the court.

The regulation of the federal government shifts the responsibility to the user. The aim is to reduce the chance of misinterpretation of lossy images by ensuring that the imaging equipment has the desired features and by providing the user with the information to make a decision. But, there is no clear specification on which the user may formulate an objective judgment of the value of using lossy schemes. The standard is also important for teleradiology applications, where there is less control of medical devices used at both ends than at a single site. The derivation of a legal standard should not depend on the court's decision, but should be a task, albeit difficult, that is undertaken with the assistance of expert medical imaging professionals.

6.8.5 Product Liability

A plaintiff who feels that he has been injured due as a result of degradation of image quality during a radiological operation may bring a suit against a vendor under product liability theory. This legal theory, which originated in California, has been in place for a number of years: it holds the vendor liable for any physical harm caused by a defective product that is "unreasonably" dangerous to the user even if the seller has made an effort in good faith to use all possible care in preparation of the product. This situation is even more complex in teleradiology, when an image is subjected to lossy compression on one system, then transmitted to another for reconstruction, and to yet a third for viewing. There is the unsettled question of who should bear the responsibility—the company whose device applies the compression, the manufacturer of the reconstruction software, or the developer of the viewing workstation. The current federal policy, which requires that images subjected to lossy compression be labeled with a caution, can help only to some extent. Thus manufacturers and developers must invest time in examining the response of their imaging processing algorithms with respect to lossy compression.

6.9 Summary and Research Directions

Despite rapid progress in mass storage density and computer network performance, the demand for transmission bandwidth and storage space in the digital radiology environment continues to outstrip the capabilities of available technologies. To overcome these two stumbling blocks, research in radiologic image compression aims to achieve a high compression ratio in representing digital images of various modalities while maintaining an acceptable image quality for clinical use.

Many studies done in the field of medical imaging indicate that it is conceivable to compress a radiologic image to a 10:1 or even higher ratio without losing its diagnostic quality. Because of the legal and medical implications of permanent loss of image quality, reversible compression is the current acceptable way to compress medical images. Nevertheless, the promise of using high performance irreversible compression to solve data storage and transmission problems has enticed medical imaging researchers and developers for years. The recent formation of certain industrial standards, such as ACR-NEMA and DICOM, and the emerging market for PACS and teleradiology, help to trigger a marked increase in the development of medical devices that use lossy coding algorithms.

The choice of a compression scheme is a complex tradeoff of system and clinical requirements. Discrete cosine transform coding, as in other digital imaging fields, is the most common approach to lossy compression in medical imaging today. Since the characteristics of radiologic images vary with modalities and applications, our discussion reveals that there are also many strong candidates in subband coding techniques, such as wavelet transforms.

Although significant progress has been made in radiologic image compression since its beginning in the last decade, many research challenges remain. First, the coming of the digital radiology environment, especially PACS and teleradiology, will continue to test the limits of disk storage and transmission bandwidth. Further improvement of existing compression techniques is thus necessary.

Second, acquisitions of 3-D and 4-D medical image sequences are becoming more usual nowadays, especially in the case of dynamic studies performed with modalities such as MRI, fast XCT, ultrasonography, nuclear medicine, or PET. Thus, another challenge is to enable multidimensional medical image coding but still provide fast response time and affordable disk space. For these new applications, parallel processing technology offers a solution to the problems inherent in manipulating and processing the significantly increased data volume. Existing image compression algorithms are optimized for sequential computing, although sporadic attempts to explore parallel compression techniques, such as full-frame DCT and parallel digital video interface compression using dedicated hardware, have reported in the literature. As the price of parallel computers is dropping, we anticipate that more effort will be spent in developing parallel compression techniques for medical applications.

It is worth noting that medical imaging scanners typically have adequate local memory space and dedicated hardware to acquire images efficiently. The critical issue of medical imaging applications is how to transmit and display the archived images promptly upon request. Hence, the focus of parallel radiologic image compression is on image decoding. This differs from other digital imaging applications, such as satellite imaging (which emphasizes fast data encoding to process the rapid arrival of satellite signals) and teleconferencing (which entails both encoding and decoding processes).

Third, it is important to develop a large and comprehensive image database that contains image sets for various modalities and diseases. The image set of each disease will cover a wide spectrum of standardized diagnostic images for that disease, with various degrees of diagnostic difficulty. This database must be established by a national committee and could be used as a universal tool for one evaluation of any image compression devices submitted to the FDA for marketing clearance.

Finally, the development of a better, and general, method for characterizing compression losses of radiologic images is urgently needed. The availability of lossy compression raises several important legal and regulatory issues that remain to be settled. For the lossy compression technology to be put into clinical environment, one crucial task is to define an objective measure of image quality, to set a legal standard for lossy compression. The traditional noise and compression ratio measurements are insufficient. They do not provide any information regarding the type of loss (e.g., spatial location or spatial frequency) that causes image unsharpness. On the other hand, besides being costly and time-consuming to perform, ROC studies are too specific to cover the wide range of medical imaging modalities and applications. Developing such a measure of radiologic imaging is not trivial: it would require the operative efforts of imaging scientists, manufacturers, and clinicians to define a general means of classifying, measuring, and evaluating the quality of radiologic images, covering not only global parameters, such as noise and compression ratio, but also local parameters, such as texture and sharpness. The standardization of an image database for radiologic image compression, augmented by recent advances in the area of *perception coding,* would shed some light on this subject.

7

Picture Archiving and Communication System (PACS) I: Infrastructure Design and Image Acquisition

7.1 Introduction

A picture archiving and communication system (PACS) consists of image and data acquisition, storage, and display subsystems integrated by various digital networks. It can be as simple as a film digitizer connected to a display station with a small image database, or as complex as a total hospital image management system. PACS developed in the late 1980s, designed mainly on an ad hoc basis to serve small subsets of the total operations of many different radiology departments. Each of these PACS modules functioned as an independent island, unable to communicate with other modules. Although they demonstrated the PACS concept and worked adequately for each of the different radiology and clinical services, the piecemeal approach did not address all the intricacies of connectivity and cooperation between modules. This weakness surfaced as more PACS modules were added to hospital networks. The maintenance, routing decisions, coordination of machines, fault tolerance, and expandability of the system became increasingly difficult problems. The inadequacy of the early design concept was due partly to a lack of understanding of the complexity of a large-scale PACS and to the unavailability at that time of certain PACS-related technologies.

PACS implementation should emphasize system connectivity. A general multimedia data management system that is easily expandable, flexible, and versatile in its programmability calls for both top-down management to integrate various hospital information systems and a bottom-up engineering approach to build a foundation (i.e., PACS infrastructure). From the management point of view, a hospital-wide PACS is attractive to administrators because it provides economic justification for implementing the system. Proponents of PACS are convinced that its ultimately favorable cost-benefit ratio should not be evaluated as a resource of the radiology department alone but should extend to the entire hospital. This concept has gained momentum. Several large hospitals have obtained funding by using this strategy and are at various stages of implementation. From the engineering point of view, the PACS infrastructure is the basic design concept to ensure that PACS includes features such as standardization, open architecture, expandability for future growth, connectivity, and reliability. This design philosophy can be realized in a modular fashion.

The PACs infrastructure provides the necessary framework for the integration of distributed and heterogeneous imaging systems and makes possible intelligent database management of all patient-related information. Moreover, it offers an efficient means of viewing, analyzing, and documenting study results, and furnishes a method for effectively communicating such results to referring physicians. The PACS infrastructure consists of a basic skeleton of hardware components (acquisition interfaces, storage devices, host computers, communication networks, display systems) integrated by standardized, flexible software subsystems for communication, database management, storage management, job scheduling, interprocessor communication, error handling, and network monitoring. The infrastructure as a whole is versatile and can incorporate rules to reliably perform not only basic PACS management operations but also more complex research job requests. The software modules of the infrastructure embody sufficient understanding and cooperation at a system level to permit the components to work together as a team rather than as individual computers connected in a network.

The PACS infrastructure is physically composed of several classes of computer systems connected by various networks. These include radiologic imaging systems, acquisition computers, the PACS controller with database and archive, and display workstations. Figure 7.1 shows the PACS components and data flow.

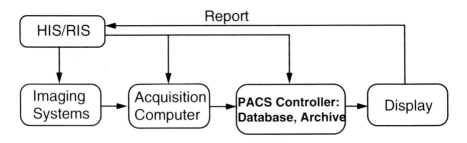

Figure 7.1 PACS components and data flow: HIS, hospital information system; RIS, radiology information system.

7.2 PACS Components

7.2.1 Data and Image Acquisition Component

The most troublesome PACS task to date has been the reliable and timely acquisition from a radiologic imaging system of images and associated study support text (information on patients, description of the study, and parameters of acquisition and image processing).

This bottleneck exists mainly because many manufacturers of imaging equipment are not prepared to follow the industry standards developed by, for example, ACR-NEMA (American College of Radiology/National Electrical Manufacturers Association), and DICOM (Digital Imaging and Communications in Medicine), as discussed later (Section 7.4.2). To circumvent these difficulties, an acquisition computer can be placed between the imaging system(s) and the rest of the PACS network, with the idea of isolating the radiologic imaging host computer from the PACS via the acquisition gateway computers. Isolation is necessary because specialized imaging device computers lack the necessary communication and coordination software that is standardized within the PACS infrastructure. Furthermore, radiologic imaging computers lack general PACS system knowledge that enables the PACS computers to cooperatively recover from various error conditions. The acquisition computer has three primary tasks: it acquires image data from the radiologic imaging system, converts the data from the equipment manufacturer's specifications to PACS standard format (header format, byte-ordering, matrix sizes) that is compliant with the proposed ACR-NEMA and DICOM data formats, and forwards the image study to the PACS controller (described later).

Connecting general-purpose PACS acquisition computers and radiologic imaging systems are interfaces of two types. With *peer-to-peer* network interfaces, which use the TCP/IP (transmission control protocol/Internet protocol) Ethernet protocol, image transfers can be initiated either by the radiologic imaging system (a "push" operation) or by the destination PACS acquisition computer (a "pull" operation). The pull mode is advantageous because if an acquisition computer goes down, images can queue in the radiologic imaging system until the acquisition computer becomes operational again, at which time the queued images can be pulled and normal image flow resumed. Assuming that sufficient data buffering is available on the imaging system, the pull mode is the preferred mode of operation because an acquisition computer can be programmed to reschedule study transfers if failure occurs (to itself or to the radiologic imaging system). If a delay in acquisition is not acceptable, studies can be rerouted to a designated backup acquisition computer on the network when the primary acquisition computer is unavailable.

The second interface type is a *master–slave* device-level connection such as the de facto industry standard, DR11-W. This parallel transfer direct memory access connection is a point-to-point, board-level interface. Recovery mechanisms again depend on which machine (acquisition computer or imaging system) can initiate a study transfer. If the acquisition computer is down, data may be lost. An alternative image acquisition method must be used to acquire these images (e.g., the technologist manually sends individual images stored in the imaging system computer after the acquisition computer is brought back up, or the technologist digitizes the digital hard copy film image). These interface concepts are described in more detail in Section 7.5.

7.2.2 PACS Controller

Imaging examinations, along with pertinent patient information, are sent from the acquisition computer, the hospital information system (HIS), and the radiology information system (RIS) to the PACS controller. The PACS controller is the engine of the PACS; its two major components are a database server and an archive system. Table 7.1 lists operations of a PACS controller. Some of the basic functions of the PACS database server are illustrated in Figure 7.2. The archive system consists of short-term, long-term, and permanent storage. These components are explained in detail in later chapters.

7.2.3 Display Stations

PACS display stations should fully use the resources and processing power of the entire PACS network. A station includes communication, database, display, resource management, and processing software. The fundamental workstation operations are listed in Table 7.2.

There are four types of display station: (1) high-resolution (2.5K × 2K) monitors for primary diagnosis, (2) medium resolution (1K × 1K) stations for referring physicians and conferences, (3) physician desktop stations (512 monitor), and (4) high-resolution, hard copy print stations. At a primary diagnosis display workstation, images are stored on fast access storage array magnetic disks. Each worksta-

Table 7.1   Operations of a PACS Controller

- Receives images of a study from acquisition computers
- Extracts text information describing the received studies
- Updates a network-accessible database management system
- Determines the workstations to which the newly generated studies are to be forwarded
- Automatically retrieves necessary comparison images from a distributed optical disk library archive system
- Automatically corrects the orientation of computed radiographic images
- Determines optimal contrast and brightness parameters for image display
- Performs image data compression
- Archives new studies onto optical disk library
- Deletes from storage on remote acquisition computers images that have been archived
- Services archive retrieval requests from workstations and other cluster controllers

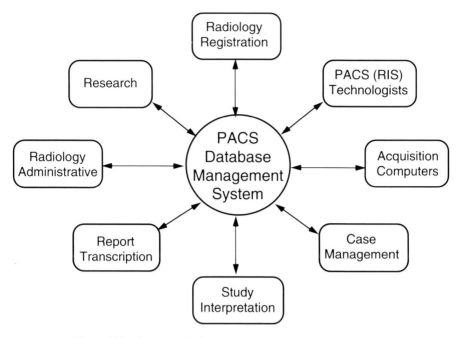

Figure 7.2   Some basic functions of the PACS database server.

tion maintains a local database for managing current cases. It also has access to the global PACS database for historical images.

7.2.4 System Networking

A basic function of any computer network is to provide an access path by which end users (e.g., radiologists and clinicians) at one geographic location can access information (e.g., images and reports) at another location. The most obvious way to characterize a radiologic location PACS network is to examine the traffic of information between various locations and users. The important networking data needed for system design include location and function of each node, frequency of informa-

Table 7.2   Operations Performed at a PACS Workstation

Operation	Description
Case preparation	Accumulation of all relevant images and information belonging to a patient examination
Case selection	Selection of cases for a given subpopulation
Image arrangement	Tools for arranging and grouping images for easy review
Interpretation	Measurement tools for facilitating the diagnosis
Documentation	Tools for image annotation, text, and voice reports
Case presentation	Tools for a comprehensive case presentation

tion passed between any two nodes, cost for transmission between nodes on various speed lines, desired reliability of the communication, and required throughput. The variables in the design include network topology, communication line capacities, and flow assignments.

Digital communication in the infrastructure design can consist of low speed (10 Mbit/s signaling rate) Ethernet, medium speed (100 Mbit/s) fiber distributed data interface (FDDI), and high speed ($\geq$155 Mbit/s) asynchronous transfer mode (ATM).

The network protocol used should be standard, for example, TCP/IP. A low speed network is used to connect the imaging devices to the acquisition computers because of the time-consuming processes performed in the imaging device. Several local Ethernets may be involved in transferring data from imaging systems to acquisition computers. Medium and high speed networks are used based on the balance of data throughput requirements and costs. A faster image network is used between acquisition computers and the PACS controller because several acquisition computers may send large image files to the controller at the same time.

Process coordination between tasks running on different machines is an extremely important issue in system networking. This coordination of processes running either on the same computer or on different computers is accomplished by using interprocessor communication methods implemented by using socket-level interfaces to TCP/IP. Commands are exchanged as American Standard Code for Information Interchange (ASCII) messages to ensure standard encoding of messages. Jobs requests are stuffed into disk resident priority queues, which are serviced by various *daemon* (agent) processes. The queue software may have a built-in job scheduler that is programmed to retry a job several times by using a default set of resources or alternative resources if a hardware error is detected.

7.3 Design Concept

Four major ingredients in the PACS infrastructure design concept are system standardization, connectivity and open architecture, reliability, and security.

7.3.1 Industry Standards

The first important rule in building a PACS infrastructure is to incorporate as many as possible of the industry de facto standards that are consistent with the overall PACS design schema. The philosophy is to minimize the development of customized software. Furthermore, use of industry standard hardware and software increases the portability of the system to other computer platforms. For example, the following industry standards should be used in the PACS infrastructure design: (1) UNIX operating system, (2) TCP/IP and DICOM communication protocols, (3) SQL (Structured Query Language) as the database query language, (4) ACR-NEMA, and DICOM standards for image data format, (5) C programming language,

(6) X Windows user interface, (7) ASCII text representation for message passing, and (8) HL7 for health care database information exchange.

The implications of using standards in PACS implementation are several. First, implementation of all future PACS components and modules is straightforward. Second, system maintenance is easier because each module looks similar to others, if not physically, then logically. Moreover, defining the PACS primitive operations serves to minimize the amount of redundant computer code within the PACS system, which in turn makes the code easier to debug, understand, and search. It is self-evident that standardizing terminology, design concepts, and so forth facilitates system understanding and documentation among all levels of developers.

7.3.2 Connectivity and Open Architecture

If two PACS modules in the same hospital cannot communicate with each other, they become two isolated systems, each with its own images and patient information, and can never be combined with other systems to form a total hospital-integrated PACS.

Open network design, which allows a standardized method for data and message exchange between heterogeneous systems, is essential. Because computer and communications technology changes rapidly, a closed architecture hinders system upgradability. For example, suppose an independent imaging console from a given manufacturer would, at first glance, make a good addition to an MR or CT scanner for viewing images. If the console has a closed proprietary architecture design, however, no components except those specified by the same manufacturer can be used to augment the system. Thus potential system upgrading and improvement are limited, and perhaps other changes as well. Considerations of connectivity are important, however, even when a small-scale PACS is planned. To be sure that a contemplated PACS is well designed and will allow future connectivity, questions such as the following should be answered with a "yes":

Can we transmit images form this PACS module to other systems and vice versa?
Does this module use a standard data and image format?
Does the machine use a standard communication protocol?

7.3.3 Reliability

Reliability is a major issue for two reasons. First, since a PACS has many components, the probability of component failure is high. Second, because the PACS manages and displays critical patient information, extended periods of downtime cannot be tolerated. In designing a PACS, it is therefore important to use fault-tolerant measures, including error detection and logging software, external auditing programs (i.e., network management processes that check network circuits, magnetic disk space, database status, processes status, and queue status), hardware redundancy, and intelligent software recovery blocks. Some recovery mechanisms that can be used include automatic retry of failed jobs with alternative resources and algorithms, and intelligent bootstrap routines (a software block executed by a computer when it is restarted) that allow a PACS computer to automatically continue operations after a power outage. Improving reliability is costly; however, it is essential to maintain high reliability of a complicated system.

7.3.4 Security

Security is an important consideration because of medicolegal issues, including particularly the need for patient confidentiality. Three major security mechanisms are account control, privilege control, and the use of views. Most sophisticated database management systems have identification and authorization mechanisms that use accounts and passwords. Application programs may supply additional layers of protection. "Privilege control" refers to granting and revoking individual users' access to specific tables, columns, or views. These security measures provide the PACS infrastructure with a mechanism for controlling access to clinical and research data. With these mechanisms, the system designer can enforce policy with respect to which persons have access to clinical studies. In some hospitals for example, referring clinicians are granted image study access only after a preliminary radiology reading has been performed and attached to the image data.

An additional security measure is the use of encryption during image and data communication. If implemented, this feature will increase the system software overhead but data transmission through open communication channels will be secure.

7.4 Two Industry Data and Image Interface Standards

Imagery and textual communications among health care information systems, have always been difficult because these components vary with platforms, modalities, and manufacturers; there have been technical obstacles, as well, to the sharing of medical imaging equipment, and picture archiving and communication systems. With the emerging of industry standards, it becomes feasible to integrate all these heterogeneous, disparate medical images and textual data. Interfacing two devices requires two ingredients, a common data format and a communication protocol. Two such major industry standards are Health Level 7 (HL7) for textual and ACR-NEMA and DICOM for image data. HL7 is a standard textual data format, whereas ACR-NEMA and DICOM include data format and communication protocols. In conforming to the HL7 standard, it is possible to share medical information between the hospital information systems, radiology information systems, and PACS. By adapting the ACR-NEMA and DICOM standard, medical images generated from a variety of modalities and manufacturers can be converted to the standardized data format. The conversion can use the data dictionary defined in the ACR-NEMA and DICOM documents (see Section 7.4.2).

7.4.1 Health Level 7 (HL7) Interface Standard

7.4.1.1 Health Level 7

Health Level 7 (HL7), established in March 1987, was organized by a user–vendor committee to develop a standard for electronic data exchange in health care environments, particularly for hospital applications. The common goal is to simplify the interface implementation between computer applications from multiple vendors. This standard emphasizes data format and protocols for exchanging certain key textual data among health care information systems, such as HIS, RIS, and PACS.

HL7 addresses the highest level (level 7) of the Open System Interconnection (OSI) model of the International Standards Organization (ISO) but does not conform specifically to the defined elements of the OSI's seventh level (see Section 8.1.2). It conforms to the conceptual definitions of an application-to-application interface placed in the seventh layer of the OSI model. These definitions were developed to facilitate data communication in a health care setting by providing rules to convert abstract messages associated with real-world events into strings of characters comprising an actual message.

7.4.1.2 An Example

Consider the three popular computer platforms used in HIS, RIS, and PACS, namely, the IBM mainframe running the VM operating system, the VAX file server running open VMS, and Sun SPARC running UNIX. Interfacing involves the establishment of data links between these three operating systems via TCP/IP communication protocol with HL7 data format at the application layer.

When an event occurs, such as a patient admission, discharge, or transfer (ADT), the IBM computer responsible for tracking this event would initiate an unsolicited message to a remote host computer (VAX) that takes charge of the next event. If the message is in HL7 format, the remote host updates its local database automatically and sends a confirmation to the sending host. Otherwise, a "rejected" message would be sent instead.

In the HL7 standard, the basic data unit is a message. Each message is comprised of multiple segments. The first segment is the message header segment, which defines the intent, source, destination and other relevant information, such as message control identification and time stamp. The other segments are event dependent. Within each segment, related chunks of information are bundled together based on the HL7 protocol. A typical message, such as patient admission, may contain the following segments:

MSH	Message header segment
EVN	Event type segment
PID	Patient identification segment
NK1	Next of kin segment
PV1	Patient visit segment

In this patient admission message, the patient identification segment may contain the segment header and other demographic information, such as patient identification, name, date of birth, and gender. The separators between fields and within a field are defined in the message header segment. Here is a sample patient identification segment:

PID||| 1234567||SMITH^ JOHN|DOE|19210131|M|||||⟨CR⟩

The data communication between a HIS and a RIS is event driven. When an ADT event occurred, the HIS would automatically send a broadcast message, confined in HL7 format, to the RIS. The RIS would then parse this message and insert, update, or remove patient demographic data in its database according to the event. Similarly, the RIS would sent an HL7-formatted ADT message, the examination reports, and the procedural descriptions to PACS. When PACS had acknowledged and verified the data, it would update the appropriate databases and initiate any required follow-up actions.

As an example, the HIS at the UCSF, which consists of an IBM main frame and eleven other computer systems, uses a custom-built interface engine called MIMP to distribute ADT data. It generates HL7-bundled messages and transfers them over the local area network to RIS. DECrad, the application running on RIS, uses the programming language environment Digital Standard MUMPS (DSM version 6.3) for the interface. This interface works for point-to-point communication. Upon receiving HL7 messages from HIS, DECrad triggers appropriate events and transfers patient data over the network to the PACS host computer (Sun SPARC). After conversion to HL7, the message can be transmitted between HIS, RIS, and PACS with a communication protocol—most commonly, TCP/IP through a network (see Section 8.1.2).

7.4.2 ACR-NEMA and DICOM Interface Standards

7.4.2.1 ACR-NEMA Standard

ACR-NEMA, formally known as the American College of Radiology and the National Electrical Manufacturers Association, created a committee to develop a set of standards to serve as the common ground for various medical imaging equipment vendors in developing instruments that can communicate and participate in the sharing of medical image information, in particular within the PACS environment. The committee, which focused chiefly on issues concerning information exchange, interconnectivity, and communications between medical systems, began work in 1982. The first version, which emerged in 1985, specifies standards in point-to-point message transmission, data formatting, and presentation, and includes a preliminary set of communication commands and data format dictionary. The second version, ACR-NEMA 2.0, published in 1988, was an enhancement to the first release. It includes both hardware definitions and software protocols, as well as a standard data dictionary. Networking issues were not addressed adequately in either version, however, and a new version was released in 1992. Because of the magnitude of changes and additions, it was given a new name: Digital Imaging and Communications in Medicine, that is, DICOM 3.0. This multivolume document is not yet complete. Although the complexity and breadth of the standards were increased by threefold, DICOM 3.0 remains compatible with the ACR-NEMA releases. One of the most distinguishing new features is a set of application message exchange and communication protocols.

The standards committee is influential in the medical imaging community. However, medical imaging equipment manufacturers were slow to respond to and comply with the ACR-NEMA standards, especially during the early years. As the specifications of DICOM 3.0 become widely accepted, manufacturers have taken a very cooperative manner and have begun to develop new versions of software equipment totally based on this standard.

While every segment of the medical imaging community is awaiting the widespread implementation of DICOM 3.0, PACS development is still handicapped with a limited set of working tools for conforming medical images to the ACR-NEMA standard. The current thought is to conform with the DICOM standard whenever possible. To facilitate conversion for modalities that meet only the ACR-NEMA standard, an ACR-NEMA-to-DICOM conversion should be developed. And for imaging modalities that do not comply with ACR-NEMA, a translator is needed to convert the manufacturer's specifications to either the ACR-NEMA or the DICOM standard. In the latter case, a set of software modules, collectively called the encoder library, is needed to convert the original image header with either the ARC-NEMA or the DICOM standard. A well-developed encoder library should reflect adherence to the following guidelines:

generic for multimodalities and imaging equipment of various vendors
portability to various hardware platforms
top-down design and modular principle in software architecture
standard programming language, like C

7.4.2.2 An Example

Let us consider an encoder for converting an imaging modality to the ACR-NEMA standard. According to the ACR-NEMA 2.0 data dictionary, each image should contain two parts: a command group and a data set. The data set can be further divided into information groups: identifying, patient, acquisition, relationship, image presentation, overlay, and image pixel data. The data in these groups, when transmitted across equipment, constitute a message.

Not every piece of header information from a modality will have a corresponding group element category specified in the ACR-NEMA format. Not every element defined in the ACR-NEMA dictionary will cover data types included in the image headers of various equipment vendors. Therefore, a minimum set of groups and a minimum set of elements within those groups as the core data structure should first be defined (see Table 7.3). In other words, all images, regardless of modality and

Table 7.3   Required Groups and Elements
in the ACR-NEMA Conversion

Group	Element	
0000	0000	(Command group)
	0001	
	0010	
	0800	
008	0000	(Identifying group)
	0001	
0009	0000	(Display shadow group)
	0001	
0010	0000	(Patient information)
0019	0000	(Raw header shadow group)
	0001	
7fe0	0000	(Pixel data group)
	0010	

manufacturer, should bear this minimum set once it has been formatted. Additional groups and elements are then defined based on the header information provided by the specific modality and the manufacturer. Additional information can be defined in two shadow groups: a display shadow group, which stores the information that is vital to support workstation display and provide fast access, and a raw header group, which retains the entire header, to permit the retrieval of data items not formatted, should this become necessary.

Additional groups and elements, such as acquisition information (group 0018), relationship information (group 0020), image information (group 0028), and overlay groups, will be applied depending on type of information provided from the manufacturer.

Applications can differ considerably with respect to the number of groups and elements to be formatted. To provide a systematic way for an encoder program to extract and map data to the ACR-NEMA format, a configuration file, which describes the included groups and elements, was developed for each modality. The encoder of a modality reads in a specific configuration file and calls various modules in its program to convert image data to the ACR-NEMA format. The last data group to be converted should be the pixel data group (7fe0), which is attached to the end of the message. In addition, for each modality, the encoders are grouped in a library with all the necessary modules for encoding. This library resides in the acquisition host computer and compiles with the host application.

The general algorithm of converting raw image data into ACR-NEMA format is as follows. First, an image is acquired from a particular modality. If it is not in the ACR-NEMA format upon arrival at the local acquisition computer, it goes through the encoding process and is converted to the standard format. After that, the formatted image is sent to the PACS controller for archiving, and, subsequently, is shipped to display workstations.

Table 7.4   Differences between ACR-NEMA 2.0 and DICOM 3.0 Standards

ACR-NEMA 2.0	DICOM 3.0
Based on an intuitive information model	Based on an explicit information model
Services provided are built into commands and descriptions of their use	Services supported are described fully in service classes
Defines a minimum for conformance, but does not describe how a claim of conformance is structured	Includes a detailed specification about how to describe conformance
Supports point-to-point communication; if it is used over networks, an interface unit (NIU) is required to support the netowrk protocol	Supports point-to-point and network commun-cations
Supports a single image per message	Supports a folder capability for multiple im-ages per message (by value or by reference)
Defines unique commands	Makes use of existing standards to define the new commands (ISO common management information service)

7.4.2.3 The DICOM 3.0 Standard

The major differences between the ACR-NEMA 2.0 and the DICOM 3.0 Standard are given in Table 7.4. In the DICOM 3.0 standard, there are two classes of information, object classes and service classes. The former include patients, modal-ities, and studies, whereas the latter include storage, query, and retrieval. Each class has a dictionary defining the attributes for proper encoding. Tables 7.5 and 7.6 list some of the object classes and service classes. The two major commands in DICOM

Table 7.5   DICOM Information
Object Classes

Composite

Computed radiograph
Computed tomogram
Digitized film image
Digital subtraction image
MR image
Nuclear medicine image
Ultrasound image
Displayable image
Graphics
Curve

Normalized

Patient
Study
Results
Storage resource
Image annotation

Table 7.6 DICOM Service Classes

Service Class	Description
Image storage	Provides storage service for data sets
Image query	Supports queries about data sets
Image retrieval	Supports retrieval of images from storage
Image print	Provides hard copy generation support
Examination	Supports management of examinations (which may consist of several series of management images)
Storage resource	Supports management of the network data storage resource(s)

are the composite and normalized commands, given in Tables 7.7 and 7.8, respectively. Each composite command is paired in the sense that a device issues a command request and the receiver responses the command accordingly. These commands are backward compatible with the earlier ACR-NEMA versions. The composite commands are generalized, whereas the normalized commands are more specific.

If an imaging device transmits data and images with a DICOM 3.0 command, the receiver must use a DICOM 3.0 command to receive the information. On the other hand, if a device transmits a DICOM 3.0 format data set with a TCP/IP communication protocol through a network, any device that connects to the network can receive the data with the TCP/IP protocol. A decoder is needed to convert the DICOM 3.0 data format for proper use. Figure 7.3 shows the procedure of converting image format to the ACR-NEMA and DICOM standards.

7.5 Image Acquisition

7.5.1 Background

Automated image acquisition from imaging devices to the PACS controller plays an important role in a PACS infrastructure. The "automatic" part is important because reliance on labor-intensive manual acquisition methods would defeat the purpose of

Table 7.7 DICOM Composite Commands

Command	Function
ECHO	Verification of connection
SEND	Transmission of an information object instance
FIND	Inquiries about information object instances
GET	Transmission of an information object instance via third-party application processes
MOVE	Similar to GET, but end receiver is usually not the command initiator
DIALOG	Communication of unformatted data
CANCEL	Handling exceptions

Table 7.8 DICOM Normalized Commands

Command	Function
M_EVENT_REPORT	Notification of information object-related event
M_GET	Retrieval of information object attribute value
M_SET	Specification of information object attribute value
M_ACTION	Specification of information object-related action
M_CREATE	Creation of an information object
M_DELETE	Delection of an information object

the PACS. However, there is no single means of enabling automated data acquisition from existing digital medical imaging systems. Based on existing manufacturers' imaging devices, we categorize the interface methods into five architectural models: sequential chain, direct interface, memory access, shared disk, and interconnected network. In the remainder of Section 7.5, we discuss the methodology,

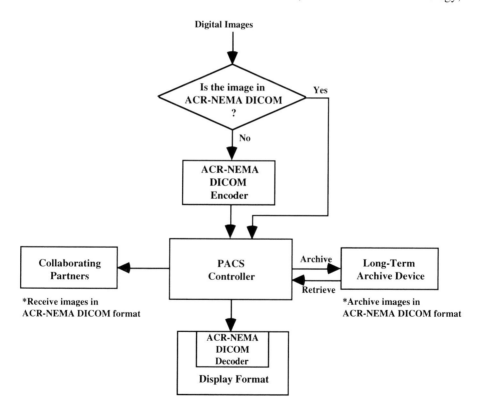

Data Encoding/Decoding to ACR-NEMA and DICOM Standards

Figure 7.3 Procedure of converting image format to the ACR-NEMA and DICOM standards.

cost, rate of data transfer, and ease of implementation of each model. An important measure of the success of an automatic acquisition is its effectiveness in ensuring the integrity and availability of patient images in PACS system. For this reason, automated fault-tolerance design in image acquisition is required. We discuss common scenarios that cause an acquisition to fail and techniques to automatically restart operations under these circumstances. The techniques include recovery from errors and traps of the acquisition process, image acquisition computer downtime, and shutdown of the medical imaging system.

7.5.2 Automated Image Acquisition Interface Methods

Generally speaking, the PACS image acquisition system consists of three major components: a medical imaging system, a computer system that acquires images from the imaging system (i.e., an acquisition computer), and an interface mechanism (hardware and software) between the imaging system and acquisition computer. The interface mechanism can be further categorized into five models: sequential chain, direct interface, memory access, shared disk, and interconnected network. Sections 7.5.2.1–7.5.2.5 illustrate the interface mechanism of each model by using manufacturers' imaging systems as examples. Each model's costs, data transfer rate, and ease of implementation are discussed.

7.5.2.1 Sequential Chain Model

In the sequential chain model, the PACS acquisition computer links a medical imaging system through a chain of interface devices provided by a manufacturer. An example of the sequential chain model is the IDNET-1 (Integrated Diagnostics Network, version 1.0) solution provided in the late 1980s by General Electric Medical Systems (GEMS) (General Electric Company, Milwaukee, WI) for acquiring CT images from the GE-9800 CT scanners. Figure 7.4 shows the schematic diagram of IDNET-1 in the total PACS context. The parallel peripheral interface (PPI) board, residing in the scanner system, functions as a virtual magnetic disk driver that reads the data from the disk of the scanner to one of the network interface equipment (NIE) units, which is separate from the scanner system. At the NIE-1 node (see Fig. 7.4), the image data and associated text data are encoded into the ACR-NEMA format and transmitted to NIE-2 using a proprietary GE data transfer protocol and a dedicated, Ethernet-based GEMS network.

The second node in the GEMS network, NIE-2, has a standard ACR-NEMA output (50-pin connector) to an ACR-NEMA interface board, which resides in a PC/AT computer. The PC/AT transmits the image data to the acquisition computer through the Ethernet with a PC Ethernet board.

Since this configuration requires several interface units, the cost of the interface is high (approximately $40,000) and the connectivity is complicated. Implementation of this configuration takes several man-months. Furthermore, it is difficult to measure the data elapse time in each interface unit, which in turn makes it hard to determine the data transfer performance precisely. Field data demonstrate that the

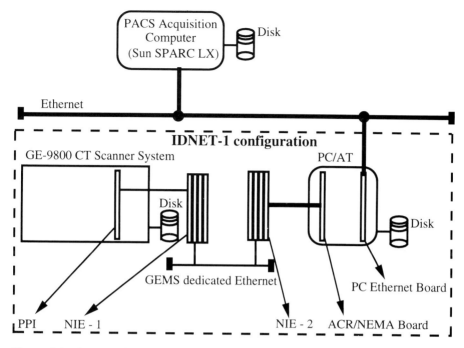

Figure 7.4 An example of the sequential chain model: image data are propagated from the scanner through the PPI, the NIE-1, the GEMS dedicated Ethernet, the NIE-2, the PC/AT, and the PACS acquisition computer.

data transfer rate between the PC/AT and the PACS acquisition computer is the most time-consuming component; between a PC/AT and a Sun minicomputer 3/260 (Sun Microsystems, Mountain View, CA), for example, this rate is about 50 Kbyte/s. The sequential chain model has the disadvantages of being costly and complex, with a low data transfer rate. Until GEMS introduced the IDNET-2, however, it was the only solution available to automatically acquire images from the GE-9800 CT scanners to the PACS. The interface configuration of IDNET-2 is simpler than that of IDNET-1. We categorize the IDNET-2 as a shared disk model.

7.5.2.2 Direct Interface Model

The direct interface model is composed of an acquisition computer connected to a medical imaging system through a set of standard electronic interface boards. An example of this model is the DR11-W interface (or SCSI interface) of the Abe–Sekkei (AS, Abe–Sekkei Inc., Tokyo, Japan) film laser digitizer (see Section 3.2.4). Figure 7.5 shows the interface configuration of this model, in which the image data from the scanner are buffered in the DR11-W interface board and transmitted to the PACS acquisition computer. The buffer size in this application is 32 kbytes. Whenever the buffer is full, the data are archived to the disk of the PACS acquisition

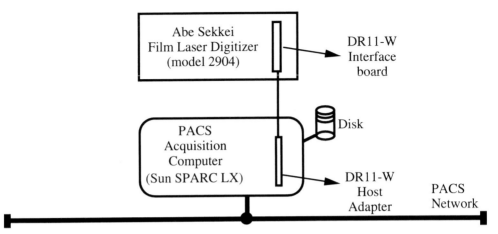

Figure 7.5 The direct interface model, showing the DR11-W interface between the Abe–Sekkei film laser digitizer and the PACS acquisition computer.

computer through the DR11-W host adapter. Other examples of this model are the SCSI data acquisition system manager (DASM) of the Fuji computed radiography (CR) system (Fuji Medical Systems, U.S.A. Inc., Stamford, CT, see Section 4.1) and the SCSI interface of the Lumiscan digitizer (Lumisys Inc., Sunnyvale, CA).

The advantages of this model are several: the interface units are commercial products, the connectivity is simple, the cost is affordable, and data throughput is fast. Integration takes approximately 2 man-weeks. The price of this type of interface devices ranges from $2000 to $8000. The transfer rate between the AS film laser scanner and the SCSI disk of a Sun SPARC LX computer shown in Figure 7.5 is greater than 1.2 Mbyte/s.

7.5.2.3 Memory Access Model

In the memory access model, a PACS acquisition computer connects to a medical imaging system through a dual-port RAM. The interface product called MegaLink, which transmits images from the Imatron Cine CT scanner (Imatron Company, Oyster Point, CA, see Section 5.2.1.5) to the PACS acquisition computer, belongs to this category. In Figure 7.6, two MegaLink bus adapter boards are linked by a pair of 25-foot ribbon cables (one for signal acknowledgment and one for data transfer). The adapter board installed in the fast reconstruction system (FRS) of the Imatron CT scanner contains 1 Mbyte of dual-ported RAM. The memory is accessible by both the FRS and the PACS acquisition computer. The FRS stores the header and reconstructed image data in this RAM, which can be accessed by the PACS acquisition computer via the MegaLink bus adapter board using the direct memory access mechanism. Simple semaphore-based interlock protocol software is used to synchronize the data transfer between the two computer systems.

The direct memory access model provides fast data throughput because the data

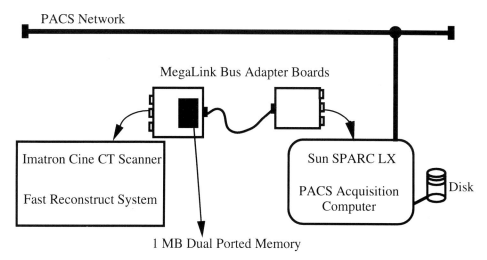

Figure 7.6 The memory access mode demonstrates the MegaLink connecting the Imatron Cine CT scanner and the acquisition computer. The acquisition computer can access the image data through the dual-ported memory.

transfer is very similar to the scenario of writing data from the CPU memory of a computer to its own disk. Field measurement for the configuration shown in Figure 7.6 is greater than 1 Mbyte/s. Since the interface devices consist of RAM memory, the cost is high (approximately $15,000). Implementation of automatic image acquisition from the Imatron CT scanner takes about 6 man-weeks.

7.5.2.4 Shared Disk Model

The shared disk model makes a disk accessible by both the PACS acquisition computer and a medical imaging system. The Siemens (both Impact and Vision models) MR scanners are examples (Siemens Medical Systems, Inc., Iselin, NJ). The Siemens MR scanner can be interfaced by using the network file system (NFS) protocol. The local disk of the imaging system can be remotely mounted by the acquisition computer through a network accessible by both computers, as shown in Figure 7.7. Thus, whenever images are available in the local disk of the imaging system, they are also available in the acquisition computer.

Of all the interface architectural models, the shared disk model has the best image data availability in the sense that no image data propagation is required. In addition, the NFS-based shared disk model is a very low cost and easily implemented configuration because the NFS feature is commonly available in most computer systems today. It takes about one man-week to complete the physical connections. The NFS-based shared disk model has a drawback, though. Any interaction between the imaging system and the acquisition computer during data transfer requires network and disk input/output (I/O) operations at the imaging computer system. Frequent I/O operations of peripheral devices, however, may cause notice-

Modality Network

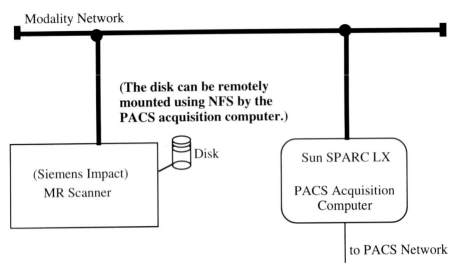

(The disk can be remotely mounted using NFS by the PACS acquisition computer.)

Disk

(Siemens Impact)
MR Scanner

Sun SPARC LX

PACS Acquisition
Computer

to PACS Network

Figure 7.7 An example of the shared disk model. The Sun computer using the network file system (NFS) protocol remotely mounts the disk, which is physically connected to the MR scanner. As a result, the acquisition computer can access the image data in the remote disk.

able performance slowdown of the imaging system. Any such interruption to the operation of the imaging system is undesirable, especially when the imaging system is in heavy clinical use.

7.5.2.5 Interconnected Network Model

The interconnected network model consists of a PACS acquisition computer and the medical imaging system host computer, which are connected in a network and communicate through standard communication protocols. GEMS's newer CT and MR scanners, such as the Hi-Speed Spiral CT and Signa 5x MR models (see Sections 5.2.1.4 and 5.5.3.4) are designed based on this model. Figure 7.8 shows the configuration of a GE imaging medical systems' interconnected network. The network follows the ISO's Open System Interconnection standard layers (see Section 8.1.2). The physical and data link layers are Ethernet, the network layer is Internet protocol (IP), and the transport layer is transmission control protocol (TCP). For the application layer, the GEMS proprietary communication programs are based on TCP/IP and a file transfer protocol (FTP). Other application layer software is the Central Test Node (CTN) software developed by Electronic Radiology Laboratory, Mallinckrodt Institute of Radiology (St. Louis, MO) based on the DICOM 3.0 standard.

Since the interconnected network model follows the industrial standards, its advantages include affordable cost, portable components, and easy implementation. The hardest part of configuring this model is laying down the network infrastructure. For an existing networking environment, this interface model can be configured with minimal effort (<1 man-week). The image data transmission performance (disk-to-disk) of this interface model ranges from 100 Kbyte/s to 400 Kbyte/s. The

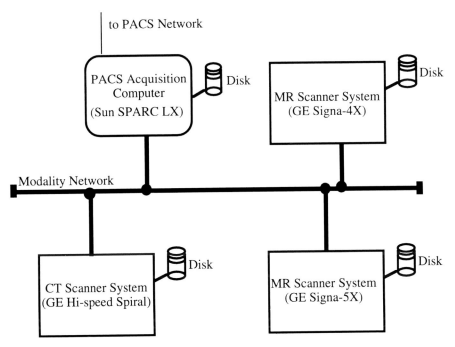

Figure 7.8   The interconnected network model. The acquisition computer acquires images from the CT and MR scanners through a standard network (Ethernet) and standard communication protocols (TCP/IP) or DICOM upper layer protocols TCP/IP.

range is so wide because its choice depends on (1) type of computer systems used (both the imaging system and acquisition computer), (2) type of system disk, (3) utilization of the network, and (4) workload of the computer systems.

Table 7.9 summarizes the five interface models according to the three parameters: costs, rate of data transfer, and time required for implementation. An example imaging system and the associated interface mechanism for each model are given.

PACS is an essential ingredient for the realization of digital radiology and hospital environment. One crucial task is to integrate image scanners and modalities of various types into the open system PACS network. Existing scanners, however, are developed based on "closed" architectural design and do not communicate with one another.

Open systems interoperability has been acknowledged to be an improtant feature in a digital medical imaging system. It can be attained only by following the standards. For this reason, the direct interface model and the interconnected network model are more favorable for designing medical imaging systems.

7.5.3 Fault-Tolerance Methods for Automated Image Acquisition

Many factors can cause an automated image acquisition system to fail. For this reason a mechanism must be designed to detect system failure and to recover from

Table 7.9 Summary of the Five Interface Models

Parameters	Model				
	Sequential Chain	Direct Interface	Direct Memory Access	Shared Disk	Interconnected Network
Cost	<$40,000	<$8000	<$15,000	$0	$0
Rate of data transfer	50 Kbyte/s	>1 Mbyte/s	>1 Mbyte/s	N/A	100–400 Kbyte/s
Time required for implementation, man-weeks	>24	2	6	11	12
Example					
Imaging system	GE CT-9800	Microscope, Abe–Sekkei Film Digitizer	Imatron CT	Siemens MR Impact	GE MR Signal 5x
Interface	IDNET-1	SCSI or DR11-W	MegaLink	NFS	Ethernet and CTN

downtime during automated acquisition. If the period of downtime is too long, the limited amount of disk space may cause the images in the imaging system to be purged before they can be acquired by the acquisition computer. In the absence of backup system to store the data, such images may be lost forever. To ensure the integrity and availability of patient images in a PACS system, automatic recovery from faults is a crucial component in the image acquisition design. In this section, we describe the major software programs involved in the acquisition computers, the common scenarios causing the acquisition process to fail, and methods for automatically recovering the operation.

7.5.3.1 *Image Acquisition Software*

In general, the image acquisition task consists of four programs (Fig. 7.9). The acquiring program receives images from the imaging system to the acquisition computer. The formatting program organizes the acquired images and the associated text information based on a standard format (e.g., DICOM). The sending program transfers the formatted image to another component of the PACS (see Fig. 7.1). This component is usually an image archiving system, but depending on the PACS architectural design, it may be an image display system as well. After the formatted image has been properly archived in the PACS controller, the deleting program erases the acquired images from the acquisition computer to free up the storage space. These four programs complete the chain of image acquisition data flow. If the chain is broken, the image acquisition task will fail to function. For simplicity, we use the term "acquisition process" to represent these four programs in the following discussions.

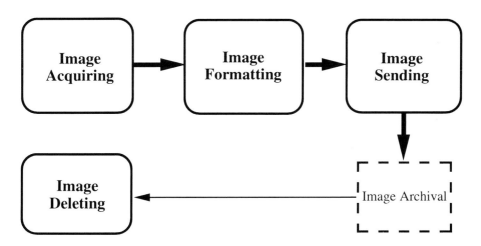

Figure 7.9   Four major software programs in the PACS acquisition computer, which complete the chain in an image acquisition task.

7.5.3.2 Acquisition Process Recovery from Errors

The acquisition process can be ended prematurely if certain fatal error conditions are encountered. Examples include I/O errors of peripheral devices and not enough CPU memory in the acquisition computer. A monitoring process is required to recover the acquisition task from faults of this type. The monitoring process should possess three functions: activation at periodic alert times, examination of the status of designated processes, and restart of the designated processes if necessary. If, for example, the monitoring process wakes up at a given time and detects that the acquisition process has been terminated; it must restart acquisition automatically. Usually, if the computer system has a clock daemon utility available, the periodical wake-up feature of the monitoring process can be replaced by the clock daemon. In this way, the user can be sure that the monitoring program will be executed periodically as long as the acquisition computer is in operation.

7.5.3.3 Acquisition Process Recovery from Traps

Occasionally, an acquisition process is terminated immediately after it has been launched by the monitoring process. If this situation occurs repeatedly (i.e., if the acquisition process is trapped), human intervention will be necessary. In the most common example of this problem, no space is left on the acquisition computer's

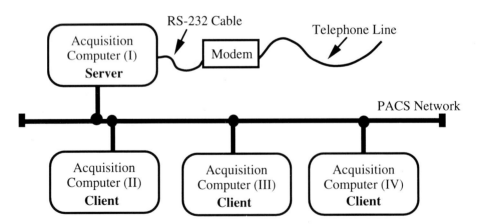

Figure 7.10 The configuration of the central dial-up and paging scheme for recovery from traps during acquisition failure. The modem is configured with the server that connects the clients with the PACS network. The clients send messages to the server through the PACS network whenever the image acquisition function is trapped. The server then sends the messages to service personnel through the modem via a pager.

disk. This fatal error condition must be addressed at once. Thus there is a need for a centralized dial-up and paging scheme to alert service personnel automatically. A typical hardware configuration of the central dial-up scheme is shown in Figure 7.10; software implementation is required, as well.

The hardware involves a computer system to be configured with a modem device that is connected to a telephone line. This central dial-up computer can be in any component in the PACS, provided it is networked with the acquisition computers and others. From the task-oriented point of view, the central dial-up computer is the server and the acquisition computers are the clients.

The software required in the server and clients mainly includes four modules: (1) sending of the service request, (2) receiving of the service request, (3) automatically dialing the pager number of the designated troubleshooter, and (4) checking the availability of the computer system network. Consider our earlier example: no disk space in the acquisition computer is available, the acquisition process is trapped, and human intervention has become necessary. In this situation, the message "no disk space" is sent from the client to the server through a network. The message contains the client computer name, the process name, and the service engineer's pager number. The computer name and the process name can be represented by numerical numbers. Each pair of numbers is then coded to become a callback number. In this way, the dial-up software module delivers the message to the engineer on call based on the pager number and the coded callback number. Besides the function of receiving request from the clients, the software checks the availability of the clients via the network. This is done because when a computer goes down, it is not available to other computers through the network.

7.5.3.4 Acquisition Computer Recovery from Downtime

The acquisition process cannot proceed if the acquisition computer goes down. There are two possibilities: either the computer can reboot itself or it can not. If the computer can reboot itself, then it can initiate an operating system kernel program, check the configured peripheral devices, and execute necessary system processes during the computer rebooting. Since the system processes can be started up in the rebooting procedures, the image acquisition programs can be launched as well. If the computer cannot reboot itself, for example, due to a power outage, then the dial-up and paging scheme can be used to request operator service.

7.5.3.5 Handling Imaging System Shutdown

When the technician who manages the imaging system is obliged to observe its operational procedure and the maintenance schedule irrespective of the ongoing acquisition process, the imaging system may shut down while image data are being transferred from the imaging system to the acquisition computer. An acquisition process that required special care whenever the technician turned the imaging system on or off would be unacceptable. Thus, the acquisition process must be transparent to the technician. To meet this requirement, the software in the image acquisition computer is designed to handle such an abrupt shutdown event. That is, code is written to impart to the system the ability to manage such error events as a broken network connection, a dropped network connection, or a connection time-out. If one of these events is detected, the acquisition process resets the uncompleted task to initial status, thus allowing the task to be processed from the beginning in the next execution. This scheme may repeatedly handle the same uncompleted task if the imaging system remains in down status. However, this mechanism ensures that the acquisition process will continue in operation whenever the imaging system is turned back on.

The integrity and availability of patient images in a PACS system very much depend on the uptime of the image acquisition process. To optimize the system uptime probability of the image acquisition process, automatic recovery schemes from faults must be implemented in the image acquisition software design. This section has presented some common scenarios that cause the acquisition task to fail and the methods used to automatically recover the operation.

7.5.4 Interface with a PACS Module

In Sections 7.5.2.1–7.5.2.5 we discussed five models of interfacing an imaging modality to the PACS acquisition computer. The last one, the interconnected network model utilizing the Central Test node software in the DICOM standard, can be used to interface a PACS module with a PACS acquisition computer. A *PACS module* is loosely defined as a self-contained PACS that has some acquisition components: a short-term archive, a database, some display stations, and a communication network linking these components. In practice, the module can function alone, as an individual unit in which the display stations show images from the acquisition components.

An example of a PACS module is the US PACS, in which several US scanners are connected to a short-term archive for up to 1–2 days of examinations. The display stations can show images from all US scanners with display format tailored for US images. There are certain advantages connecting the US PACS module to a hospital-integrated PACS (HI-PACS). First, US images can be appended into the same patient's image and data folder to form a complete file, then sent to the PACS database for long-term archiving. Second, US images can be shown with other modality images in the PACS general display workstations for cross-modality comparisons. Third, some other modality images can also be shown in the US module's specialized workstations. In this case, care must be taken because the specialized workstation (e.g., a US workstation) may not have the full capability for displaying images from other modalities. For these reasons, there are advantages to integrating the US PACS module into a hospital-wide PACS. A preferred method for interfacing a PACS module to the HI-PACS is to treat the module as an imaging acquisition

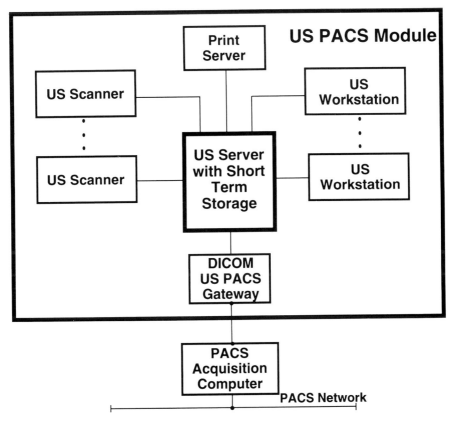

Figure 7.11   Interface of a PACS module to an acquisition computer; this example features a US PACS module.

device and use the interconnected network model for the linkage. We use the US PACS module as an example.

Figure 7.11 shows the general connection of the US PACS module to a PACS acquisition computer via a DICOM gateway. Each patient image file in the US server contains the full-sized color or black and white images (compressed or original), thumbnail (quarter-sized) images for indexing, and image header information for DICOM conversion. In the DICOM gateway, several processes are running concurrently. The first one is a daemon constantly checking for new US examinations arriving from scanners. When one is found, the device sends to a second process to convert the file to the DICOM format. Because a color US image file is normally large (see Sections 5.4.2.4 and 6.7), a third process compresses it to a smaller file, normally with a 3:1 ratio. The gateway generates a DICOM *send* command to transmit the compressed DICOM file to the acquisition computer, using DICOM TCP/IP protocols.

In the acquisition computer, several daemons are running concurrently also. The first is a DICOM gateway routine that checks for the DICOM *send* command from the gateway. Once the *send* has been detected, the second daemon checks the proper DICOM format and saves the information in the acquisition computer. The third daemon queues the file to be stored by the PACS controller's long-term archive.

To request other modality images from a US workstation, the patient's image file is requested from the PACS long-term archive. The archive transmits the file to the acquisition computer, which sends it to the US PACS gateway. The US gateway computer transmits the file to the US workstation.

Other important PACS modules that can be interfaced to the HI-PACS are the nuclear medicine PACS module and the emergency room PACS module. The requirement for the interface in these modules is a built-in DICOM gateway with the DICOM commands for communication and DICOM format for the image file.

7.6 Image Preprocessing

After being sent from the imaging device to the acquisition computer, but before being archived in the PACS controller, an image goes through a preprocessing step. There are two categories of preprocessing function. The first is related to the image format—for example, a conversion from the manufacturer's format to DICOM. This type of preprocessing involves mostly data format conversion and was described in Section 7.4. The second type of preprocessing prepares the image for an optimal viewing at the display station. To achieve optimal display, an image should have proper size, good initial display parameters (e.g., a suitable lookup table), and proper orientation; any distracting background should be removed. Preprocessing function is modality specific in the sense that each imaging modality has a specific set of preprocessing requirements. Some preprocessing functions may work well for certain modalities but poorly for others. In the remainder of this chapter we discuss preprocessing functions according to each modality.

7.6.1 Computed Radiography (CR)

7.6.1.1 Reformatting

A CR image can have three different sizes (given here in inches) depending on the type of imaging plates used: $L = 14 \times 17$, $H = 10 \times 12$, or $B = 8 \times 10$. These plates give rise to 2140×1760, 2010×1670, and 2000×2510 matrices, respectively. Since display monitor screens vary in pixel sizes, a reformatting of the image size from these three dimensions may be necessary to fit a given monitor. In the reformat preprocessing function, since both the image and the monitor size are known, a mapping between the size of the image and the screen is first established. We use as an example two of the most common screen sizes: 1024×1024 and 2048×2048. If the size of an input image is larger than 2048×2048, the reformatting takes two steps. First a two-dimensional bilinear interpolation is performed to shrink the image at a 5:4 ratio in both directions; this means that an image size of $2000 \times$

2510 is reformatted to 1600 × 2008. Second, a suitable number of blank lines is added to extend the size to 2048 × 2048. If a 1024 × 1024 image is desired, a further subsampling ratio of 2:1 from the 2048 image is performed.

For imaging plates that produce pixel matrix sizes smaller than 2048 × 2048, the image is extended to 2048 × 2048 by adding blank lines and then subsampling (if necessary) to obtain a 1024 × 1024 image.

7.6.1.2 Removing Unexposed Background

The second CR preprocessing function is to remove the image background due to X-ray collimation. In pediatric images and in extremity images, collimation can result in the inclusion in the image of significant white background that should be removed to reduce the amount of unwanted background light in the image during soft copy display.

An algorithm that removes image background begins by searching for the raw edges (left, right, top, and bottom) of the radiation field. The raw edge points are those with a standard deviation in the desired direction exceeding an empirically determined threshold. The raw edge points are searched to find the outer corners of the rectangular radiation field. These boundaries are tested to see whether any portion of the radiation field has been excluded (i.e., left outside the boundaries). This test also is based on standard deviations of gray values, a parameter dependent on body region and amount of collimation, in which the background and the radiation field are characterized by low deviations and higher deviations, respectively. If necessary, error correction is carried out by extending the boundary in the appropriate direction to include the previously excluded portion of the radiation field. Finally, the correct contour is constructed as a collection of left, right, top, and bottom edges of the radiation field. Areas outside are set to the darkest gray level.

If the imaging plate is not placed under the patient properly (if it lies, e.g., at a slant angle with respect to the patient's body axis), the exposed field may not be a rectangle. The algorithm should have the ability to detect this situation and correct for the search of the edges accordingly. Figure 7.12 shows a CR image before and after the background removal.

After background removal, the image size will be different from the standard *L, H, B* sizes. To center an image such that it occupies the full monitor screen, it is sometime advantageous to automatically zoom and scroll the image from which background has been removed for an optimal display. Zoom and scroll functions are standard image processing functions and are discussed later (Section 9.3.2.1).

7.6.1.3 Automatic Orientation

The third CR preprocessing function is automatic orientation. "Properly oriented" means that when displayed on a monitor, the image appears in the conventional way expected by a radiologist about to read the hard copy image from a light box. Depending on the way the imaging plate is placed under the patient, there are eight

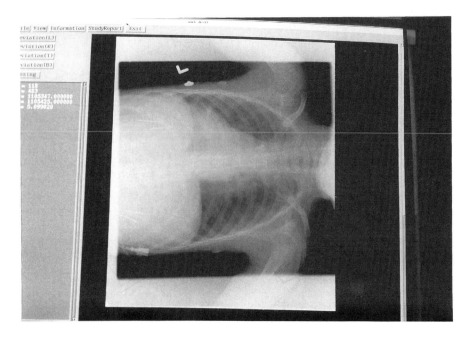

(A)

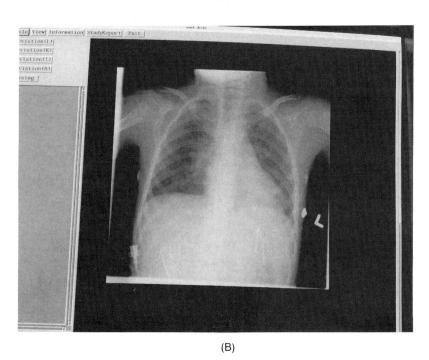

(B)

Figure 7.12 A pediatric CR chest image with the background removal and automatic orientation. (A) The original CR image: sideways and with some X-ray collimation background (white). (B) The same CR image, after background removal, is rotated automatically to the proper orientation. The lookup table is also adjusted for optimal display.

Source: Courtesy of Jianguo Zhang.

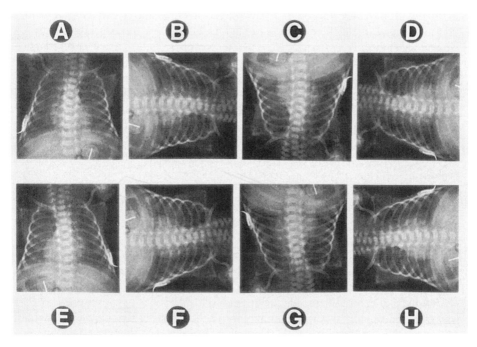

Figure 7.13   Eight possible orientations of an AP chest image: the automatic rotation program determines the body region shown and adjusts it to the proper orientation.
Source: Courtesy of Ewa Pietka.

possible orientations (Fig. 7.13). An image can be oriented correctly or rotated 90° clockwise, 90° counterclockwise, or 180°. In each case, the image can also be y-axis-flipped.

The algorithm first determines from the image header the body region contained in the image. Three common body regions are chest, abdomen, and hand. Let us first consider the automatic orientation of the anterior–posterior (AP) or PA chest images.

For AP or PA chest images, the algorithm searches for the location of three characteristic objects: spine, abdomen, and neck or upper extremities. To find the spine and abdomen, horizontal and vertical pixel value profiles (or line scans), evenly distributed through the image, are taken. The average density of each profile is calculated and placed in a horizontal or a vertical profile table. The two tables are searched for local maxima to find a candidate location. Before a decision is made regarding which of the two possible (horizontal or vertical) orientations marks the spine, however, it is necessary to search for the densest area that could belong to either the abdomen or the head. To find this area, an average density value is computed over two consecutive profiles taken from the top and bottom of both tables. The maximum identifies the area to be searched. From the results of these scans and computations, the orientation of the spine is determined to be either horizontal or vertical.

A threshold image (threshold at the image's average gray value) is used to find the location of the neck or upper extremeities along the axis perpendicular to the spine. The thresholding marks the external contours of the patient and separates them from the patient background (area that is exposed but is outside the patient). Profiles of the threshold image are scanned in a direction perpendicular to the spine (identified earlier). For each profile, the width of the intersection between the scan line and the contour of the patient is recorded. Then the upper extremities for an anterior–posterior (AP) or posterior–anterior (PA) image are found on the basis of the ratios of minimum and maximum intersections for the threshold image profiles. This ratio also serves as the basis for distinguishing between AP (or PA) from lateral views.

The AP and PA images are oriented on the basis of the spine, abdomen, and upper extremity location. For lateral chest images, the orientation is determined by using information about the spine and neck location. This indicates the angle that the image needs to be rotated (0°, 90° counterclockwise, or 180°).

For abdomen images, again there are several stages. First the spine is located by using horizontal and vertical profiles, as before. The average density of each profile is calculated, and the largest local maximum defines the spine location. At the beginning and end of the profile making the spine, the density is examined. Higher densities indicate the subdiaphragm region. The locations of the spine and abdomen determine the angle at which the image is to be rotated.

For hand images, the rotation is performed on a threshold image: a binary image in which all pixel values are set at zero if they are below the threshold value and at one, otherwise. To find the angle (90° clockwise, 90° counterclockwise, or 180°), two horizontal and two vertical profiles are scanned parallel to the borders. The distances from the borders are chosen initially as one-fourth of the width and height of the hand image, respectively. The algorithm then searches for a pair of profiles: one that intersects the forearm and a second that intersects at least three fingers. If no such pair can be found in the first image, the search is repeated. The iterations continue until a pair of profiles (either vertical or horizontal), meeting the above-mentioned criteria, is found. On the basis of this profile pair location, it is possible to determine the angle at which the image is to be rotated.

7.6.1.4 Lookup Table Generation

The fourth preprocessing function for CR images is the generation of a lookup table. The CR system has a built-in automatic brightness and contrast adjustment; since CR is a 10-bit image, however, it requires a 10- to 8-bit lookup table for mapping onto the display monitor. The procedure is as follows. After background removal, the histogram of the image is generated. Two numbers, the minimum and the maximum, are obtained from the 5 and the 95% points on the cumulative histogram, respectively. From these two values, one computes the two parameters in the lookup table: level = (maximum + minimum)/2, and window = (maximum − minimum). This is the default linear lookup table for displaying the CR images.

For CR chest images, preprocessing at the acquisition device (or the exposure itself) sometimes results in images that are too bright or lack contrast, or both. For these images, several piecewise-linear lookup tables can be created to adjust the brightness and contrast of different tissue densities of the chest image. These lookup tables are created by first analyzing the image gray level histogram to find several key breakpoints. These breakpoints serve to divide the image into three regions: background (outside the patient, but still within the radiation field), radiographically soft tissue region (skin, muscle, fat, overpenetrated lung), and radiographically dense tissue region (mediastinum, subdiaphragm, underpenetrated lung).

From these breakpoints, different gains can be applied to increase the contrast (gain or slope of the lookup table > 1) or reduce the contrast (gain or slope < 1) of each region individually. In this way, the brightness and contrast of each region can be adjusted dependent on the application. If necessary, several lookup tables can be created to enhance the radiographically dense and soft tissues, with each having different levels of enhancement. These lookup tables can be easily built in and inserted into the image header and applied at the time of display to enhance different types of tissues.

7.6.2 Digitized X-Ray Images

Digitized X-ray images share some preprocessing functions with the CR: reformatting, background removal, and lookup table generation, for example. Each of these algorithms requires some modifications, however. Most X-ray film digitizers are 12 bits and allow the user to specify a field in the film to be digitized; as a result, the digitized image differs from the CR image in three aspects. First, the size of the digitized image can have various dimensions instead of just three. Second, there will be no background in the digitized image because the user can effectively eliminate it by positioning the proper window size during digitizing. Third, the image is 12 bits instead of 10 bits. For reformatting, the mapping algorithm therefore should be modified for multiple input dimensions. No background removal is necessary, although the zoom and scroll functions may be still needed to center the image and occupy the full screen size. The lookup table parameters are computed from 12 instead of 10 bits. Note that no automatic orientation is necessary, since the user will have oriented the image properly during the digitizing.

7.6.3 Sectional Images: CT, MR, and US

In sectional imaging, the only necessary preprocessing function is lookup table generation. The two lookup table parameters, window and level, can be computed from each image (either 8 or 12 bits) in a sectional examination similar to that described in the case of the CR image. The disadvantages of taking this approach are twofold: inspection of many images in a sectional examination can turn out to be a very time-consuming process, and a lookup table is needed for each image. The requirement for separate lookup tables will delay the multiple image display on the screen because the display program must perform a table lookup for each image. A method of circumventing the many-lookup-tables drawback is to search the corresponding histograms for the minimum and maximum gray levels of a collection of images in the examination and generate a single lookup table for all images. For US, this method works well because the US signals are quite uniform between images. In CT, several lookup tables can be generated for each region of the body for optimal display of lungs, soft tissues, or bones. This method in general works well for CT. This method does not work well for MR, however, because each lookup table is generated for a pulse sequence and the strength of the body or surface coil can vary from section to section, creating variable histograms for each image. Automatic lookup table generation of a set of MR images remains a challenging research topic.

8

Picture Archiving and Communication System (PACS) II: Communications and Databases

8.1 Background in Communications

8.1.1 Terminology

Communication is the movement of information from one place to another, usually by way of media of some type. Media may be either bound (cables) or unbound (broadcast). *Analog* communication systems encode the information into some continuum (video) of signal (voltage) levels. *Digital* systems encode the information into two discrete states ("0" and "1") and rely on the collection of these binary states to form meaningful data. A communication standard encompasses detailed specifications of the media, the explicit physical connections, the signal levels and timings, the packaging of the signals, and the high level software necessary for the transport. A video communication standard describes the characteristics of composite video signals including interlace or progressive scan, frame rate, line and frame retrace times, number of lines per frame, and number of frames per second. In a PACS, the soft copy display is video signals; depending on the types of monitor used, these video signals will follow certain standards.

In digital communications, the packaging of the signals to form bytes, words, blocks, and files is usually referring to as a communication protocol. *Serial* data transmission moves digital data, one bit at a time, over a single wire or pair of wires. This single bit stream is reassembled into meaningful byte/word/block data at the receiving end of a transmission.

On the other hand, *parallel* data transmission uses many wires to transmit bits in parallel. Thus, at any moment in time, a serial wire has only one bit present, but a set

Table 8.1 Five Commonly Used Network Topologies

Topology	In PACS Applications	Advantages	Disadvantages
Bus	Ethernet	Simplicity	Difficult to trace problems when a channel fails
Tree	Video broadband headend	Simplicity	Bottleneck at the upper level
Ring	Fiber distributed data interface	Simplicity; no bottleneck	In a single ring, the network fails if the channel between two nodes fails
Star (Hub)	ATM switch	Simplicity; easy to isolate a fault	Bottleneck at the hub
Mesh		Immunity to bottleneck failure	Complicated

of parallel wires may have an entire byte or word present. Consequently, parallel transmission effects an n-fold increase in transmission speed, where n is the number of wires used.

In applications that call for maximum speed, *synchronous* communication is used. That is, the two communication nodes share a common clock and data are transmitted in a strict way according to this clock. *Asynchronous* communication, used when simplicity is desired, relies on start and stop signals to identify the beginning and end of data packets. Accurate timing is still required, but the signal encoding allows a wide variance in the timing on the different ends of the communication line. We will discuss the asynchronous transfer mode (ATM) technology in Section 8.1.3.3.

In digital communication, the most primitive protocol is the RS-232 asynchronous standard for point-to-point communication, promulgated by the Electronic Industries Association (EIA). This standard specifies the signal and interface mechanical characteristics, gives a functional description of the interchange circuits, and lists application-specific circuits. This protocol is mostly used for peripheral devices (e.g., the track ball or mouse in a display workstation). Current digital communication methods are mostly networking. Table 8.1 lists the five popular network topologies and Figure 8.1 shows their architectures. The bus, ring, and star architectures are most commonly used in PACS applications. A network that is used in a local area (e.g., within a building or a hospital) is called a local area network, or LAN. If it is used outside of a local area, it is called a metropolitan area network (MAN) or wide area network (WAN) applies otherwise, depending on the area covered.

8.1.2 Network Standards

The two most commonly used network standards in PACS applications are the DOD standard developed by the U.S. Department of Defense, and the OSI (Open Systems Interconnect) developed by the ISO (International Standards Organization). As

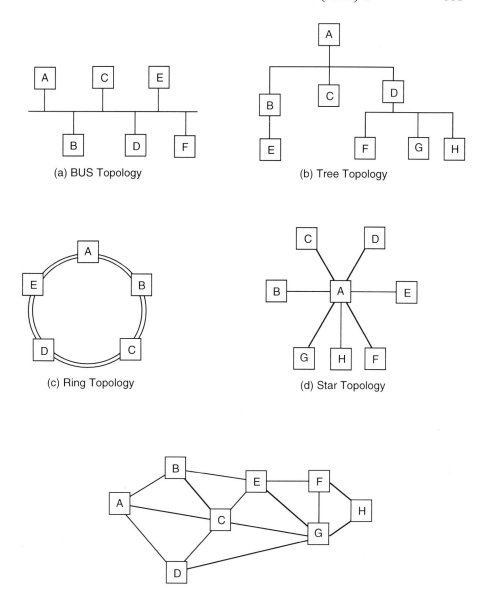

Figure 8.1   Five commonly used network topology architectures.

shown in Figure 8.2, the former has four-layer protocol stacks and the letter with seven-layer stacks. In the DOD protocol stack, the FTP (file transfer protocol) and the TCP/IP (transmission control protocol/Internet protocol) are two popular communication protocols used widely in the medical imaging field. The seven layers in the OSI protocols are defined in Table 8.2.

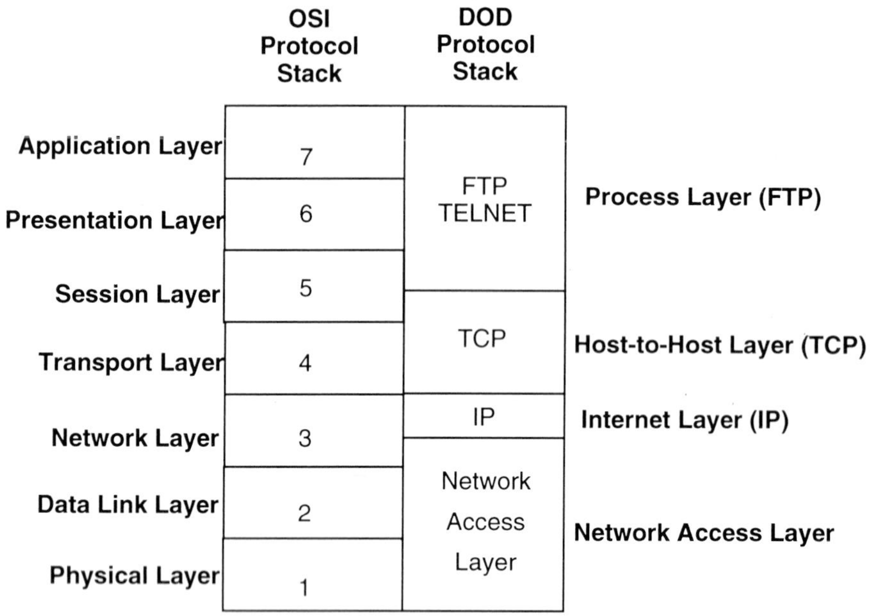

Figure 8.2 Correspondences between the seven-layer OSI and the four-layer DOD communication protocols.

We now discuss an example of how data is sent from one node to another node in a network through the DOD TCP/IP protocol. Figure 8.3 shows the procedure: the steps by which a block of data is transmitted with protocol information are listed at the left. First, the block of data is separated to segments of data, whereupon each segment is given a TCP header, then an IP header, and finally a packet header. The packet of encapsulated data is then sent, and the process is repeated until the entire block of data has been transmitted. The encapsulated procedure is represented by the boxes on the right. In the TCP/IP protocols, the overheads in transmission are the TCP header, the IP header, and the packet header.

Table 8.2 The Seven-Layer Open Systems Interconnect (OSI) Protocols

Layer	Protocol	Definition
7	Application layer	Provide services to users
6	Presentation layer	Transformation of data (encryption, compression, reformatting)
5	Session layer	Control applications running on different workstations
4	Transport layer	Transfer of data between endpoints with error recovery
3	Network layer	Establish, maintain, and terminate network connections
2	Data link	Medium access control: network access (collision detection, token passing) and network control
		Logical links control: send and receive data messages or packets
1	Physical layer	Hardware layer

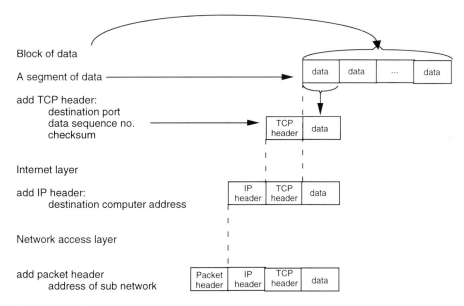

Figure 8.3 Example of sending a block of data from one network node to another with the TCP/IP protocol.

8.1.3 Network Technology

Now we turn to three commonly used network technologies in PACS applications: the Ethernet, fiber distributed data interface (FDDI), and asynchronous transfer mode (ATM), which are used for low speed, medium speed, and high speed communications, respectively. All three technologies can run on TCP/IP communication protocols.

8.1.3.1 Ethernet

Ethernet (luminiferous ether), which is based on IEEE standard 802.3, Carrier Sense Multiple Access with Collision Detection (CSMA/CD), uses the bus topology (see Fig. 8.1). It operates at 10 Mbit/s either on a half-inch coaxial cable, twisted-pair wires, or fiber-optic cables. Data are sent out in packets to facilitate the sharing of the cable. All nodes on the network connect to the backbone cable via Ethernet taps. New taps can be added anywhere along the cable, and each node possesses a unique node address that allows routing of data packets by hardware. Each packet contains a source address, a destination address, data, and error detection codes. In addition, each packet is prefaced with signal detection and transmission codes that ascertain status and establish the use of the cable. For twisted-pair cables, the Ethernet concentrator acts as the backbone cable.

As with all communication systems, the quoted operating speed represents the raw throughput speed of the communication channel—in this case a coaxial cable with a base signal of 10 Mbit/s. The Ethernet protocol calls for extensive packaging of the data. Since a package may contain as many as 1500 bytes, a single file is usually broken up into many packets. This packaging is necessary to allow proper sharing of the communication channel. It is the job of the Ethernet interface hardware to route and present the raw data in each packet to the necessary destination computer. The performance of a typical Ethernet network with multiple connections in various communication models, as used in PACS is analyzed later (see discussion in connection with Fig. 8.16). With more than four connections, the transmission rate stays at about 60 Kbyte/s. In PACS applications, Ethernet is best for transmitting images from an imaging device to the acquisition computer and for complete system backup purposes. Not only is the very mature, low cost, Ethernet technology ideal as a backup system, but high speed is not required to transmit images to the acquisition computer because the process of imaging acquisition is slow.

A recent development is the concept of fast Ethernet or the Ethernet hub, in which all Ethernet connections go through the Ethernet hub, which has the capacity to process each transmission with 10 Mbit/s. As a result, each node can experience a true 10 Mbit/s specification throughput.

8.1.3.2 FDDI (Fiber Distributed Data Interface)

FDDI is a fiber-optic token ring LAN running at 100 Mbit/s. The FDDI runs on two rings, one transmitting in the clockwise direction and the other counterclockwise. The second ring is used as a backup. Figure 8.4a shows the double FDDI ring. In case one connection fails, the double ring can revert to a single ring and the FDDI can continue operating (Fig. 8.4b). FDDI can be used as a medium speed communication application, for example, from the acquisition computer to the PACS controller.

8.1.3.3 ATM (Asynchronous Transfer Mode)

Both Ethernet and FDDI are designed for LAN applications. The current concept in radiologic image communication is that no physical or logical boundaries should exist between LANs and WANs. For this reason, ATM for both LANs and WANs has become the emerging technology. ATM is a method for transporting information that splits data into fixed-length cells, each one consisting of 5 bytes of ATM transmission protocol header information and 48 bytes of data information. ATM operates from 155 Mbit/s at optical carrier level 3 (OC3), and potentially into the gigabit (10^9 bits) range with OC48, 2.5 Gbit/s. Based on the virtual circuit-oriented, packet-switching theory developed for telephone circuit switching applications, ATM systems are designed in the star topology, in which an ATM switch serves as a hub. Figure 8.5 shows an example of the use of an ATM switch to achieve both WAN and LAN communication.

At Mount Zion Hospital, two miles away from the University of California at San Francisco, an ASX 200 ATM switch (FORE, Warrendale, PA) is connected to a SPARC20 computer (Sun Microsystems) with an S-bus ATM adapter board

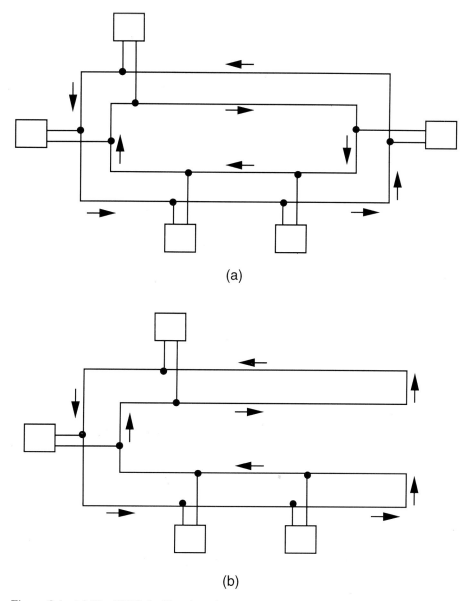

Figure 8.4 (a) The FDDI double token ring. (b) If one node fails, the double ring reverts back to a single ring and the FDDI can continue operating.

(FORE) using two multimode optical fibers. The ASX 200 ATM switch is connected to the ATM main switch at Pacific Bell in Oakland, California, via single-mode optical fibers.

At the University of California at San Francisco (UCSF), another ASX 200 ATM switch (see Fig. 8.6 bottom) is connected to SPARC 10, 20, and 690 multiprocessor

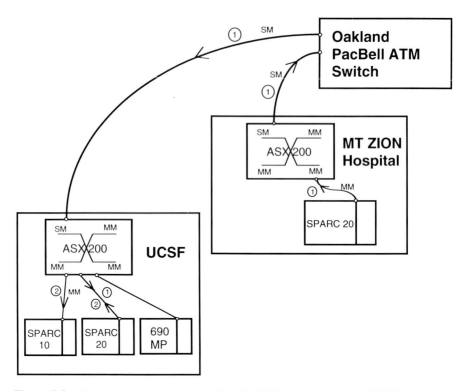

Figure 8.5 Experimental setup using multimode (MM) and single-mode (SM) fibers for the asynchronous transfer mode (ATM) (OC-3 specification, 155 Mbit/s transfer rate) wide area network (WAN) and local area network (LAN) throughput test between University of California, San Francisco and Mount Zion Hospital, using the ATM switch of Pacific Bell (PacBell) in Oakland. Path 1 is for WAN performance measurement, path 2 for LAN performance measurement; for both WAN and LAN measurement, paths 1 and 2 are combined.

(MP) computers using multimode optical fibers. A SPARC20 computer was used to simulate the acquisition computer at Mount Zion Hospital; SPARC20 and 690 MP computers were used to simulate the display workstation computer and the PACS controller computer at UCSF, respectively. During the experiment, connection(s) were turned on and off as needed. The ATM WAN and LAN throughputs were measured under various conditions.

The ATM WAN performance can be measured by activating only the path marked with a 1 in Figure 8.5. ATM LAN performance can be measured by activating only the path marked 2 in Figure 8.5. The performance of both networks can be measured by activating paths 1 and 2 simultaneously. The simulation used the following parameters: image buffer size, 128K bytes; measurement, from computer memory to computer memory; data set size, 256 Mbyte; communication protocol, TCP/IP.

Table 8.3 shows that the ATM WAN performance is about 60.64 Mbit/s, and for the ATM LAN it is 66.64 Mbit/s (or close to 40% of the 155 Mbit/s signaling rate).

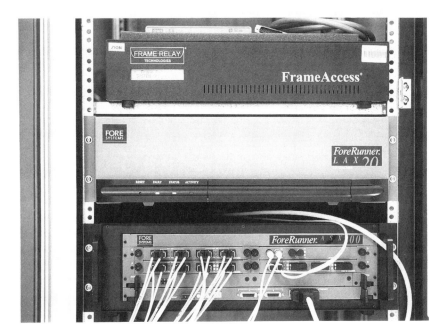

Figure 8.6 Stacked WAN and LAN components: frame access for T1; LAX20, ATM Ethernet LAN; ASX2000, ATM WAN.

When combining the WAN and the LAN concurrently, performance decreases by 46% and 73%, respectively, but the aggregate performance reaches 77 Mbit/s.

8.1.4 Connecting Networks Together

Communication protocols set up standards to pass data from one node to another node in a network. To connect different networks, additional devices are needed, namely, a repeater, a bridge, a router, and a gateway.

Table 8.3 Asynchronous Transfer Mode Optical Carrier
Level 3 Performance Statistics

Path	Performance (Mbit/s)		
	Wide Area Network	Local Area Network	Aggregate
1: From Mount Zion Hospital SPARC20 to UCSF SPARC20	60.64		60.64
2: From UCSF SPARC20 to UCSF SPARC10		66.64	66.64
1 and 2 concurrently	28.16	48.80	76.96

Table 8.4 Communication Devices
for Internetwork Connection

Device	Protocol Layer*	Network Connections
Repeater	Physical (1)	Similar network but different media
Bridge	Data link (2)	Similar network
Router	Network (3)	Similar or not similar network
Gateway	Application (7)	Different network architecture

* Numbers in parentheses give OSI layers as defined in Table 8.2.

A *repeater* passes data bit by bit in the physical layer. It is used to connect two networks that are similar but use different media; for example, a thinnet (see Section 8.2.1) and a twisted-pair Ethernet might be connected by means of hardware in layer 1 of the OSI standard. A *bridge* connects two similar networks (e.g., Ethernet to Ethernet or FDDI to FDDI) by both hardware and software in layer 2. A *router* directs packets by using network layer protocol (layer 3); it is used to connect two or more networks, similar or not (e.g., to transmit data between WAN, MAN, and LAN). A *gateway,* which connects different network architectures (e.g., RIS and PACS), uses the application level (level 7) protocol. A gateway is usually a computer with dedicated communication software. Table 8.4 compares these four communication devices.

8.2 Cable Plan

8.2.1 Networking Cables

This section describes several types of cable used for networking. The generic names have the form "10 Base X," where 10 means 10 mbit/s and X represents media type as specified by IEEE standard 802.3, because some of the cables were developed for Ethernet use.

10 Base5, also called thicknet or thick Ethernet, is a coaxial cable terminated with N series connectors. 10 Base5 is a 10 MHz, 10 Mbit/s network medium with a distance limitation of 500 meters. This cable is typically used as a Ethernet trunk or backbone path of the network. Cable impedance is 50 ohms (Ω).

10 Base2, also called thinnet or cheaper net, is terminated with BNC connectors. Also used as an Ethernet trunk or backbone path for smaller networks, 10Base2 is a 10 MHz, 10 Mbit/s medium with a distance limitation of 185 m. Cable impedance is 50 Ω.

10 BaseT, also called unshielded twisted pair (UTP), is terminated with AMP 110, or RJ-45 connectors following EIA standard 568. With a distance limitation of 100 m, this low cost cable is used for point-to-point applications such as Ethernet and copper distributed data interface (CDDI), not as a backbone. Categories 3, 4, and 5 UTP can all be used for Ethernet, but category 5, capable of 100 MHz and 100 Mbit/s, is recommended for medical imaging applications.

Fiber-optic cables normally come in bundles of 1 to 216 fibers. Each fiber can be either multimode (62.5 μm in diameter) or single mode (9 μm). Multimode, normally referred to as 10 BaseF, is used for Ethernet, FDDI, and ATM (see Section 8.1.3).

The Single mode is used for longer distance communication. 10 BaseF cables are terminated with SC, ST, SMA, or FC connectors, but usually ST. For Ethernet applications, single mode has a distance limitation of 2000 meters and can be used as a backbone segment or point to point. 10 BaseF cables are used for networking. Patch cords are used to connect a network with another network, or a network with an individual component (e.g., imaging device, image workstation). Patch cords usually are AUI (Attachment Unit Interface, DB 25), UTP, or short fiber-optic cables with the proper connectors.

Air-blown fiber (ABF) is a new technology that makes it possible to use compressed nitrogen to "blow" fibers as needed through a tube distribution system (TDS). Tubes come in quantities from 1 to 16. Each tube can accommodate bundles from 1 to 16 fibers, either single mode or multimode. The advantage of this type of system is that fibers can be blown in as needed once the TDS has been installed.

Video cables are used to transmit images to high resolution monitors. For 2K systems, 50 Ω cables are used: RG 58 for short lengths or RG 214U for distances up to 150 feet. RG 59, a 75 Ω cable used for 1K stations, can run distances of 100 feet.

8.2.2 The Hub Room

A hub room contains routers, bridges, repeaters, fanouts, switches, and other networking equipment for connecting and routing/switching information to and from networks. This room also contains the center for networking infrastructure media such as thicknet, thinnet, UTP, and fiber-optic patch panels. Patch panels, which allow the termination of fiber optics and UTP cables from various rooms in one central location, usually are mounted in a rack. At the patch panel, networks can be patched or connected from one location to another or by installing a jumper from the patch panel to a piece of networking equipment. One of the main features of the hub room is its connectivity to various other networks, buildings, and rooms. Air conditioning and backup power are vital to a hub room to provide a fail-safe environment. If possible, semi-dust-free conditions should be maintained.

Any large network installation needs segmented hub rooms, which may span different rooms and or buildings. Each room should have multiple network connections and patch panels that permit interconnectivity throughout the campus. The center or main hub room is usually called the network distribution center (NDC). The NDC houses the main routers, bridges, switches, and concentrators. It should be possible to connect via a computer to every network within the communication infrastructure from this room. From the NDC, the networks span to a different building containing a room called the building distribution frame (BDF). The BDF routes information from the main subnet to departmental subnets, which may be located on various floors within a building. From the BDF, information can be routed to an intermediate distribution frame (IDF), which will route or switch the network information to the end users.

Each hub room should have a predetermined path for cable entrances and exits. For example, four 3-inch sleeves (two for incoming and two for outgoing cables) should be installed between the room and the area the cables are coming from, to allow a direct path. Cable laddering is a very convenient way of managing cables throughout the room. The cable ladder is suspended from the ceiling, which allows the cables to be run from the 3-inch sleeves across the ladder and suspends the cables down to their end locations. Cable trays can also be mounted on the ladder for separation of coaxial, UTP, and fiber optics. In addition to backup power, access to emergency power (provided by external generators typically in a hospital environment) is necessary. The room should have a minimum of two dedicated 20 A, 120 V quad power outlets—more may be required, depending on the room size. Figure 8.7 shows the generic configuration of hub room connections.

8.2.3 Cables for Input Sources

Usually, an imaging device is already connected to an existing network with thicknet, thinnet, fiber-optics, or twisted-pair media. A tap of the same medium type can be used to connect an acquisition computer to this network, or, the aid of a repeater may be required, as in the following example. Suppose a CT scanner is already on a thinnet network, and the acquisition computer has access only to twisted-pair cables in its neighborhood. The system designer might select a repeater residing in a hub room that has an input of thinnet and an output of UTP to connect the network and the computer. When cables must run from a hub room to an acquisition device area, it is always advisable to lay extra cables at the time of installation, since this is easier and less expensive than pulling the cables later to clear the way for an upgrade.

When installing cables from the IDF or BDF to areas housing acquisition devices planned for Ethernet use at a distance less than 100 meters, a minimum of one category 5 UTP per node and four strands of multimode fiber per imaging room (CT, MR, CR) is recommended. If the fiber-optic broadband video system (see Section 8.3.2) is also planned, an additional multimode fiber-optic cable should be allocated for each input device. With this configuration, the current Ethernet technology is fully utilized and the infrastructure still has the capacity to be upgraded to accept any protocols that may be encountered in the future.

8.2.4 Cables for Image Distribution

Cable planning for input devices and image distribution differs in the sense that the former is ad hoc—that is, most of the time the input device already exists, and there is not much flexibility in the cable plan. On the other hand, image distribution requires planning because the destinations usually do not have existing cables. In planning the cables for image distribution, the horizontal run and the vertical run should be considered separately. The vertical runs, which determine several strategi-

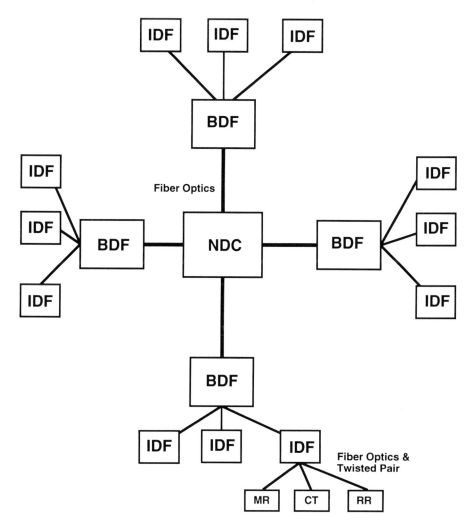

NDC: Network DistributionCenter
BDF: Building Distribution Frame
IDF: Intermediate Distribution Frame
MR: Magnetic Resonance Imaging
CT: Computerized Tomography Imaging
RR: Reading Room

Figure 8.7 Generic configuration of hub room connections based on a network distribution center (NDC), building distribution frame (BDF), and intermediate distribution frame (IDF) from which the image acquisition devices and image workstations are connected.

cal risers by taking advantage of existing telecommunication closets, usually are planned first. From these closets vertical cables are run for the connection to various floors. Horizontal cables are then installed from the closets to different hub rooms, to NDC, to BDF, to IDF, and finally to the image workstation areas. All cables at the workstation areas should be terminated with proper connectors and should have enough cable slack for termination and troubleshooting.

Horizontal run cables should be housed in conduits. Since installing conduits is expensive, it is advisable whenever possible to put in a larger conduit than is needed initially, to accommodate future expansion. Very often, the installation of conduits calls for drilling holes through floors and fire walls (core drilling). Drilling holes in a confined environment like a small telephone cable closet in a hospital is a tedious and tricky business. Extreme care must be exercised. It is important to check for the presence of any pipes or cables that may embedded in the concrete. In addition, each hole should be at least three times the size of the diameter of the cables being installed, to allow for future expansion and to meet fire code regulations. The following tips also will be useful when planning the installation of cables.

1. Always look for existing conduits and cables, to avoid duplication.
2. If possible, use Plenum cables (fire retardant) for horizontal runs.
3. When installing cables from a BDF to multiple IDFs or from an IDF to various rooms, use fiber whenever possible. If the distance is long and future distribution to other remote sites through this route is possible, install at least twice as many fibers as planned for the short term.
4. Label all cables and fibers at both ends with meaningful names that will not change in the near future (e.g., room numbers, building/floor number).

8.3 Video Broadband Communication System

8.3.1 Broadband System

A broadband video communication system employs single or double cables that can be tapped anywhere along the cable length for immediate two-way access to information. The term "broadband" refers to the transmission of information over a wide band of radio frequencies. Information is encoded and modulated to the RF range (5–450 MHz), and demodulated and decoded at the receiving end, very much the same as in cable television technology.

In particular, a broadband communication system in the context of digital image networks uses a mix of modulation, encoding, and channel allocation to create a two-way communication system that allows both digital and analog information transfer. The capability of transmitting both digital and analog information in a single cable makes the broadband system very attractive to a digital radiology department.

8.3.1.1 Broadband Video

Video information is presented at the display monitor of an imaging device or a workstation as RS-170 analog signals. To place this baseband (base frequency, 30 frames of 525-line video per second) signal onto the broadband cable, the signal must first be frequency-modulated onto a broadband channel. Television channels are simply numerical designators for particular frequency bands on a broadband system. Each channel actually occupies 6 MHz of radio frequency signal some-where between 5 and 450 MHz. Only 4.2 MHz of the 6 MHz channel is used for video signal; the remaining 1.8 MHz serves as a buffer or guard between adjacent channels. Video modulators take the RS-170 signal and modulate it onto a broadband carrier operating within the specified band. This signal is then placed on the broadband cable and mixed with the other channels present.

At the receiving end of the system, a television tuner (broadband demodulator) simply tunes to the appropriate RF channel and demodulates the video information back into RS-170 video, which can be displayed on a video monitor. Theoretically, video information can occupy the entire 5–450 MHz spectrum, thus yielding 74 possible channels. The use of conventional broadcast video equipment allows the use of the predefined television channel system, resulting in a total of 60 available channels. Thus, as many as sixty $512 \times 512 \times 8$ images can be transmitted in a single cable at any instant of time.

8.3.1.2 Broadband Digital

Digital information travels in a broadband cable much as a video signal travels. In this case, the digital information is first encoded as voltage changes, and then it is modulated onto one or more video channels. Unlike video, a single digital signal requires a rather small band of the available channel. For example, a 19.2 Kbaud terminal theoretically requires only a 19.2 kHz channel; thus a 4.2 MHz video channel can accommodate the communication requirement of 200 terminals. Figure 8.8 shows the digital and video channel designations in a typical broadband communication system.

8.3.1.3 Two-Way Broadband Communication

Central to the design of a broadband system is the idea of a central retransmission facility (CRF: sometimes called the head end). This facility allows the use of a single-cable broadband system or two-way communication. The CRF resides at one end of the cable system. The cable system branches out from the CRF in a tree pattern (see Fig. 8.1b) with the CRF at its root. Components such as taps and frequency dividers are designed to allow free flow of certain frequency ranges only in certain directions. Thus, the term *inbound* refers to signals moving toward the CRF and *outbound* refers to signals moving away from the CRF.

In a single-cable system, the frequency spectrum is divided into a return band and a forward band, separated by a guard band. Transmitting devices always transmit toward the CRF using the return band. At the CRF, a channel in the return band is received, and its frequency is shifted by a frequency translator to a higher frequency channel in the forward band. This frequency-shifted signal is then retransmitted outbound from the CRF in the forward band. The outbound signals are available at any tap by way of a demodulator tuned to this higher frequency on the cable tree.

This split-frequency scheme for two-way communication can be applied to both video and digital information. Consider the RS-232 connection, which has both transmit and receive data lines. To use these connections on a broadband system, the

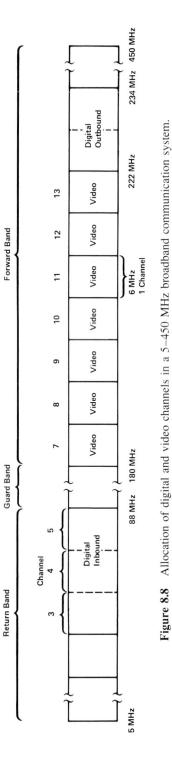

Figure 8.8 Allocation of digital and video channels in a 5–450 MHz broadband communication system.

314

RS-232 connector is plugged into a modulator/demodulator box (modem) that contains both transmit and receive electronics. Each modem has its own unique address and, when in operation, is logically connected to another modem via broadband cable. This logical connection is established by modem hardware or software switches. When a keypress is made on a broadband-connected terminal, the RS-232 signals go out the transmit line of the RS-232 cable to the modem. This signal is packaged along with a source and destination address. The packet containing the data and the addresses is then encoded and modulated onto a low frequency carrier. The low frequency signal, in turn, is placed on the broadband cable, where it travels inbound and is received by the CRF. The frequency translator at the CRF adds a fixed-frequency offset to the signal (e.g., 216 MHz) and retransmits the higher frequency signal outbound. This outbound signal is received by all the modems on the network, but the packet source modem also listens to the message and verifies that it was retransmitted properly. This talk-low, listen-high strategy allows full-featured bidirectional communication. As mentioned, video information can be transmitted in a similar fashion except that no CRF is required if the transmission is unidirectional communication.

The discussion so far has concentrated on a single-cable system. Dual-cable systems are similar in architecture but have the advantage that one cable can be designated inbound and the other outbound. The CRF has only to amplify inbound signals and route them to the outbound cable, without recourse to frequency shifting. In this way, the effective bandwidth of the cable system is doubled (i.e., a full 450 MHz for inbound and 450 MHZ for outbound).

8.3.2 Fiber-Optic Broadband Video Communication System

8.3.2.1 Background

This section gives an example of the use of a fiber-optic broadband video communication system for real-time monitoring of patient CT/MR studies in a large imaging center with multiple CT and MR scanners. The system allows a technologist to transmit CT/MR images to a radiologist in real time for immediate consultation while the patient is being scanned. The radiologist, viewing the images generated during the examination without being physically in the scanner room, can instruct the technologist to continue, change the protocol, or abort the study. The radiologist can also monitor multiple scanners with the broadband system.

Traditional broadband systems use coaxial cable, which has high signal loss and therefore limits the distance between input image source and output viewing station. The fiber-optic broadband system minimizes signal loss and can potentially connect scanners with a radius of 5.0 km.

8.3.2.2 Modeling

To design a fiber-optic broadband video network, we first derive a model to describe the signal loss characteristics due to various components in the communication system. The model

$$SL = F(B, D, M, C, W, TR) \tag{8.1}$$

describes the signal loss SL of the image during the transmission as a function of the image bandwidth B, the distance between two nodes D, the mode of the fiber M, the fiber connector type C, the wavelength of the light W, and the characteristics of the optical transmitter–receiver pair TR. As a first approximation, we assume that F is a linear combination of all these variables.

In this model, the losses associated with D, M, C, and W can be measured through the existing fiber-optic cables using an optical time domain reflectometer (OTDR). The CT/MR images output video signal have a known bandwidth, which is approximately 25 MHz with a horizontal scan rate of 33.36 kHz (1120 lines). The total video signal loss that is acceptable for a system in clinical use is -20 dB based on visual inspection. From this information the optical transmitter–receiver pair can be specified for this system. Unfortunately, the "off the shelf" optical transmitter–receiver pair currently available can accommodate only a 10 MHz video signal bandwidth. Therefore, it is necessary to reduce the bandwidth of the transmitted video signal from 25 MHz to 10 MHz in two stages. First, the video signal is reduced from 25 MHz to 10 MHz; then the 10 MHz video signals are transformed to optical signals for transmission. This can be accomplished by using a fiber-optic laser transmitter tuned to 10 MHz (X285TV-V5, Meret, Inc, Santa Monica, CA). The result is equivalent to passing the image through a low pass filter, hence degradation of image quality is minor.

8.3.2.3 The Video Communication System

The multiplexed broadband video communication system is an established means of image transmission. The term "multiplexed" refers to the method of modulating and combining multiple baseband (single video) signals into a composite broadband signal, effectively using a single-broadband (relatively wide bandwidth) channel to transmit multiple-baseband (relatively narrow bandwidth) channels.

Real-time video images (10 MHz) are transmitted from CT/MR scanners to the head end, where they are converted to specific ranges of radio frequencies and distributed to receivers in a similar manner to that found in cable television technology. The communication medium used is either a multimode (shorter distance) or a single-mode (longer distance) fiber-optic cable. The $512 \times 512 \times 8$ (CT) and $256 \times 256 \times 8$ (MR) pixel images can be assigned to a given channel (10 MHz in bandwidth) in the 5–450 MHz frequency range. The video signal at the scanner is converted from an electrical to an optical signal before being transmitted to a head end. When the video signal is received at the head end, it is converted back from an optical to an electrical signal. Here, it is multiplexed (modulated and combined) with the other scanner video signals, creating a multiplexed, broadband video signal.

Next, the broadband signal is converted from an electrical to an optical splitter, where the signal is distributed to all monitoring stations. Here at the monitoring station, the optical broadband signal is converted back to an electrical signal, demodulated (i.e., channel is selected), and displayed on a viewing monitor.

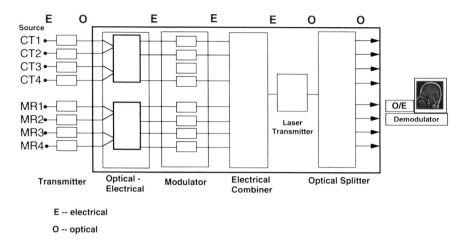

Figure 8.9 Detailed schematic diagram of a fiber-optic broadband system with a connection to eight CT/MR scanners and eight monitoring stations.

Each monitor station consists of an optical receiver, a demodulator (channel selector), and a modified Conrac 1023-line, progressive scan, 8-bit video monitor (Duarte, CA). Figure 8.9 shows the details of the video communication system for eight scanners and eight remote monitoring stations. Monitoring stations are placed in such clinical locations as the thoracic, neuro, abdominal, musculoskeletal, gastro-intestinal, genitourinary, and pediatric radiology reading rooms. Figure 8.10A shows how a monitoring station can be connected with a high resolution video tape recording system for video image archive. Figure 8.10B illustrates displays on two remote monitoring stations: two different images from two MR scanners are shown simultaneously and in real time.

8.3.2.4 Clinical Operation

In any of the monitor stations, a radiologist/physician, by selecting the proper channel assigned to the scanner, can view a patient's CT/MR examination in real time while the study is being performed. The radiologist can communicate with the technologist by telephone to monitor the examination.

This fiber-optic broadband communication system has the two advantages of being inexpensive and capable of transmitting images from many sources in real time. The system can be used primarily as a CT/MR examination monitoring system. The system has some disadvantages, however. First, image quality may not be sufficient for primary diagnosis because the image transmitted to the video monitor is of a lower bandwidth. Second, images appearing on the monitor are volatile and therefore cannot be stored or retrieved later.

To obtain temporary image archiving, this system can be connected to a high resolution video tape recording system (Ampex XVR-80, San Fernando, CA). This

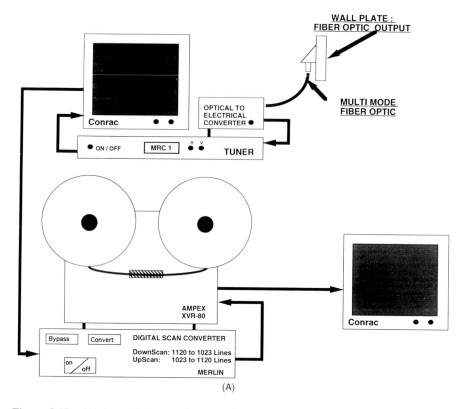

Figure 8.10 (A) A monitoring station turned to the MR scanner (MRC1) is connected to a high resolution video tape recording system for archive. (B) Two monitoring stations at UCSF showing two different images from two MR scanners (MRC1, and MRC2), simultaneously and in real time. Each station is tuned to a different channel.

video recorder coupled with Merlin Engineering's DownScan Converter (Palo Alto, CA), can be connected to any of the monitoring stations to record images from any of the scanners. The resolution of the images saved in this video recorder is equivalent to what appeared on the monitor.

8.4 Digital Communication Networks

8.4.1 Background

Within the PACS infrastructure, the digital communication network is responsible for transmission of images from acquisition devices to the PACS controller and then to display stations. First, images are transmitted from imaging modality devices to image acquisition computers, where the images are staged and reformatted. The

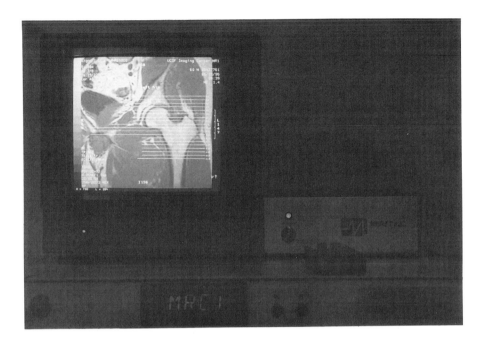

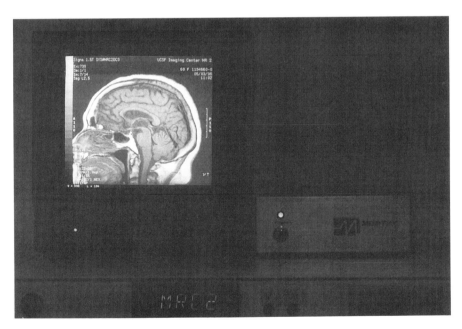

(B)

Figure 8.10   (*continued*)

Table 8.5 Characteristics of Image Transmission in a Radiology Department

	Image Modality Device to Acquisition Computer	Acquisition Computer to PACS Controller	PACS Controller to Display Stations
Speed requirement	Slow: 100 Kbyte/s	Medium: 200–500 Kbyte/s	Fast: 4 Mbyte/s
Technology	Ethernet	Ethernet/FDDI/ATM	ATM
Signaling rate	10 Mbit/s	100 Mbit/s	155 Mbit/s
Cost per connection	1 unit	1–10 units	10 units

reformatted images are sent to the PACS controller, where they are archived permanently on optical disks and categorized in the image database. After images have been categorized, they are transmitted to output stations for either soft copy or hard copy display. Many computers and processors are involved in this image communication chain: some have high speed communication protocols and some do not. Therefore, in designing this network, several communication technologies must be used to accommodate the various computers and processors. The ultimate goal is to have an optimal image throughput in a given clinical environment.

Table 8.5 describes the image transmission rate requirements of a modern radiology department. Transmission from the imaging modality device to the acquisition computer is slow because the imaging modality device is generally slow in generating images. The medium speed requirement from the acquisition computer to the PACS controller reflects the dependence, as a rule, of the type of acquisition computer selected on the characteristics of the imaging modality device computer system or protocols. Typically, the processors used in imaging modality devices do not normally make use of high speed communication protocols. High speed communication between the PACS controller and image display stations is necessary, however, because radiologists and clinicians must access images at a rapid rate: 4 Mbyte/s, equivalent to the transfer of a 2048 × 2048 × 8 bit conventional digitized X-ray image in one second, is the average tolerable waiting time for the physician.

8.4.2 Design Criteria

The five design criteria for the implementation of digital communication networks are speed, standardization, fault tolerance, security, and component cost.

8.4.2.1 Speed of Transmission

From Table 8.5, it is seen that Ethernet should be used as the communication protocol (slow speed) between imaging modality devices and acquisition computers. For image transfer between acquisition computers and the image archive servers, FDDI (medium speed) or ATM should be used if the acquisition computer supports the technology; otherwise, Ethernet hub is acceptable. For image transfer between the PACS controller and an image display station, ATM should be used.

8.4.2.2 Standardization

The throughput performance for each of the three networks described earlier (Ethernet, FDDI, and ATM) can be tuned through the judicious choice of software and operating system parameters. For example, the throughput of TCP/IP networks can be increased by enlarging the TCP send and receive space within the UNIX kernel for Ethernet, FDDI, and ATM network circuits. Alternatively, transmission speed may be enhanced by increasing the memory data buffer size in the application program. The altering of standard network protocols to increase network throughput between a client–server pair can be very effective. The same strategy may prove disastrous in a large communication network, however, since it interferes with network standardization, making it difficult to maintain and service the network. All network circuits should use standard TCP/IP network protocols with a standard buffer size (e.g., 8192 bytes).

8.4.2.3 Fault Tolerance

Communications in the PACS infrastructure should have a backup. All active fiber-optic cables have a duplicate, as does the Ethernet backbone (thicknet and twisted pair). Since the standard TCP/IP protocol can be used over all three networks (Ethernet, FDDI, and ATM), if the higher speed network circuit (ATM or FDDI) fails, the socket-based communications software immediately switches over to the next fastest network, and so forth, until all network circuits have been exhausted. The global Ethernet backbone, through which every computer on the PACS network is connected, is the ultimate backup for the entire PACS network.

8.4.2.4 Security

There are normally two cable systems in an imaging network. The first comprises the cables leased or shared with the campus, or hospital, network authority (CNA). In this case, users should abide by the rules established by the CNA. Once these cables have been connected, the CNA enforces its own security measures and provides service and maintenance.

The second cable system consists of the departmental or internal PACS cables, which are enclosed in conduits with terminations at the hub rooms. The hub rooms should be locked, and no one should be allowed to enter without authorization from a departmental or PACS official.

The global Ethernet should be monitored around the clock with a LAN analyzer. The FDDI and ATM are closed systems and cannot be tapped in. All hospital personnel can access the network to view patients image displays at a work station, similar to the setup at a film library or film light box. Only authorized users are allowed to copy images and to deposit information into the image database through the network.

8.4.2.5 Costs

The digital communication network is designed for clinical use and should be built as a very robust system with redundancy. Cost, although of importance, should not be compromised in the selection of components. Of the three network technologies mentioned, if we consider Ethernet to have a unit cost, then FDDI and ATM would have a cost of 10 units for each computer connection.

8.4.3 Network Models in a PACS Environment

It is advantageous at this point to introduce some network models as a means of measuring the performance of a digital network in a PACS environment. In this discussion, we consider an Ethernet bus topology with eight nodes running TCP/IP protocols used on a server–client basis in which a client node initiates the transfer of image data to a server node. Figure 8.11 shows the topology. The four most commonly occurring cases in a PACS environment are the bidirectional model, the parallel model, the centralized model, and the relay model.

8.4.3.1 Bidirectional Model

Bidirectional communication between two nodes (A and B) is shown in Figure 8.12. Two communication processes, in which one process sends image data from node A to node B while another sends image data from node B to node A, run concurrently.

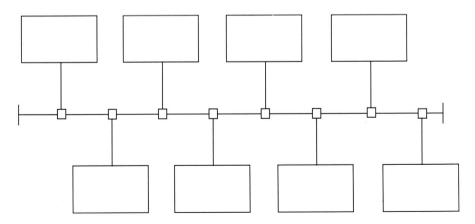

Figure 8.11   An eight-node Ethernet bus topology.

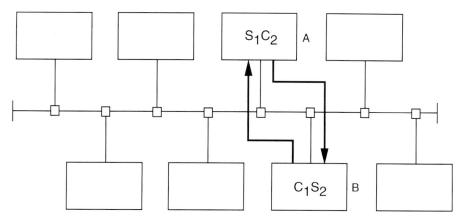

Figure 8.12   The bidirectional model with two communication processes (C, client; S, server) running at each node.

The average transfer rate can be measured using different combinations of the eight nodes. This model resembles the communication between two gateway computers.

8.4.3.2 Parallel Model

In the parallel model, the network is shared by mutually exclusive pairs of nodes. Each pair of nodes runs a client–server process that is independent of processes from other pairs of nodes. Four server–client couples can be arranged using eight nodes, and image transfer can be initiated in sequence one pair at a time. The change in transfer rate of the first pair is measured as the workload of the network increases. Figure 8.13 shows the configuration of the parallel model, which resembles four imaging modalities transmitting images to four acquisition computers.

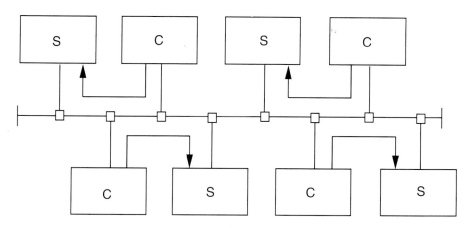

Figure 8.13   The parallel model with four pairs of client (C) and server (S) processes.

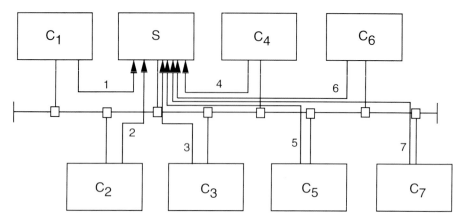

Figure 8.14 The centralized model with one centralized server (S) and seven clients (C_1–C_7). Processes are added successively from 1 to 7.

8.4.3.3 Centralized Model

In the centralized model, image transfer is initiated between two nodes: client 1 and the central server. Transmission processes between the remaining nodes and the central server are added successively. The degradation in network performance, as measured at the server, is due to the increasing load of the number of processes in the network. The central server in the centralized model shown in Figure 8.14 simulates the PACS controller, whereas each client represents an acquisition computer.

8.4.3.4 Relay Model

The relay model (Fig. 8.15) resembles a network in an actual PACS environment. Node A is the PACS controller, which functions both as servers and as clients. Other client nodes function as the acquisition computers, and server nodes function as the display workstations. During the simulation there is a transfer of images between two nodes, A and client 1. Image communication processes between other nodes and node A are successively added.

8.4.3.5 Simulation Data

Figure 8.16 shows some simulation data of the parallel, centralized, and relay models based on some IBM PC and Sun computers of the early 1990s. The simulation results demonstrate the following. First, PACS applications realize only 10–30% of the specific network bandwidth. Second, the transfer rate of each individual process decreases with increasing number of connections, but in most cases the

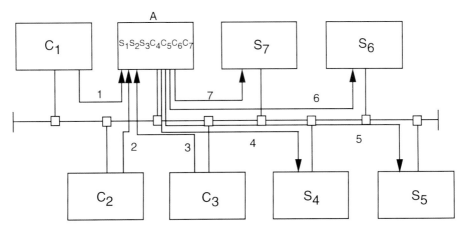

Figure 8.15   The relay model, with node A functional as the PACS controller, C_1, C_2, and C_3 as acquisition computers, and S_4, S_5, S_6, and S_7 as workstations. Processes are added successively from 1 to 7.

overall throughput increases. With this background in network communications, we can discuss the actual PACS network.

8.4.4 PACS Network Design

PACS networks are either external or internal. External networks have minimum security and are connected to information systems, imaging devices, and worksta-tions from the outside world. Internal networks, which have maximum security and are accessible only through layers of security measures, are networks connecting to components within the PACS controller. Another look at Figure 7.1 will emphasize that all networks except those inside the PACS controller are external networks.

8.4.4.1 External Networks

Manufacturer's Image Acquisition Device Network

Major image manufacturers have their only networks for connecting imaging de-vices for better image management. Examples are the General Electric Medical Systems Genesis network and Sienet of Siemens Medical Systems for connecting the respective vendor's CT and MR scanners. Most of these networks are Ethernet based; some use the TCP/IP protocols, and others use proprietary protocols for higher network throughput. If such a network is already in existence, the acquisition computer must be connected to this manufacturer's acquisition device network before CT and MR images can be transmitted to the PACS controller (see again Figs. 7.7 and 7.8). This network has no security with respect to the PACS infrastruc-

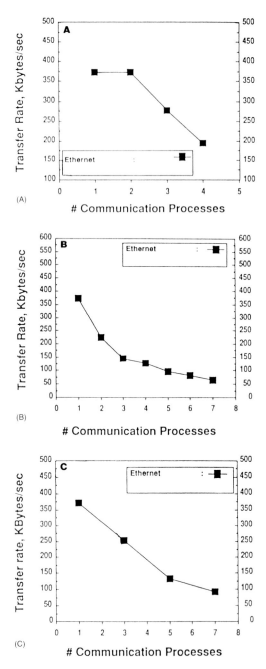

Figure 8.16 Simulation results of the (A) parallel, (B) centralized, and (C) relay models based on an Ethernet bus topology running TCP/IP protocols with early 1990s IBM PC and Sun computers. Buffer size is 2 Kbytes, and measurement is from computer memory to computer memory. Ethernet performance decreases drastically from 365 Kbyte/s to 60 Kbyte/s when the number of server–client pairs increases from one to seven. This result clearly shows the limits of the Ethernet's usefulness as an image communication network when number of connections becomes large.

ture because every user with a password can access the network and obtain all information passing through it.

Hospital and Radiology Information Networks

Hospital and university campuses usually have a campus network authority that operates the institutional network. Among the information systems that go through this network are the HIS and the RIS. Since PACS requires data from both HIS and RIS, this portion of the PACS network is maintained by the campus network authority, over which the PACS network has no control. For this reason, as far as the PACS infrastructure design is concerned, the hospital network is an external network of the PACS.

Research and Other Networks

One major function of PACS is to allow users to access the wealth of the PACS database. A PACS network connection can be set up for connecting research equipment to the PACS. Research equipment should allow access to the PACS database for information query and retrieval. In the PACS infrastructure design, this type of research network is considered an external network.

The Internet

A network carrying information from outside the hospital or the campus through the Internet is considered to be an external network in the PACS infrastructure design. Such a network carries supplemental information for the PACS, ranging from electronic mail and library information systems to files available through FTP.

Display Workstation Networks

Sometimes it is advantageous to have display workstations of similar nature to form a subnetwork for the sharing of information. For example, workstations in a hospital intensive care unit can form an ICU network and neuro workstations can form a neuro network. These display workstation networks are open to all health care personnel to use, and therefore only a minimum security can be imposed. Too many restrictions would deter the users from logging on. However certain layers of priority can be imposed; for example, some users may be permitted to access information but not to deposit it.

8.4.4.2 Internal Networks

A PACS internal network, on the other hand, has maximum security. Data inside the internal network are considered to be clinical data to be archived; they cannot be corrupted. Both image and textual data from acquisition devices and other information systems coming from all the external networks just described except those of display workstations must go through a gateway computer, where data are checked and scrutinized for authenticity before they are allowed to be deposited in the

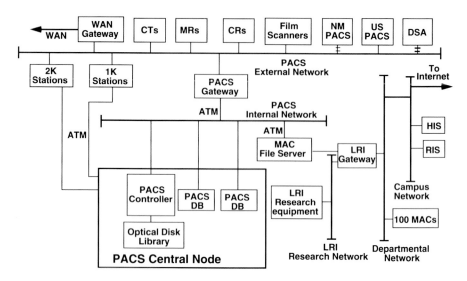

Figure 8.17 Network architecture for the Department of Radiology at the University of California, San Francisco.

internal network. Firewall machines are sometimes incorporated into the gateway computer for this purpose. Only the PACS manager is authorized to allow data to be deposited in the internal network.

8.4.4.3 An Example

The PACS network at the University of California at San Francisco (Fig. 8.17) is an example of a comprehensive PACS. In this architecture, there are several external networks: a wide area network (WAN), the campus network, a departmental network, the Laboratory for Radiological Informatics (LRI) research network, the Internet, the PACS external network, and workstation networks.

Wide Area Network (WAN)

The WAN is used to connect UCSF main campus radiology department with radiology departments from affiliated hospitals and clinics in the San Francisco Bay area. The standard connection is the T1 line (Fig. 8.6 top: Frame Access) with 1.5 Mbit/s and the ATM OC3 with a transmission rate of 155 Mbit/s (Fig. 8.6: bottom, ASX 200).

The Departmental Ethernet

The departmental Ethernet connects 150 Macintosh users in the department. This network is mainly for file transfer and electronic mail, and as a connection to the department image file server, which allows Macintosh users access to the PACS image database and the RIS database. This network is connected to the Laboratory for Radiological Informatics research network through a bridge that allows Macintosh users access to images generated from research equipment. Macintosh users can also have access to the Internet through the campus network. HIS, RIS, and digital voice information are transmitted to the PACS controller first through the campus network and then through the departmental network.

LRI Research Network

The Laboratory for Radiological Informatics research network connects all research equipment in the laboratory, including laser film scanners, laser film printers, images processing computers, research image file servers, display workstations, and the PACS image file server. It also connects to the departmental Ethernet through a bridge.

PACS External Network

The PACS external network connects all digital image acquisition devices in the department, including CTs, MRs, CRs, film digitizers, and the nuclear medicine and US PACS modules. All clinical viewing stations either 1K or 2K are also connected through this network. The WAN ATM gateway and the T1 lines are connected to this network via a router and an ATM gateway computer.

PACS Internal Network

The PACS internal network is a secured network that connects the PACS controller and the PACS database to the PACS external network. The router and the firewall machine protect the internal network by screening all incoming information to the PACS controller. The internal network transmits image files from the PACS image database to the 1K and 2K display stations for clinical use. Macintosh users can also access image files from the PACS controller through the departmental Macintosh image server.

8.4.5 Teleradiology Network Design

In the preceding discussion of PACS network design, we mentioned the PACS external networks. One component in the external network is image and textual information originating outside a local hospital or campus. Such data are essential to teleradiology applications. In Sections 8.4.5.1 and 8.4.5.2 we discuss the various communication methods in teleradiology under the category of WAN.

8.4.5.1 Teleradiology

Technologies used in teleradiology are very similar to those in PACS. Teleradiology can be as simple as sending CT, MR, or US images from an examination site to a radiologist's home for quick review, or as complicated as setting up a large-scale

Table 8.6 Wide Area Network
(WAN) Technology

- DS-0: 56 Kbit/sec
- DS-1 dial-up: 56 Kbit/s to 24 × 56 = 1.344 Mbit/s
- DS-1 Private line (T1): 1.544 Mbit/s
- DS-3 Private line (T3): 28 DS-1 = 45 Mbit/s
- ISDN: 56 Kbit/s–1.544 Mbit/s
- ATM (OC-3): 155 Mbit

Note: DS, digital service; ISDN, integrated service digital network; ATM, asynchronous transfer mode; OC-3, optical carrier level 3.

image and data communication network between referring sites and expert centers. The former application requires minimum WAN technology. In the latter, which is our focus here, the expert center can have the capability of performing telediagnosis, teleconsultation, and telemanagement [these functions are mentioned in ascending order of complexity of technology requirements]. In teleradiology, image compression is a very important factor in keeping costs of communication as low as possible.

Generally speaking, there are five steps in teleradiology: acquiring images from a scanner to the acquisition computer (Section 7.5.2), reformatting (Section 7.4.2), transmission and archiving (Section 8.5), and display (Section 9.1). Table 8.6 shows currently available WAN technology. Table 8.7 compares the costs of the DS-0 and the T1.

There are three possible input methods in teleradiology: a laser film scanner (Section 3.2.4), frame grabber (or video digitizer, see Section 3.2.1.3), and direct digital output with ACR-NEMA or DICOM image format (Section 7.4.2). Depending on the input method, and the tradeoff between speed and cost, there are several choices in communication technology for teleradiology application.

Table 8.7 Cost and Speed Comparison
between DS-0 and T1

Installation, Charges, Speed	Network Lines	
	T1	DS-0
Modem (2)	$12,000	$400
Ethernet converter (2)		
T1 installation	$ 2,500	$100
Total	$14,500	$500
Monthly charge*	$ 600	$ 30
Per call charge*	No	20¢/min, 6 A.M.–6 P.M.
		15¢/min, 6 P.M.–6 A.M.
Speed	200 seconds†	30 × 200 seconds

* Within the San Francisco Bay Area, first quarter, 1995 prices.
† Based on one CT exame, 40 slices (20 MBytes), 50% efficiency, no compression.

8.4.5.2 Communication Methods in Teleradiology

Figure 8.18 shows some teleradiology communication methods. Communication using the T1 line calls for two major components at each node: a multiplexer and a CSU/DSU (channel service unit/data service unit) (see Table 8.7) for the cost). The

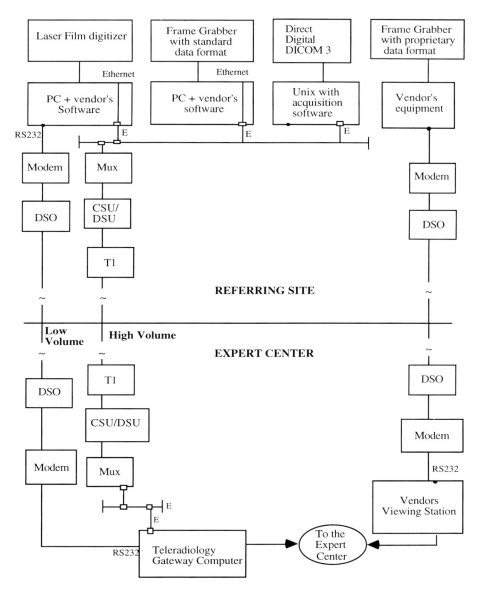

Figure 8.18   Communication methods in teleradiology: CSU/DSU, channel service unit/ data service unit; Mux, multiplexer.

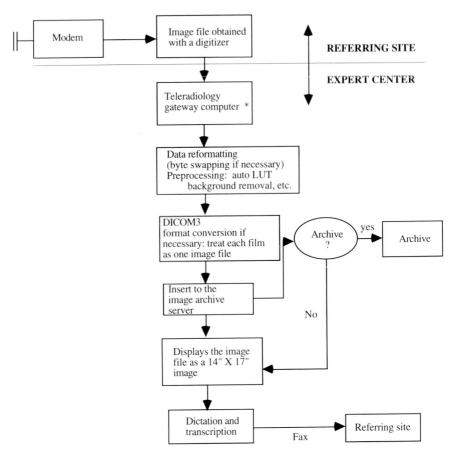

* The gateway computer also performs bookkeeping functions.

Figure 8.19 Example of data flow at the expert center in a teleradiology communication network.

DS-0 needs only a modem at each node. Figure 8.19 shows an example of how the expert center described here handles the images received.

8.4.6 Telepathology and Teleradiology

Telepathology is the transmission of digital microscopic images through a WAN. In telemedicine applications, telepathology and teleradiology can be combined into one system. Figure 8.20 shows an example of a generic combined telepathology and teleradiology system; its major components and their functions are described as follows:

1. A 1K film scanner for digitization.
2. A 512-line display system for quality control.

3. A personal computer (PC) with four functions:
   (a) (for the teleradiology application) software for image acquisition, input patient data, and data communication
   (b) (for the telepathology application) software for automatic focusing, x–y stage motion, color filter switching, and frame grabbing
   (c) a database for managing images and textual data
   (d) a standard communication protocol for LAN and WAN
4. A light microscope with automatic focusing; an x–y stepping motor controlled stage; red, green, and blue color filters; and a CCD camera.
5. Standard communication hardware for LAN and WAN.
6. Communication carrier (e.g., T-1 or ISDN).
7. The display station at the expert site should be able to display a 1K × 1K monochromatic image, and 512 color images with standard user interface. It needs a local database to manage the local data. The display station should be able to control the motion of the microscopic stage as well as the automatic focusing.

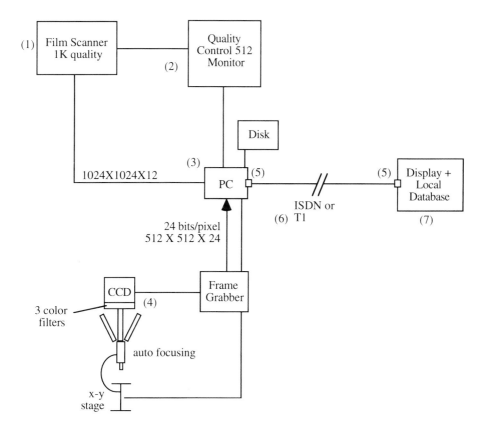

Figure 8.20 A combined teleradiology and telepathology system for the transmission of image and textual data. ISDN, integrated service digital network.

8.5 The PACS Central Node

The PACS central node, the engine of the PACS (see Figs. 7.1 and 8.17), has two components: the PACS controller and an image storage management system. The former, consisting of the hardware and software architecture, directs the data flow in the complete PACS using interprocess communication among major processes. The latter provides a hierarchical image storage management system for short-, medium-, and long-term image archiving. Sections 8.5.1 and 8.5.2 describe the design concept and implementation strategy of the PACS central node.

8.5.1 Design Concept

Two major aspects should be considered in the design of the image storage management system: data integrity, which promises no loss of images once received by the PACS from the imaging systems; and system efficiency, which minimizes access time for images at the display stations. Now we turn to some major issues in storage management system design.

8.5.1.1 Local Storage Management via PACS Intercomponent Communication

To ensure data integrity, the PACS always retains two copies of an individual image on separate storage devices until the image has been archived successfully to the long-term storage device (e.g., an optical disk library). Figure 8.21 shows the various storage subsystems in the PACS. This backup scheme is achieved via the PACS intercomponent communication, which can be broken down as follows:

- *At the radiologic imaging device.* Images are not deleted from the imaging device's local storage unless technologists have verified the successful archiving of individual images via the PACS terminals. In the event of failure of the acquisition process or of the archive process, images can be re-sent from these imaging systems to the PACS.
- *At the acquisition computer.* Images acquired in the acquisition computer remain on its local magnetic disks until the archive subsystem has acknowledged to the acquisition computer that a successful archive has been achieved. These images are then deleted from the magnetic disks residing in the acquisition computer, so that storage space from these disks can be reclaimed.
- *At the PACS central node.* Images arriving in the archive server from various acquisition nodes are not deleted until they have been successfully archived to the optical storage. On the other hand, all archived images are stacked in the archive server's cache magnetic disks and will be deleted based on aging criteria (e.g., number of days ago an examination was performed; discharge or transfer of a patient).
- *At the display station.* Images stored in the designated display station will remain there until the patient is discharged or transferred. Images in the PACS archive can be retrieved from any display station via PACS intercomponent communication.

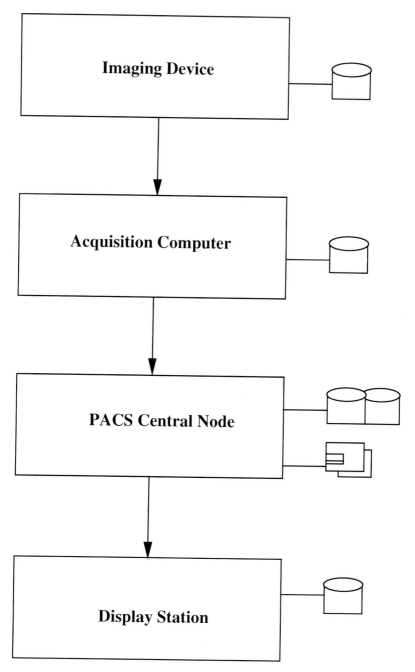

Figure 8.21   Various storage subsystems in the PACS to ensure data integrity. Until an individual image has been archived in the permanent storage (optical WORM), two copies of it are retained on separate storage (magnetic) devices.

Table 8.8 Multiple Storage in the Storage Management System

Level	Storage Medium	Location	Purpose	Optimal Capacity (GByte)
1	Redundant array of inexpensive disks (RAID): temporary storage	PACS controller (archive server)	Provides immediate access to both current and selected historical images	10–30
2	Magnetic disks: temporary storage	Archive subsystem (archive server)	Provides fast retrieval of current images	10
3	Magneto-optical disks: temporary longer	Archive subsystem (optical disk library)	Provides retrieval of historical images	500
4	Write Once Read many disks (WORM)	Archive subsystem (optical disk library)	Provides retrieval of historical images	1000–3000

8.5.1.2 *Multiple Storage Media*

The storage management system in the PACS central node can have storage media of four types: (1) a redundant array of inexpensive disks (RAID) for immediate access for current image, (2) magnetic disks for fast retrieval of cached images, (3) erasable magneto-optical disks for temporary long-term archive, and (4) write once, read many (WORM) disks in the optical disk library, which constitute the permanent archive. All local magnetic disks in the radiologic imaging systems and the acquisition computers are used for storing newly acquired images. These images are deleted once they have been successfully archived to the WORM disks. Table 8.8 shows the configuration of these multiple-level storage media.

Low speed disk I/O has been a major obstacle to the quick retrieval of high volume image data from the PACS storage devices. Service delay at the display stations due to access latency on images certainly reduces user confidence, hence diminishes acceptance of the PACS. A solution for improving data access from storage media is the RAID technology introduced in late 1980s. This technology uses a disk striping technique to bind multiple disks so that data can be broken down into "chunks" and distributed evenly across the striped disks. Since RAID disks support concurrent access to segmented data, their aggregate I/O performance improves.

8.5.2 System Configuration

The archive system consists of four major components: an archive server, a database system, an optical disk library, and a communication network (Fig. 8.22). Attached to the archive system through the communication network are the acquisition computers and the display stations. Images acquired by the acquisition computers

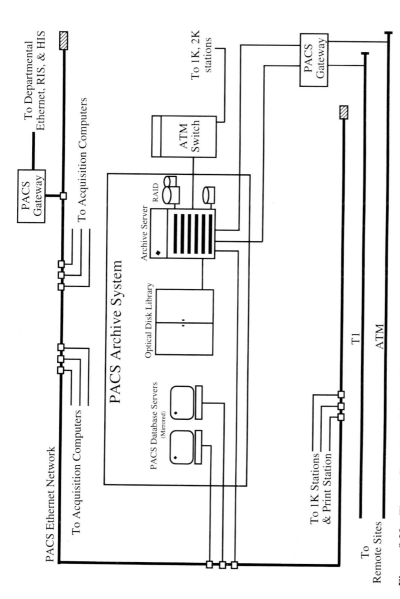

Figure 8.22 The configuration of the archive system and the PACS network. A server machine connected to an optical disk library serves as an archive server, two host computers serve as a mirrored database system, a global Ethernet network interconnects all PACS components, and a high speed ATM network connects the archive server to 1K and 2K display stations, providing fast image display. In addition, the archive server is connected to remote sites, the hospital information system (HIS), and the radiology information system (RIS) via departmental and campus Ethernet networks, T1 lines, and the asynchronous transfer mode (ATM) network.

337

from various radiologic imaging devices are transmitted to the archive server, from which they are archived to the optical disk library and routed to the appropriate display stations.

8.5.2.1 The Archive Server

The archive server should be powerful, with multiple central processing units (CPUs), small computer systems interface (SCSI) data buses, and network interfaces (Ethernets and ATM). With its redundant hardware configuration, the archive server can support multiple processes running simultaneously, and image data can be transmitted over different data buses and networks. In addition to its primary function of archiving images, the archive server acts as a PACS controller, mastering the flow of images within the entire PACS from the acquisition computers to various destinations such as the display stations or the print station.

The archive server uses its large capacity RAID or magnetic disks as a data cache, capable of storing 2 weeks' worth of images acquired from different radiologic imaging devices. As an example, a 13.6 Gbyte RAID can hold simultaneously up to 500 computed tomography (CT), 1000 magnetic resonance (MR), and 500 computed radiography (CR) studies. In this example, each CT or MR study consists of a complete sequence of slice images from one examination, and each CR study consists of one exposure. The calculation is based on the average study sizes in the field, in megabytes: CT, 11.68; MR, 3.47; CR, 7.46. The magnetic cache disks configured in the archive server should sustain high data throughput for the read operation, which provides fast retrieval of recent images from these RAID or magnetic disks instead of the slower optical disks.

8.5.2.2 The Database System

The database system should comprise redundant database servers, running identical reliable commercial database systems (e.g., Sybase, Oracle), with Structured Query Language (SQL) utilities. The system should have a mirroring effect, duplicating the data in the two database servers. The data can be queried from any PACS computer via the communication networks. The mirroring feature of the system provides the entire PACS database with uninterruptible data transactions that guarantee no loss of data in the event of system failure or disk crash.

Besides its primary role of image indexing to support the retrieval of images, the database system should be interfaced with the radiology information system (RIS) and hospital information system (HIS), allowing the PACS database to collect additional patient information from these two health care databases.

8.5.2.3 The Optical Disk Library

The optical disk library should consist of multiple optical drives and disk controllers, which allow concurrent archival and retrieval operations on all its optical drives. The library should have a large storage capacity, in the terabyte range (1 Tbyte = 10^{12} bytes), and should support both erasable and WORM optical disks in a mixed-media mode. Redundant power supply is essential for uninterrupted operation.

The average overall throughputs for read and write operations between the magnetic disks of the archive server and the optical disks can reach 1.0 Mbyte/s.

8.5.2.4 The Communication Network

The PACS archive system should connect to both the local area network and the wide area network. The PACS LAN can have a two-tiered communication network composed of Ethernet and ATM networks. The WAN provides connection to remote sites and can consist of T1 lines and ATM transport.

The PACS LAN uses the high speed ATM to transmit high volume image data from the archive server to 1K and 2K display stations. The low cost standard Ethernet is used for interconnecting PACS components to the image server, including acquisition computers, RIS and HIS, and 1K and 2K display stations. The Ethernet is also used as a backup of the ATM. Failure of the ATM automatically triggers the archive server to reconfigure the communication network so that images will be transmitted to the 1K and 2K display stations over the Ethernet.

8.5.3 System Software

All software implemented in the archive server should be coded in a standard programming language—for example, C on the UNIX open systems architecture. In the archive server, processes of diverse functions run independently and communicate simultaneously with other processes using client–server programming, queuing control mechanisms, and job prioritizing mechanisms. Figure 8.23 shows the interprocess communications among the major processes running on the archive server and Table 8.9 describes the functions of these processes.

Major tasks performed by the archive server include image receiving, image stacking, image routing, image archiving, studies grouping, platter management, RIS interfacing, PACS database updating, image retrieving, and image prefetching. Sections 8.5.3.1–8.5.3.10 describe the functionality carried out by each of these tasks.

8.5.3.1 Image Receiving

Images acquired from various radiologic imaging devices in the acquisition computers are converted into ACR-NEMA or DICOM data format. From these acquisition computers, the reformatted images are transmitted to the archive server via the Ethernet or ATM by using client–server applications over standard TCP/IP protocols. The archive server can accept concurrent connections for receiving images from multiple acquisition computers.

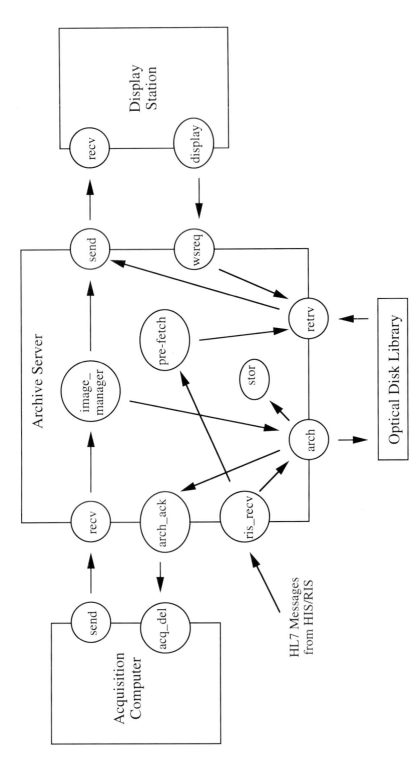

Figure 8.23 Interprocess communications among the major processes running on a PACS archive server: HL7, Health Level 7; other symbols defined in Table 8.9.

Table 8.9 Processes in the Archive Server

Process	Description
arch	Copy images from magnetic disks to erasable optical disks (before patient discharge) and from erasable optical disks to WORM disks (at patient discharge); update PACS data base; notify stor and *arch_ack* processes for successful archiving.
arch_ack	Acknowledge acquisition computers for successful archiving.
acq_del	Process at acquisition computers; delete images from local magnetic disks
image_manager	Process image information; update PACS data base; notify *send* and *arch* processes.
pre-fetch	Select historical images and relevant text data from PACS data base; notify *retrv* process.
recv	Receive images from acquisition computers; notify *image_manager* process.
ris_recv	Receive Health Level 7 messages (e.g., patient admission, discharge, and transfer; examination scheduling; impression; diagnostic reports) from the RIS; notify *arch* process to group and copy images from erasable optical disks to WORM disk (at patient discharge, notify *pre-fetch* process (at scheduling of an examination), or update PACS database (at receipt of an impression or a diagnostic report).
retrv	Retrieve images from optical disks; notify *send* process.
send	Send images to destination stations.
stor	Manage magnetic storage of the archive server.
wsreq	Handle retrieve requests from the display process at the *display* stations.
display	Acknowledge archive server for images received.

8.5.3.2 *Image Stacking*

Images arrived in the archive server from various acquisition computers are stacked in its local magnetic disks. The archive server holds as many images in its 10–30 Gbyte magnetic disks as possible and manages them on the basis of aging criteria. During a hospital stay, for example, images belonging to a given patient remain on the archive server's magnetic disks until the patient is discharged or transferred. Thus all recent images that are not already in a display station's local storage can be retrieved from the archive server's high speed magnetic disks instead of the low speed optical disks. This feature is particularly convenient for radiologists or referring physicians who must retrieve images from different display stations.

8.5.3.3 *Image Routing*

Images that have arrived in the archive server from various acquisition computers are immediately routed to their destination display stations. The routing process is driven by a predefined routing table composed of parameters including examination type, display station site, radiologist, and referring physician. All images are classified by examination type (1-view Chest, CT-Head, CT-Body, etc.) as defined in the RIS, and the destination display stations are classified by location (Chest, Pediatrics, CCU, etc.), as well as by resolution (1K or 2K). The routing algorithm performs table lookup based on the aforementioned parameters and determines an image's destination(s).

Images are transmitted to the 1K and 2K stations over either Ethernet LAN or ATM, and to remote sites over dedicated T1 lines or the ATM WAN.

8.5.3.4 Image Archiving

Images arriving in the archive server from various acquisition computers are copied from temporary storage on magnetic disks to the erasable optical disks for longer term storage. When transfer to the optical disks is complete, the archive server will acknowledge the corresponding acquisition computer, allowing that system to delete the image from its local storage and reclaim its disk space. In this way, the PACS always has two copies of an image on separate magnetic disk systems until the image is archived to an optical disk.

Images that belong to a given patient during a hospital stay will be scattered across the erasable optical disks and will remain on these disks until the patient is discharged or transferred.

8.5.3.5 Studies Grouping

During a hospital stay, a patient may have different examinations on different days. Each of these examinations may consist of multiple studies. Upon discharge or transfer of the patient, images from these studies are grouped from the erasable optical disks and copied contiguously to a single WORM disk or to consecutive WORM disks for permanent storage. Once these images have been archived permanently, they are removed from the erasable optical disks, permitting storage space on the erasable disks to be reclaimed.

8.5.3.6 Platter Management

Studies grouping allows all images belonging to a patient during a hospital stay to be archived contiguously to optical disk(s). Platter management, on the other hand, manages the storage space reserved in the WORM disks for future images in case a patient revisits or is readmitted. In this way, images of a patient from multiple hospital visits can be accumulated on a single WORM disk or on consecutive disks, reducing excess disk swapping and, consequently, minimizing retrieval time for these images. It is expensive, however, to preallocate storage space on an optical disk for a particular patient. To minimize the disk space preallocated for individual patients, the storage management software should allow the PACS archive process to group multiple optical disks into one volume. In addition to saving disk space, logically grouping consecutive optical disks into one volume can reduce disk swapping time, hence speeding up the retrieval time for images resident on different disks in the same volume. Figure 8.24 illustrates the studies grouping and platter management mechanisms.

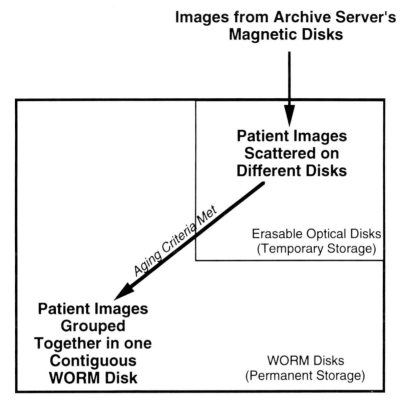

Figure 8.24 Studies grouping and platter management: current images are copied from the magnetic disks of the archive server to erasable optical disks; when an aging criterion is met (e.g., a given patient is discharged or transferred), images belonging to that patient are grouped and copied contiguously to WORM disks for permanent storage.

8.5.3.7 RIS and HIS Interfacing

The archive server accesses the HIS/RIS through a PACS gateway computer. The HIS/RIS relays a patient admission, discharge, and transfer (ADT) message to PACS only when a patient is scheduled for an examination in the radiology department, or when a patient in the radiology department is discharged or transferred. Forwarding ADT messages to PACS not only supplies patient demographic data to the PACS but also provides knowledge the archive server needs to initiate the prefetch, studies grouping, and platter management mechanisms. Exchange of messages among these heterogeneous computer systems should be in Health Level 7 (HL7) standard data format using TCP/IP protocols on a client–server basis.

In addition to receiving ADT messages, PACS receives examination data and diagnostic reports from the RIS. This information is then used to update the PACS database, which can be queried and reviewed from any display station.

8.5.3.8 PACS Database Updates

Data transactions performed in the archive server, such as insertion, deletion, selection, and update, are carried out using SQL utilities in the database. Data in the PACS database are stored in predefined tables, with each table describing only one kind of entity. For example, the patient description table consists of master patient records, which store patient demographics; the study description table consists of study records describing individual radiological procedures; the archive directory table consists of archive records for individual images; and the diagnosis history table consists of diagnostic reports of individual examinations. These tables are updated by individual PACS processes running on the archive server with information extracted from image headers or RIS interface to reflect any changes of the corresponding tables.

8.5.3.9 Image Retrieving

Image retrieval takes place at the display stations. The display station is connected to the archive system through the communication networks. The optical disk library in the archive system configured with multiple optical drives can support concurrent image retrievals from multiple optical disks. The retrieved data are then transmitted from the optical disk library to the archive server via the SCSI data buses.

The archive server handles retrieve requests from display stations according to the priority level of these individual requests. Priority is assigned to individual display stations and users based on different levels of needs. For example, highest priority is always granted to a display station that is used for primary diagnosis or is in a conference session or at an intensive care unit. Thus, in effect, a display station used exclusively for research and teaching purposes is compromised to allow "fast service" to radiologists and referring physicians in the clinic for immediate patient care.

The archive system should support image retrievals at 2K display stations for online primary diagnosis, 1K stations for ICU and review stations, and Macintosh stations for personal offices throughout the hospital. To retrieve images from the optical disk library, the user at a display station can activate the retrieval function and request any number of images from the archive system.

8.5.3.10 Image Prefetching

The prefetching mechanism is initiated as soon as the archive server detects the arrival of a patient via the ADT message from HIS/RIS. Selected historical images, patient demographics, and relevant diagnostic reports are retrieved from the optical disk library and the PACS database. Such data are distributed to the destination display station(s) prior to completion of the patient's current examination. The prefetch algorithm is based of predefined parameters such as examination type, disease category, radiologist, referring physician, location of display station, and the number and age of the patient's archived images. These parameters determine which historical images should be retrieved.

8.5.4 System Operations

The archive system should operate 24 hours a day, 7 days a week. All operations should be software driven and automatic; the system should not require any manual-operated procedures. Full disks removed from the library are managed by the PACS database and can be reinserted as needed for retrieval of historical images. The only nonautomatic procedure is the addition of new or removal of old optical disks to make room for new disks from the optical disk library; such media must be manually inserted into or removed from the library.

A fault-tolerant mechanism in the archive system should be established to ensure data integrity and minimize system downtime. Major features of this mechanism include the following:

1. An uninterruptible power supply (UPS) system, which protects all archive components, including the archive server, database servers, and optical disk library, from power outages.
2. A mirrored database system, which guarantees data integrity.
3. Multiple optical drives and robotic arms, which provide uninterruptible image archival and retrieval in the event of operation failure of a single optical drive or robotic arm.
4. A central monitoring system, which automatically alerts quality control staff via RS-232 terminals and pagers to salvage any malfunctioning archive components or processes.
5. Spare parts for immediate replacement of any malfunctioning computer components, which may include network adapter boards, SCSI controllers, and the multi-CPU system board (archive server).
6. A 4-hour turnaround manufacturer's on-site service, which minimizes system downtime due to hardware failure of any major archive component.

8.6 Interface with HIS and RIS

8.6.1 Background

Access to an external information system can be designed in three different ways with varying degrees of complexity. The interface of HIS, RIS, and PACS utilizes all three methods.

8.6.1.1 Terminal Emulation

A system that emulates the terminal of a remote host computer allows the user to perform any of its functions. For example, the user at a PACS workstation can emulate the RIS terminal by viewing the diagnostic reports for a specific patient.

The user can also perform any RIS administration function, such as scheduling a new examination, updating patient demographics, or recording a film movement. However, this method provides no data exchange or system integration. The user is therefore required to master different database systems and interfaces. In addition, RIS and HIS cannot emulate the PACS terminal, since the configuration of PACS is too specific.

8.6.1.2 Database-to-Database Transfer

A database-to-database transfer allows two or more information systems to share a subset of information by storing in their local databases some data provided through the communications network by remote information systems. This operation includes making the external data meaningful to the local information systems. Some software is required, however, because before storage, the data must be reformatted according to the local conventions for data representation. The database-to-database method is most often used to share information between HIS and RIS.

8.6.1.3 Heterogeneous Distributed Database System

It is possible to provide a single interface and language to access data distributed in several heterogeneous database systems; the data appear to the user to be managed by a single integrated database. A query protocol is responsible for analyzing the requested information, identifying the databases required to answer it, fetching the information, assembling the results, and presenting this material to the user. Ideally, all this is done transparently and without affecting the autonomy of each database system. Currently available commercial database management products do not provide the possibility of sharing information or communicating with database management systems of other types, however, and as a result the requirements for transparency and uncompromised autonomy are not easy to achieve.

8.6.2 HIS and RIS

A hospital information system (HIS) is a computerized management system for handling three categories of tasks in a hospital environment: the support of clinical and medical patient care activities in the hospital, the administration of the hospital (financial, personnel, payroll, bed census, etc.), and the management and control operations to assist in long-range planning and evaluation of hospital performances and costs. Radiology information systems (RIS) was originally a component of HIS. Later, independent RIS was developed, probably because of the limited ability of HIS to support the handling of information related to the radiology department. The RIS is designed to support both administrative and clinical parts of a radiological department, to reduce administrative overhead, and to improve the quality of radiological examination delivery. Therefore, RIS mostly manages general radiology patient demographics and billing information, procedure descriptions and scheduling, diagnostic reports, patient arrival scheduling, film location, film movement, and examination room scheduling. The RIS configuration is very similar to the HIS but is on a smaller scale. The RIS equipment consists of a departmental computer with peripheral devices such as alphanumeric terminals, printers, and bar code readers. Most independent RISs are autonomous systems with limited access to HIS. However, some HISs offers embedded RIS subsystems with a higher degree of integration.

8.6.3 Reasons for Interfacing PACS with HIS and RIS

In a hospital environment, interfacing the PACS, RIS, and HIS has become necessary to enhance four functions described in Sections 8.6.3.1–8.6.3.4.

8.6.3.1 Diagnostic Process

The diagnostic process at the PACS display station includes not only the recall of images illustrating the case of interest but also the display of textual information describing patient history and studies. Along with the image data and the image description, a PACS should provide all related text information acquired and managed by the RIS and the HIS in a way that is useful to a radiologist during the diagnostic process. RIS and HIS information such as clinical diagnosis, radiological reports, and patient history are indeed necessary at the PACS workstation to complement the images of the cases being viewed.

8.6.3.2 PACS Image Management

Some information provided by the RIS can be integrated into PACS image management algorithms to optimize the routing of the image data on the network to the requesting locations (see Section 8.5.3.3). In the PACS database, which stores huge volumes of data, a sophisticated image management system is required to handle these image data.

8.6.3.3 RIS Administration

Planning of a digital-based radiology department requires the reorganization of some administrative operations carried out by the RIS. For example, the PACS will need to be able to share some information, such as the image archive status and the image data file. RIS administration operations would also benefit from interfacing to the HIS by gaining access to some knowledge about patient admission, discharge, and transfer (ADT).

8.6.3.4 Research and Teaching

Much research and teaching in radiology involves mass screening of clinical cases and determining what constitutes a normal versus an abnormal condition for a given patient population. The corresponding knowledge includes diverse types of information that need to be correlated, such as image data, results from analyzed images, medical diagnosis, patient demographics, study description, and various patient conditions. Some mechanisms are needed to access and to retrieve data from either the HIS or the RIS during a search for detailed medical and patient information related to image data. Cooperation between diverse medical database systems such as HIS, RIS, and PACS is therefore critical to the successful management of research and teaching issues in radiology.

8.6.4 Some Rules

To interface the HIS, RIS, and PACS, some basic rules must be followed.

1. Each system (HIS, RIS, PACS) remains unchanged in its configuration, data, and functions performed.
2. Each system is hardware- and software-extended, to allow communication with other systems.
3. Only data are shared; functions remain local. For example, RIS functions cannot be performed at the PACS or the HIS workstation. Keeping each system specific and autonomous will simplify the interface process, since database updates will not be allowed at a global level.

Based on these rules, successfully interfacing HIS, RIS, and PACS includes the following steps:

1. Identify the subset data that will be shared with the other systems. Access rights and authorization problems are solved during this process.
2. Convert the data to a standard form (e.g., HL7). This step, which consists of designing a high level presentation, solving data inconsistencies, and naming conventions, can be accomplished by using a common data model and data language, and by defining rules of correspondence between various data definitions.
3. Define the protocol of data transfer (e.g., using TCP/IP or DICOM TCP/IP).

8.6.5 Common Data in HIS, RIS, and PACS

The system software in the PACS archive server described in Section 8.5.3 requires certain data from HIS and RIS. This store of data is necessary for the archive server to archive images and associated data in the optical disk library properly and to distribute them to the display workstation in a timely manner. Figure 8.25 illustrates information common to the HIS, RIS, and PACS. Table 8.10 describes the data definition, the origin and the destination, and the action that triggers the system software functions.

8.6.6 Implementation of the RIS–PACS Interface

Two methods of implementing the RIS–PACS interface are trigger mechanisms and the query protocol. These approaches are discussed in turn.

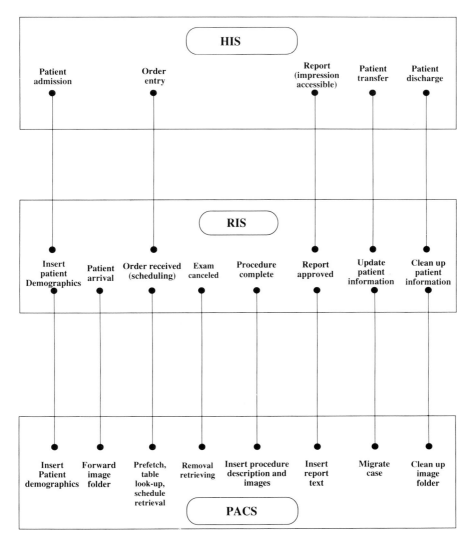

Figure 8.25   Information transfer from the HIS to the RIS, and from the RIS to the PACS.

8.6.6.1 Trigger Mechanism Between Two Databases

In HL7 format the PACS is notified of the following events when they occur in the RIS: ADT, order received, patient arrival, examination canceled, procedure complete, and report approved. The application level of the interface software waits for the occurrence of one of these events and triggers the corresponding data to be sent. The communication level transfers the HL7 file to the PACS image file server using two processes *send* (to PACS) and *ris_recv*. The PACS image file server receives this file and archives it in the database tables for subsequent use. Figure 8.26 shows the trigger mechanism interface. The trigger mechanism is used when a small

Table 8.10 Information Transferred Between the HIS, RIS, and PACS Triggering Events in the PACS File Server

Events	Message	From	To	Action	Location
1. Admission	Previous images/ reports	HIS/RIS	PACS file server	Preselected images and reports transferred from permanent optical archive to workstations	WS at FL, RR
2. Order entry	Previous images/ reports	RIS	File server, scanner	Check event 1 for completion	WS at FL, RR
3. Arrival	Patient arrival	RIS	File server, scanner	Check events 1 and 2 for completion	WS at FL, RR
4. Examination	New images	Scanner	RIS, file server	New images to Folder Manager;* WS	Temporary optical archive; WS at FL, RR
5. Dictation	"Wet" reading	RR	Digital dictaphone	Dictation recorded on DD, digital voice to Folder Manager* and to WS	DD; WS at FL, RR
6. Transcript	Preliminary report	RR	RIS, file server	Prelim report to RIS, temporary optical archive and to WS, dictation erased from DD	RIS; temporary optical archive; WS at FL, RR
7. Signature	Final report	RR	RIS, file server	Final report to RIS, to WS, and to temporary optical archive; preliminary report erased.	RIS: temporary optical archive; WS at FL, RR
8. Transfer	Patient transfer	RIS	File server	Transfer image files	WS at new location
9. Discharge	Images, report	HIS/RIS	File server	Patient folder copied from temporary optical archive to permanent optical archive, patient folder erased from WS	WS at FL, RR; temporary and permanent optical archive

* See Section 9.5.1.2

Note: DD, digital dictaphone; FL, floors in the ward; RR, reading rooms in the radiology department; WS, workstations.

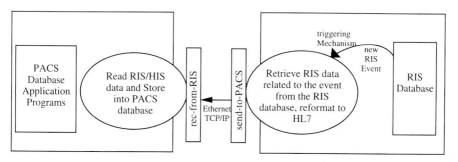

Figure 8.26 RIS and PACS interface architecture implemented using a database-to-database transfer with a trigger mechanism.

amount of predefined information from RIS needs to be available in the PACS in a systematic and timely fashion. In addition to requiring storage overhead in both databases, this method is tedious for information updating and unsuitable for user queries.

8.6.6.2 Query Protocol

The query protocol allows access to information from the HIS, RIS, and PACS databases by using an application layer software on top of these heterogeneous database systems. From a PACS workstation, users can retrieve information uniformly from any of these systems and automatically integrate the data to one answer. The application layer software should utilize the following standards:

SQL as the global query language
relational data model as the global data model
TCP/IP communication protocols
HL7 data format

Figure 8.27 illustrates the query protocol.

8.7 Interface with Other Medical Databases

8.7.1 Other Medical Databases

The many functions of a radiology specialist in a large medical center include consulting with primary and referring physicians on the proper radiological procedures for patients, performing the procedures, reading images from the procedures, and dictating and confirming reports. Referring physicians review images with the radiologists and receive consultation. Based on these radiological images, reports, and consultations, the requesting physicians prescribe the proper treatment plan for their patients. The radiologists also use the images from the procedures and the corresponding reports to train fellows, residents, and medical students.

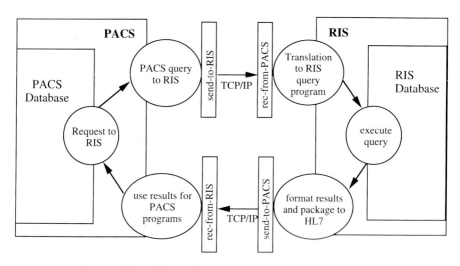

Figure 8.27   RIS and PACS interface with a query protocol.

In their practice, radiologists often request from medical records other necessary patient information (e.g., demographic data, laboratory tests, consultation reports from other medical specialists). Radiologists also review literature from the library information systems and give *formal rounds* to educate colleagues on radiological procedures and new radiological techniques. Thus, the practice of radiology requires integrating various types of information—voice, text, medical records, images, and video recordings—into proper files. These various types of information exist on different media and are stored in data systems of different types. The advance of computer and communication technologies allows the possibility of integration of these various types of information to facilitate the practice of radiology. We have already discussed two such information systems, namely, HIS and RIS.

8.7.2 Multimedia in the Radiology Environment

"Multimedia" has different meanings depending on the context. In the radiology environment, the term refers to the integration of medical information related to radiology practice. This information is stored in various databases in voice form or as text records, images, or video. Patient demographic information, clinical laboratory test results, pharmacy information, and pathological reports are stored in the HIS. The radiological images are stored in the PACS optical disk library archiving system, and its corresponding reports are stored in the reporting system of the RIS. The electronic mail and files are stored in the personal computer system database. The digital learning files are categorized in the learning laboratory or the library in the department of radiology. Some of these databases may exist in a primitive way in the sense that the digital and communication technology used is primitive; others—PACS, for example—can be very advanced. Thus, the challenge of developing multimedia in the radiology environment is to establish infrastructure for the seamless integration of this medical information by means of blending different technologies, while providing an acceptable data transmission rate to various parts of the department and to various sites in the hospital. Once the multimedia infrastructure has been established, various medical information can exist as modules and be interfaced to this infrastructure In the multimedia environment, radiologists (or their medical colleagues) can access this information through a user-friendly, inexpensive, efficient, and reliable interactive workstation.

RIS, HIS, electronic mail, and files involve textual information running to 1K or 2K bytes. Although developing interface to each information system is tedious, the technology involved is manageable. On the other hand, PACS contains image files that can be in the neighborhood of 20–40 Mbytes. The transmission and storage requirements for PACS are manyfold that of text information. For this reason, PACS becomes central in developing multimedia in the radiology environment. Figure 8.28 illustrates the concept of multimedia in the radiology environment.

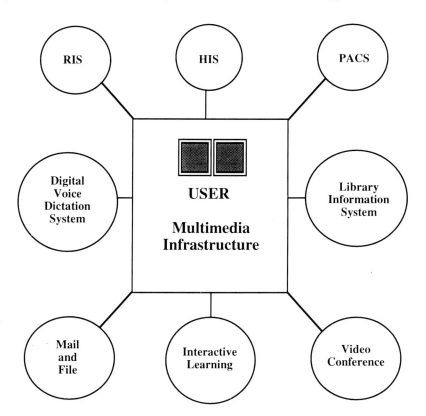

Figure 8.28 Concept of multimedia in the radiology environment. User can use single or multiple monitors; multiple database can be accessed at a desktop workstation.

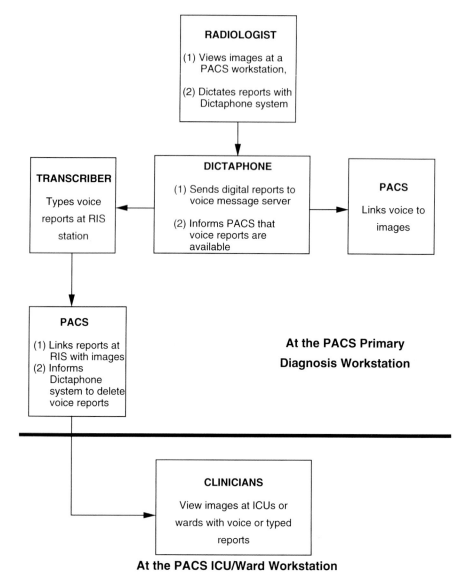

Figure 8.29 Operational procedure when a digital voice system is connected with the PACS.

8.7.3 Integration of Heterogeneous Databases: Digital Voice with PACS

For multimedia to operate effectively in the radiology environment, at least five heterogeneous databases must be integrated, namely, the HIS, RIS, PACS, electronic mail and file, and digital voice dictation systems. In Section 8.6 we described the

HIS–RIS interface. In this section, we describe the digital voice system. Discussion of electronic mail and files is deferred until Chapter 9.

Typically, radiological reports are archived and transmitted independently from the image files. They are first recorded on an audiocassette recorder from which a textual form is transcribed and inserted into the RIS several hours later. The interface between the RIS and the PACS allows for sending and inserting these reports into the PACS database, from which a report can be displayed at the PACS workstation upon request by a user. This process is not efficient because the delay imposed by the transcription prevents the textual report from reaching the referring physician in a timely manner.

Figure 8.29 shows a method of interfacing a digital voice system directly to the PACS database. The concept of interfacing these systems is to have the digital voice database associated with the PACS image database; thus before the written report becomes available, the referring physician can look at the images and listen to the report simultaneously. Following Figure 8.29, the radiologist views images from the PACS workstation and uses the digital dictaphone system to dictate the report, which is converted to a digital format and stored in the voice message server. The voice message server in turn sends a message to the PACS data service, which links the voice with the images. The referring physicians at the workstation in, for example, an intensive care unit, request certain images and at the same time listen to the voice report through the voice message server linked to the images. Later, the transcriber transcribes the voice using the RIS. The transcribed report is inserted into the RIS database server automatically. The RIS server sends a message to the PACS database server. The latter appends the transcribed report to the PACS image file and signals the voice message server to delete the voice message. Note that although the interface is between the voice database and the PACS database, the RIS database also comes into the picture.

Picture Archiving and Communication System (PACS) III: Display and Information Retrieval

9.1 Soft Copy Display Workstations

At this point we have discussed all the components in the PACS data flow (Fig. 7.1) except the display. It is from this component that the user interprets the images, along with relevant data forming the diagnostic report that feeds back to the hospital and radiology information systems (HIS, RIS). Although soft copy display is the major emphasis in PACS, a hard copy on film is useful during the interim period between semidigital and fully digital operation. A display workstation allows radiologists and referring physicians to review multimodality digital images. The conventional method of reviewing radiologic images is to use films hung on an alternator or a light box. Table 9.1 shows the characteristics of a typical alternator. Since the advantages of an alternator are its large surface area, high luminance, and convenience in use, the ideal design for a soft copy display workstation incorporates the function and convenience of the alternator.

In this chapter, the term "soft copy workstation," "display workstation," and "imaging workstation" are used interchangeably. "Workstation" alone is reserved for a host computer (e.g., a Sun SPARC station) that controls image display.

An imaging workstation consists of three major components: image buffer and processing hardware, display monitors, and storage devices. A communication network and application software connects these components with the PACS controller, as described in Section 8.5. The image buffer and processing hardware are responsible for transforming the image data for visualization on the display monitors. Storage devices used to meet the high capacity, high performance requirements of the imaging display applications include Winchester disks, parallel transfer disks,

Table 9.1 Characteristics of a Typical Alternator

Dimensions (in.)		Table Height	Number of Panels	Viewing Capability				
Width	Height			Number of Visible Panels	Viewing Surface per Panel (height × width)	Average Luminance	Viewing Height (from table top to top of lower panel)	Time Required to Retrieve a Panel
72–100	78	30–32	20–50	2 (upper and lower)	16 × 56 to 16 × 82 inches	500 ft-L*	32 + 16 inches	6–12 seconds

* One foot-lambert (ft-L) = 3.426 cd/m².

and optical disks. The communication network is used for transmitting images into and out of the display workstation.

9.1.1 Image Buffer and Processing Hardware; Special-Purpose Image Processors

In the hardware configuration most prevalent for imaging workstations today, a special-purpose image buffer and processing hardware (or image processor) are connected to a workstation. The image processors may be board-level units that plug directly into the host computer's general-purpose bus (such as VME, S-bus) or they may be chassis-level products that communicate with the host computer via a host bus adapter. A typical image processor consists of an image memory (or frame buffer), a pixel processor, and a video output processor (Fig. 9.1). These components share a common image transfer bus to realize high speed transfer of data.

Image memory is needed in addition to the main CPU memory on the host computer because the CPU memory normally lacks the capacity and speed to store and process image data. Ideally, the image memory should be addressable in linear, two- or three-dimensional modes to eliminate address calculation overhead otherwise necessary for pixel and voxel data access. The pixel processor performs arithmetic operations on the data copied from the image memory. These operations include point functions, such as image addition, subtraction, and merge; geometric functions, such as magnification; statistical functions, such as histograms; and transformation functions, such as lookup table operations. Optional hardware compo-

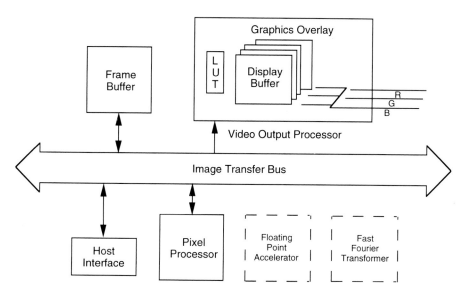

Figure 9.1 Simplified hardware configuration for a typical image processor controlled by a host computer (or workstation). Components enclosed by dashed lines are needed for high power image processing (see Section 9.1.4).

nents often available to speed up image processing computations include floating point accelerators and fast Fourier transform coprocessors. The video output processor normally contains three channels of image output to provide either one 24-bit, full-color image or three 8-bit, gray scale images. In addition to providing the image channels, a well-designed system also supplies an alpha channel for graphics overlay.

9.1.2 Display Monitors

The video output processor generates picture signals, which are used to drive a display device. Today, the cathode ray tube (CRT) monitor is still the predominant display device because of its overall superiority in image quality compared with liquid crystal screens, light valves, and flat-panel displays, and so on. Since the image quality of the visualized data can affect the interpretation of the data, the CRT display monitors play a crucial role in the formation of visual information. The characteristics of the video display monitor that affect visual quality are scanning techniques, resolution, phosphor characteristics, luminance and contrast, and color display.

9.1.2.1 Scanning Techniques

CRT display utilizes the raster scanning method in which the electron beam scans the CRT screen in a fixed pattern of closely spaced parallel lines (see Section 3.2.1). These lines are usually horizontal, and scanning proceeds from the top to the bottom of the screen. The beam current is either "on–off" or continuous, to produce a monochrome or a gray scale picture, respectively. There are two modes of scanning: interlaced and progressive. An interlaced frame is displayed in two steps. For example, in the American standard, the even lines are painted ($\frac{1}{60}$ second), then the odd lines fill the gaps ($\frac{1}{60}$ second) to comprise a complete picture frame in a total of $\frac{1}{30}$ second, or 30 Hz. The progressive scan consists of painting the image from left to right and top to bottom continuously. In progressive scans the trend is to use a monitor that is operating between 60 and 72 frames per second (Hz). It is commonly accepted now that to eliminate flicker, 72 Hz progressive scans should be used in medical imaging applications.

9.1.2.2 Phosphor

Visible light is produced by the phenomenon called cathodo-luminescence in which high energy electrons excite phosphors deposited on a screen plate. As the excited electrons in the phosphor return to the ground state, light is emitted whose intensity is proportional to the electron beam current. More than 50 different types of phosphor are available and are listed in the P number register provided by the Electronic Industries Association (EIA). Crystalline materials most commonly used as phosphors are based on zinc sulfide, although recently there has been increasing usage of rare-earth-activated oxides and oxysulfides. The important factors to consider in selection of phosphors are luminous conversion efficiency, decay time, color, and longevity. A large number of phosphors can convert 10–20% of electron beam energy into light. These efficiencies are remarkably high, with a magnitude of 10 or more times those used in other types of display device, which is one of the reasons for the continued predominance of CRT technology.

Phosphor decay times may vary from less than a microsecond to a few seconds. The longer persistence phosphors can be used to reduce flicker by allowing significant integration of temporal variations in luminance. This practice works well for stationary images but causes smearing in dynamic images. Phosphors of almost any emission color may be selected from the visible light spectrum. The conversion efficiency is degraded as the excitation increases. Most phosphors have a practical lifetime of several thousand hours. To prolong phosphor longevity, the screen-saver feature (in which the electron beam is automatically shut off after a certain period of user input inactivity) is often installed in workstations.

Phosphor selection criteria involve the following considerations (see Table 9.2).

1. Phosphor steady state color: during excitation, the phosphor should acquire a slight blue tint to resemble the hue of the radiograph. The relative percentage of the primary colors presented in a given color can be found from the CIE chromaticity diagram (promulgated by the Commission Internationale de L'Eclairage— the International Lighting Commission).
2. Phosphors with light scintillation decay times shorter than the field refresh rate of an interlacing scan (16.7 ms) or the frame refresh rate of progressive scan (33.3ms) will cause an annoying flicker effect of the static image. To minimize flicker, the phosphorescence decay time chosen for the phosphor should be longer than the scanning refresh rate.
3. Light output efficiency provides a scale of efficiency for a given input beam current. A phosphor with a low efficiency (relative to P4) needs a larger beam current to produce the same light output influence (intensity). A larger beam current, however, reduces the life expectancy of the electron beam in the monitor.

Table 9.2 Specifications of Three Popular Phosphors Used in Display Monitors

Phosphor*	Primary Color (%)			Decay Time (ms)	Efficiency (relative to P4)
	Red	Green	Blue		
P4	27	30	43	0.100	1.00
P40	26	33	41	>100.0	0.76
P164	27	29	44	>100.0	0.60

* From EIA registry.

9.1.2.3 Coating of the Glass Tube

Some computer terminals use an antiglare coat or screen to minimize the glare due to the reflection from the glass tube. The currently available antiglare coating is not suitable for use in image display monitors, however, because it reduces resolution. Some removable antiglare screens are being tested to determine the tradeoff between minimizing reflection and lowering resolution (see Section 9.2.1).

9.1.2.4 Resolution

The display screen contains a layer of phosphor 10 μm or less thick. The pixel size is limited by the spot size of the electron beam. The spot, which has a Gaussian-like current distribution over a cross-sectional area, is usually defined as the width between points at which the beam current has dropped to a certain fraction, such as $1/e$ ($\approx 37\%$) of its maximum value. The beam spot diameter increases linearly as the square root of the beam current. The minimum diameter to which this spot size can be reduced is dictated by the beam current required to produce acceptable phosphor brightness. Therefore, there is a tradeoff between resolution and image brightness.

The resolution of a display monitor is most commonly specified in terms of number of scan lines. For example, a "1K monitor" has 1024 raster lines; "2K" means 2048 lines. In the strict sense of the definition, however, it is not sufficient to specify spatial resolution simply in terms of raster lines because the actual resolving power of the monitor may be less. Consider a digitally generated line pair pattern (black and white lines in pairs). The maximum displayable number of these line pairs on a 1K monitor is 512. However, the monitor may not be able to resolve 1024 alternating black and white lines in the vertical direction if the electron beam spot is out of focus or the contrast/brightness is set too high, causing the adjacent raster lines to overlap. Horizontal resolution has no relation to the number of raster lines; rather, it is limited by the beam spot size and is dependent on how quickly the beam current changes according to the driving video signals (see Section 3.2.1.2).

Several techniques are available for the measurement of resolution. The simplest and most commonly used method employs a test pattern that consists of varying widths of line pair objects in vertical, horizontal, and sometimes radial directions (refer again to Fig. 2.3). It should be noted that this visual approach measures the resolution of the total display–perception system, including the visual acuity of the observer, and therefore it is prone to subjective variations.

Other techniques include the shrinking raster test, the scanning spot photometer, the slit analyzer, and measurement of the modulation transfer function (MTF) (Section 2.5.1.4). One additional noteworthy issue is that resolution is a function of location on the screen. In general, the defocusing effect increases as the electron beam moves away from the center of the screen. Therefore, resolution specification must be accompanied by data concerning where on the screen the measurement was taken, as well as the luminance of the screen.

9.1.2.5 Geometric Distortion

Soft copy display using a CRT monitor can create certain geometric distortions; among these are pincushion, barrel, nonlinearity, hooks and flagging, line pairing, and ringing. The *pincushion* effect, common in large screens, is characterized by nonlinear inward edges, whereas a *barrel*, the manifestation of nonlinear outward edges, can be the result of overcorrection for pincushion distortion. *Nonlinearity* is noticeable when a large circle is flattened or stretched in the monitor display. *Hooks* (*flagging*) usually are presented as a bending of the upper left-hand corner of the screen on the edge of the raster scan. *Line pairing*, a bunching of horizontal scan lines, which show up as bright and dark regions, happens most often on interlaced monitors. *Ringing* is seen as a series of dark- and light-shaded bands that appear at the left of the screen and disappear after a small distance away from the edge. Geometric distortion on a monitor does happen from time to time. Therefore calibration during preventive maintenance with a standard phantom (e.g., the SMPTE described in Figure 6.12) is necessary.

9.1.2.6 Luminance and Contrast

Luminance measures the brightness in candelas per square meter (cd/m^2) or in footlamberts (ft-L): 1 ft-L $= 3.426$ cd/m^2. Luminance is a function of the electron beam current and the conversion efficiency of the phosphor. There is more than one definition for contrast and contrast ratio. The one that is most often used for contrast C is the ratio of the difference between two luminances to one of the two luminances, usually the larger,

$$C = \frac{L_B - L_O}{L_B} \tag{9.1}$$

$$C = \frac{L_O - L_B}{L_0} \tag{9.2}$$

where L_O is the luminance of the object and L_B is the luminance of the background.

Contrast ratio C_r is frequently defined as the ratio of the luminance of an object to that of the background. This is expressed by:

$$C_r = \frac{L_{max}}{L_{min}} \tag{9.3}$$

where L_{max} is the luminance emitted by the area of the greatest intensity and L_{min} is the luminance emitted by the area of least intensity.

Because of the particular nature of the phosphors and their optical transparency, the screen acts as a high efficiency reflector that scatters back 25–75% of the incident light. The light emitted from the phosphor is viewed against this reflected light. The contrast ratio, therefore, depends not only on the luminance of the CRT image but on the intensity of the ambient light as well. For instance, in bright sunlight the display surface can have an apparent luminance of 3×10^4 cd/m^2. To achieve a contrast of 10, the luminance of the cathodo-luminescence must be 3×10^5 cd/m^2, which is extremely high even for a high efficiency phosphor.

9.1.2.7 *Just Noticeable Differences (JND)*

The luminance of the CRT affects the physiological response of the eye in perceiving image quality (spatial resolution and subject contrast). Two characteristics of the visual response are acuity, or the ability of the eye to detect fine detail, and the detection of luminance differences (threshold contrast) between the object and its background. Luminance differences can be measured by using an absolute parameter—just noticeable differences (JNDs) or a relative parameter—threshold contrast (TC)—related by:

$$TC = JND/L_B \tag{9.4}$$

where L_B is the background luminance.

The relationship between the threshold contrast and the luminance can be described by the Weber–Fechner law. When the luminance is low (1 ft-L), in the double-log plot, the threshold contrast is a linear function of luminance, with a slope of -0.5 sometime referred as the Rose model.* When the luminance is high, the threshold contrast is governed by the Weber model, which is a constant function of the luminance, again in the double-log plot. In the Rose model region, when the object luminance L_O is fixed, the JND and the background luminance L_B are related by

$$JND = k_1 L_O (L_B)^{1/2} \tag{9.5}$$

In the Weber model region, we write

$$JND = k_2 L_O (L_B) \tag{9.6}$$

where k_1 and k_2 are constants.

In general, the detection of small luminance differences by the visual system is dependent on the presence of various noises measurable by their standard deviations, in particular:

- the fluctuations in the light photon flux
- the noise from the display monitor
- the noise in the visual system

Thus, the value of JND depends on L_O and L_B, which in turn are affected by the environment, the state of the display monitor, and the conditions of the human observer.

9.1.2.8 *Color CRT*

Although the majority of radiographic images are monochromatic, Doppler US, nuclear medicine, and PET images use colors for enhancement. Also, recent devel-

---

* $TC = -0.5L_B$ in the double-log plot, or $TC = k(L_B)^{-1/2}$ in the standard plot.

opments in image-guided therapy and minimum invasiveness surgery use extensive color graphics superposed on monochromatic images. The oldest and still most widely used design of color CRT is the shadow mask. It consists of three electron guns, a shadow mask with circular holes, and a phosphor screen. The phosphor screen has arrays of "triads," each consisting of the phosphors of three primary emission colors, namely, red, green, and blue. The guns are positioned in a triangular or delta form—the so-called delta gun. The geometrical relationship of delta gun, shadow mask, and screen is such that the beam from each gun strikes only one type of phosphor in the triad. The other two types of phosphor are masked from the gun by the shadow mask. Since the beams are made larger than the holes, a beam will completely fill the corresponding hole to transfer the maximum energy to the phosphor. Three guns can independently modulate the beam current to produce the desired color mixture for each triad.

In the recent years, shadow mask and gun design has been improved to meet the increasing demands of the high brightness, high resolution market in such applications as large-scale PC board design, detailed CAD/CAM, and computer graphics. The current trend is to place guns in line to achieve better tracking of the beam, thus improving the hit rate of the proper color phosphor. The shadow mask may be either slotted or circular with the corresponding screen, with color triads laid down as vertical stripes or as circular dots, respectively. To display a color image, three image memories (R, G, B) are needed. As shown in Section 9.1.1, a composite video controller combines these three memories to form a color display (see Fig. 9.1).

9.1.3 Image Storage Devices

Requirements placed on the storage device in PACS display are stringent. The sheer volume of data calls for a large capacity, in excess of gigabyte range, and increasing demands for image processing and graphics at interactive speed require a very high throughput capability. Magnetic disks that allow an average input/output transfer rate of 1–2 Mbyte/s from the disk to the video display are the common storage medium for images. To achieve higher I/O rates, two types of high speed image storage can be used. One is the random access memory, which is connected directly to the image processor or the host computer bus. RAM image storage has a very fast input/output rate, but is volatile and expensive. The second type is the magnetic disk array, which is slightly slower than the RAM but is permanent and less expensive (see Section 8.5.1.2).

9.1.3.1 Random Access Memory

Random access memory is used as a buffer in an imaging workstation. However, because RAM is expensive, the nominal size of the RAM memory in a workstation is about 32—128 Mbyte, which will allow the storage 8–32 images, 2048 × 2048 × 8. The RAM memory is used as a buffer in the sense that a set of images is first loaded from the disk storage to the RAM. From there, one image at a time is transferred to a video buffer of VRAM (video RAM). The VRAM, which has a much higher input/output rate than the RAM and is even more costly, is connected to the video monitor through a fast D/A converter. Upon performance of the digital-to-analog conversion, the image is displayed on the video monitor. This architecture allows for the rapid display of an image on the video monitor.

9.1.3.2 Parallel Transfer Disks and Disk Arrays

A parallel transfer disk (PTD) or disk array can achieve data transfer rates between the disks and the display memory in the neighborhood of 10 Mbyte/s. The PTD allows multiple read/write heads to simultaneously transfer data. The disk array, on the other hand, configures multiple conventional magnetic disks in parallel. Two common approaches for the disk array are software striping and hardware paralleling. In software striping, the disks are connected to the system bus through traditional controllers. Blocks of data are segmented and moved to and from the disk drives in parallel. Data segmentation and recombination are handled by the software. In the hardware approach, a parallel drive array controller simultaneously manages multiple disk drives. For example, eight enhanced small device interface (ESDI) disk drives, each capable of transferring data at 2.5 Mbyte/s and storing 1.2 Gbyte can be configured in parallel to deliver a transfer rate of 20 Mbyte/s with a total storage capacity of 9.6 Gbyte. Disk arrays are sometimes referred to (see RAID, Section 8.5.1.2).

9.1.4 Image Workstations

Image workstations can be loosely categorized into six types based on their applications. Thus there are diagnostic, review, analysis, digitizing and printing, interactive teaching, and editorial and research workstations.

9.1.4.1 Diagnostic Workstation

A diagnostic workstation is used by the radiologists for making primary diagnoses. The components in this type of workstation should be of the best quality possible. If the workstation is used for displaying projection radiographs, multiple 2K monitors are needed. On the other hand, if the workstation is used for CT and MR images, multiple 1K monitors will be sufficient. A diagnostic workstation requires a digital dictaphone to report the findings. The workstation provides software to append the report to the images. In addition to having all the image processing functions described in Section 9.3, the diagnostic workstation requires a rapid ($\approx 1-2$ s) image retrieval time. Figure 9.2 shows a two-monitor 2K display station at UCSF. The station is based on the Sun SPARCserver 470 computer and two 21-inch diagonal 2K portrait mode monitors (UHR-4820P MegaScan display system, E-Systems, Littleton, MA). Each 2K station has a parallel transfer disk with 5.2 Gbyte formatted storage, which can display a $2048 \times 2048 \times 12$-bit image in 1.5 seconds (Storage Concepts, Irvine, CA).

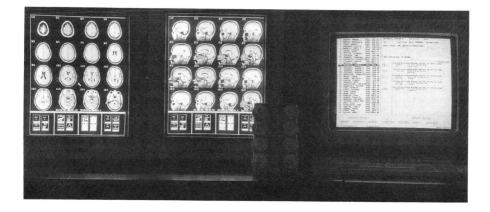

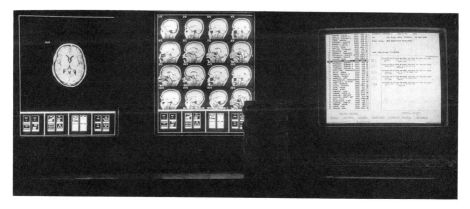

Figure 9.2 Two-monitor 2K display workstation showing two sets of MR neurological images. (A) Patient directory (left) and study list (right) are shown on the text monitor. Image processing functions are controlled by the icons located at the bottom of the 2K monitor screens and by external knobs. (B) An enlarged image (left) appears during operation in cine mode; the right monitor display remains intact.

9.1.4.2 Review Workstation

A review workstation is used by radiologists and referring physicians to review cases in the hospital wards. The dictation or the transcribed report should be available, with the corresponding images. A review workstation may not require 2K monitors, since images might have been read by the radiologist from the diagnostic workstation and the referring physicians will not be looking for every minute detail. Diagnostic and review workstations can be combined as a single workstation sharing both diagnostic and review functions like an alternator. Figure 9.3 shows a two-monitor 1K (1600-line) display station used in the intensive care units at UCSF. This workstation consists of a Sun SPARC 20 workstation with two gigabyte

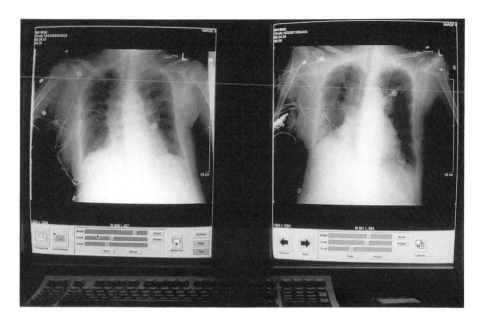

Figure 9.3   Two-monitor 1K (1600 line) display ICU workstation showing two CR images. Left-hand monitor shows the current image; all previous images can be accessed within one second on the right hand monitor by clicking the two lower left icons (Previous and Next). Image processing functions are controlled by the icons located at the bottom of the screens.

magnetic disks, two GXTurbo video display boards, and two 1600 × 1024 display monitors.

9.1.4.3 Analysis Workstation

Analysis workstations differ from the diagnostic and review workstations in that the former are used to extract useful parameters from images. Some parameters are easy to extract from a simple region of interest (ROI) operation, as described in Section 9.3; others (e.g., blood flow measurements from DSA, 3-D reconstruction from sequential CT images) are computation intensive and require an analysis workstation with a more powerful image processor and high performance software. Figure 9.4 shows what an analysis workstation can display (see color plate; see also Section 11.2.3).

9.1.4.4 Digitizing and Printing Workstation

The digitizing and printing workstation is for radiology department technologists or film librarians who must digitize historical films, and films from outside the department. The workstation is also used for converting soft copy images to hard copy. In addition to the standard workstation components already described, this workstation requires a laser film scanner (see Section 3.2.4), a laser film imager (see Section

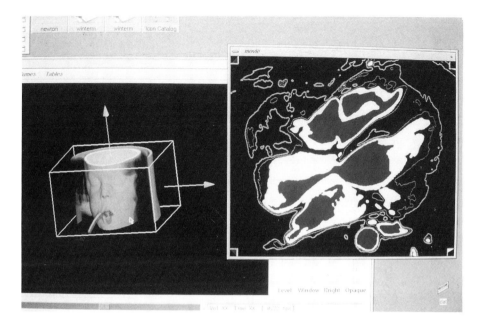

Figure 9.4 High end analysis workstation (Reality Station, ONYX) at UCSF showing 3-D rendering of a CT examination of a child's head and simulated blood flow (blue) in the four chambers of her heart. (See color plate.)

Source: (Courtesy of SiliconGraphics Computer Systems, Mountian View, CA, S. Wong and E. Grant).

9.4), and a paper printer. The paper printer is used for pictorial report generation (see Section 9.3.3) from the diagnostic, review, and editorial and research workstations. A 1K display monitor for quality control purposes would be sufficient for this type of workstation.

9.1.4.5 Interactive Teaching Workstation

A teaching workstation is used for interactive teaching in the department. It emulates the role of a teaching library but with more interactive features. Figures 9.5 and 9.6 show a digital mammography teaching workstation from VICOM (Fremont, CA) and workstation architecture, respectively.

9.1.4.6 Editorial and Research Workstation

An editorial and research workstation, used by physicians to generate lecture slides, teaching and research materials, and reports with images, includes the functions in the PC or the Macintosh personal computer. This workstation uses the paper printer mentioned in connection with the digitizing and printing workstation to generate pictorial report. Section 9.6 describes the architecture of a physician's desktop workstation in more detail.

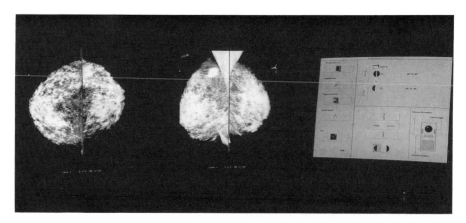

Figure 9.5   Four mammographs from a 2K digital mammography teaching workstation: *left,* left and right craniocaudal views, *middle,* left and right mediolateral oblique views. *Right:* Text monitor with icons for image display and manipulation at this workstation.

Image workstations, which directly interact with radiologists and physicians, are the most important component in a PACS. To design them effectively, a thorough understanding of the clinical operating environment requirements is necessary.

9.2 Ergonomics of Image Workstations

Among the factors in the ergonomics of an image workstation relating to perceived image quality are lighting conditions, glare, and acoustic noise due to hardware.

9.2.1 Glare

Glare, the most frequent complaint among the workstation users, is the sensation produced within the visual field by luminance that is sufficiently greater than the luminance to which the eyes are adapted to cause annoyance, discomfort, or loss in visual performance and visibility (see Section 9.1.2.6 on luminance and contrast).

Glare can be caused by reflections of electric light sources, windows, and light-

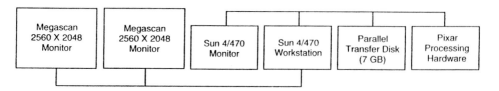

Figure 9.6   Architecture of the 2K digital mammography teaching workstation. In this design, the Sun 4/470 is the host computer and the Pixar is the image processor. The parallel transfer disks allow 1–2 seconds display time for a 2K image.

colored objects, including furniture and clothing. The magnitude of the sensation of glare is a function of the size, position, and luminance of a source, the number of sources, and the luminance to which the eyes are adapted at the moment. It may be categorized according to its origin: direct or reflected glare. Direct glare may be caused by bright sources of light in the visual field of view (e.g., sunlight and lightbulbs). Reflected glare is caused by light reflected from the display screen (see Section 9.1.2.3 on coating of the glass tube). If the reflecitons are diffuse, they are referred to as veiling glare.

Image reflections are both distracting and annoying, because the eye is induced to focus alternately between the displayed and reflected images. Reflected glare can be reduced by increasing the display contrast, by wearing dark-colored clothing, by correctly positioning the screen with respect to lights, windows, and other reflective objects, and by adjusting the screen angle.

Further reduction of glare can be achieved by etching the screen glass, by treating the glass with antireflective coatings, or by superimposing on the screen antireflection filters such as micromesh, circular polarizers, and neutral density filters with antireflective coatings. Etching the glass reduces reflection by scattering the reflected light, thus giving reflected objects a more diffuse and less conspicuous appearance. Since the light emitted from the display phosphors is also dispersed, image sharpness may be compromised. Coating of the screen with a thin film of antireflective agent such as Lambda-4 usually does not diminish the image sharpness. The coating layer, however, can be easily and permanently smeared with fingerprints. Antireflection filters reduce the perceived glare by attenuating the reflected light more than the light emitted from the CRT, since the reflected light must pass through the filter twice. Using antireflective technqiues, objective methods can be derived to measure luminance, modulation transfer function, contrast, and glare, as well as subjective evaluation of the brightness, sharpness, contrast, color, and glare. On the average, the order of preference is: gray antireflection filter, micromesh filter, circular polarizer, blue antireflection filler, etched plastic filler, and no filter.

9.2.2 Ambient Illuminance

An important issue related to the problem of glare is proper illumination of the workstation area. Excessive lighting can increase the readability of documents but can also increase the reflected glare, while sufficient illumination can reduce glare but make it difficult to read source documents at the display workstation.

Ergonomic guidelines for the traditional office environment recommend a high level of lighting: 700 lux (an engineering unit for lighting) or more (Cushman, 1987). A survey of 38 computer-aided design (CAD) operators who were allowed to adjust the ambient lighting indicated that the median illumination level is around 125 lux (125 at keyboard, etc.) with 90% of the readings falling between 15 and 505 lux (Heiden, 1984). These levels are optimized for CRT viewing but certainly not for reading written documents. An illumination of 200 lux is normally considered inadequate for an office environment. Another study suggests a lower range (150–

400 lux) for tasks that do not involve information transfer from paper documents. At these levels, lighting is sufficiently subdued to permit good display contrast in most cases. A higher range (400–550 lux) is suggested for tasks that require the reading of paper documents. Increasing ambient lighting above 550 lux reduces display contrast appreciably. If the paper documents contain small and low contrast print, 550 lux may not provide adequate lighting. Such cases may call for supplementary special task lighting directed at the document surface only. This recommendation is based on the conditions needed to read text, not images, on a screen. Another recommendation specifies the use of a level of ambient illumination equal to the average luminance of an image on the display workstation screen (Horii, 1992).

9.2.3 Acoustic Noise Due to Hardware

An imaging workstation often includes components like parallel transfer disks, image processors, and other arrays of hardware that produce heat and require electric fans for cooling. These fans often produce an intolerably high noise level. Even for a low noise host computer attached to the display workstation, it is recommended that the computer be separated from the display workstation to isolate noise that would affect human performance.

As personal computers become more and more common, the computer, the terminal, and the display monitor become an integrated system insofar as they are connected by very short cables. Most imaging workstations utilize a personal computer as the host, however, and because of the short cabling, the host computer and the image processor wind up in the same room as the terminal, display monitors, and the keyboard. Failure of the image workstation designer to consider the consequences of having all these units together creates a very noisy environment at the imaging workstation, and it is difficult for the user to sustain concentration during long working shifts. Care must be exercised in designing the workstation environment to avoid problems due to acoustic noise from the hardware.

9.3 Image Processing and Display Functions

9.3.1 Image Enhancement Functions

Image processing is used at the display workstation to improve the diagnostic value of the images. This section discusses some commonly used image processing functions for enhancing radiology diagnosis. Image processing functions are different from preprocessing functions (see Section 7.6) in the sense that preprocessing does not alter the appearance of the image, whereas processing will.

9.3.1.1 Outlining

Let $f(x,y)$ be the gray level of a pixel located in (x,y). The absolute partial differences

$$|\Delta_x f| = K|f(x + 1,y) - f(x,y)| \tag{9.7}$$

$$|\Delta_y f| = K|f(x,y + 1) - f(x,y)| \tag{9.8}$$

measure the rate of change of gray level (or the gradient) at the pixel *(x,y)* in the horizontal and vertical directions respectively, where K is a constant. An image sensitive to both horizontal and vertical directions can be measured by using the maximum absolute partial difference as follows:

$$\text{MAX}\Delta = \max(|\Delta_x f|, |\Delta_y f|) \tag{9.9}$$

Figure 9.7 shows an example of applying Eqs. (9.7), (9.8), and (9.9) to a digitized chest radiograph (Fig. 9.7A); the results are shown in Figures 9.7B, C, and D, respectively. It should be pointed out that "outlining" only enhances the visual appearance of objects of interest in an image; it does not extract the boundary coordinates that are sometimes necessary to define a region of interest.

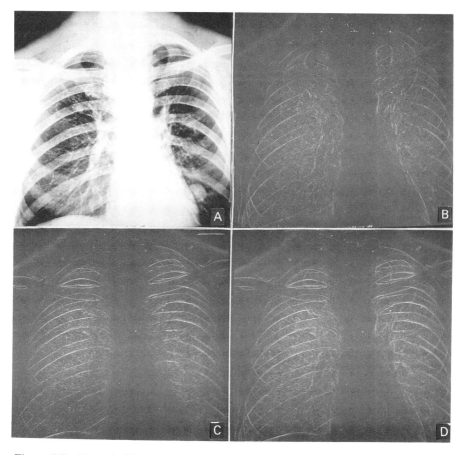

Figure 9.7   Example illustrating the principle of outlining: (A) a digitized chest X-ray, (B) $\Delta_x f$, (C) $\Delta_y f$, (D) MAX Δ.

9.3.1.2 Boundary Detection

During an image review session it is sometimes desirable to measure parameters (e.g., average gray level, shape, geometry) of a region of interest in the image. To do so, we first extract the boundary of the ROI. When the region or object of interest has more than one boundary, the procedure is called *segmentation*.

Two steps are involved in boundary detection: determination of a cutoff gray level of the ROI and a boundary search. A cutoff gray level can be determined by using either the histogram method or an approach that often is more subjective, namely, defining the object boundary as one or more preset gray levels in an image.

In the histogram method, a CT image (e.g., Fig. 9.8A) is analyzed to produce a histogram (Fig. 9.8B), which includes the object of interest as well as the background. Boundary detection is initiated by defining the cutoff gray level of the ventricles and the brain (outlined in Fig. 9.8C) as the gray level value at the troughs: a and b in histogram of Figure 9.8B.

Once the cutoff gray level is known, the coordinates of the boundary can be obtained by a programmed search in the vicinity of the object of interest. The procedure starts by an automatic search of a pixel whose value is equal to the cutoff gray level value. Once identified, this pixel becomes the first boundary pixel of this ROI, and its (x,y) coordinates are recorded. Its eight adjacent neighbors are searched systematically, one by one, to determine the best candidate for the next boundary pixel. The search follows the scheme:

$$
\begin{array}{ccc}
3 & 2 & 1 \\
4 & * & 8 \\
5 & 6 & 7
\end{array}
$$

where * is the current boundary pixel, and the numerals are the order of the search.

The criteria used to determine the best candidate are closeness of pixel value to the cutoff boundary value and present status as a boundary pixel. The best candidate becomes the second boundary pixel, and the procedure is repeated until all the boundary pixels of the object have been located and recorded. In general, the boundary of an object of interest is always a closed curve.

9.3.1.3 Deblurring

Occasionally, an image is blurred as a result of an imperfection that comes about during the radiographic acquisition procedure. If the blur is not severe, it is possible to sharpen the image by using a deblurring procedure.

The most popular deblurring technique is based on the assumption that the picture has been blurred by a process that satisfies the two-dimensional diffusion equation. Thus to deblur the image, one can apply the following approximate equation:

$$ f \doteq 2\bar{f} - \bar{f}_{av} = (\bar{f} - \bar{f}_{av}) + \bar{f} \tag{9.10} $$

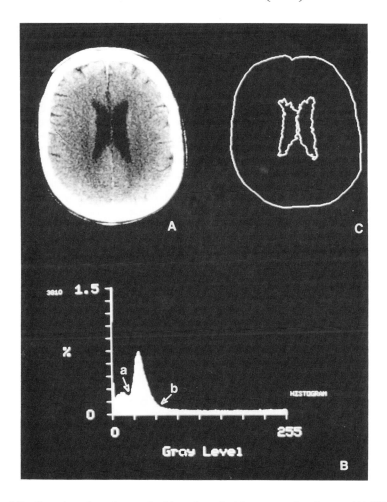

Figure 9.8 Boundary detection method based on the histogram of an image: (A) CT head image, (B) histogram of the CT head image, (C) outlines of the brain and the ventricles using the boundary detection method.

where $\bar{f}$ is the blurred image, f is the deblurred image, and

$$\bar{f}_{av} = \frac{1}{5} \nabla^2 \bar{f} + \bar{f} \qquad (9.11)$$

is the five-point average of $\bar{f}$, and

$$\nabla^2 \bar{f} = -4\bar{f}(x,y) + \bar{f}(x - 1,y) + \bar{f}(x + 1,y) \qquad (9.12)$$
$$+ \bar{f}(x,y - 1) + \bar{f}(x,y + 1)$$

is the Laplacian operator.

To obtain a sharper image f from an image $\bar{f}$, therefore, one can take the differ-

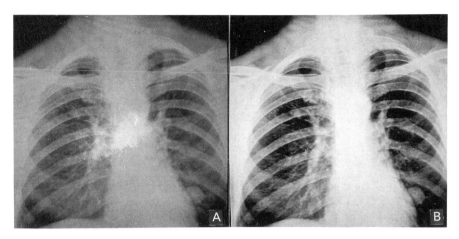

Figure 9.9   Example illustrating the deblurring process: (A) blurred image obtained from Figure 9.7A by using a Gausian smooth filter and (B) the deblurred image using Eq. (9.10).

ence between this image $\bar{f}$ and its average image $\bar{f}_{av}$ and then add the difference to $\bar{f}$. Intuitively, the difference between $\bar{f}$ and $\bar{f}_{av}$ yields the high frequency content of the original image f, which was lost during the imperfect image acquisition process.

As an example, consider Figure 9.9A, which is the blurred image $\bar{f}$ obtained from Figure 9.7A using a Gaussian distribution filter (see Section 9.3.1.5 on filtering). If one computes $2\bar{f} - \bar{f}_{av}$, the resulting deblurred image f is as shown in Figure 9.9B. It is seen immediately that the deblurred image (Fig. 9.9B) has better quality than the blurred image (Fig. 9.9A), but it is still not as good as the original image (Fig. 9.7A).

9.3.1.4. Noise Cleaning

Radiologic images often suffer from various types of noise. One common type is TV "snow or "salt and pepper" noise, in which the gray levels of some points have been randomly increased or decreased. Such noise can be reduced by local averaging of the image using Eq. (9.11), but this process is undesirable because it produces a blurring effect. Instead, one can use a nonlinear process that replaces a point with the average of its neighbors, provided the point differs from most or all of its neighbors by a significant amount (i.e., above a threshold or below a threshold). If such a process still has a blurring effect on edges where the gray level is changing rapidly, one can use an edge sensitive operator (e.g., the absolute partial difference: Eq. 9.9) to detect the presence of edges of objects of interest. And at edge points, one can average only the neighbors that lie in the direction along the edge detected by the edge-sensitive operator.

Figure 9.10A shows a chest image superposed by the salt-and-pepper noise. Figure 9.10B demonstrates how this noise can be minimized by using a median filter operation (see next section).

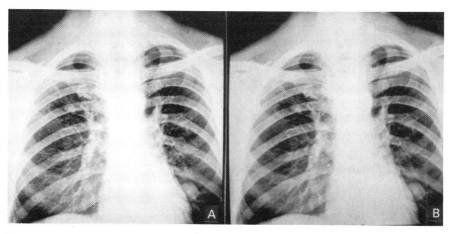

Figure 9.10 (A) Salt-and-pepper noise (small dots) is introduced in a chest pulmonary arteriogram randomly. (B) A 3 × 3 medium filter is used to minimize the salt-and-pepper noise; observe, however, that the image is not as sharp as the original image (A).

9.3.1.5 Filtering

Filtering can be used to smooth an image or to sharpen it, regardless of whether the image is represented in the spatial domain or in the frequency domain (see Section 2.4).

Spatial Domain

Smoothing is usually performed to get rid of image noise. In the method for smoothing an image represented by eq. (9.11), the image $\bar{f}$ is smoothed by replacing each pixel value with the average gray level of the four adjacent neighbor pixels and itself. The resultant image $\bar{f}_{av}$ is smoother than $\bar{f}$. Another smoothing filter in the spatial domain is the median filter, which replaces the pixel value by the median pixel value of certain neighbor pixels. The result shown in Figure 9.10B is an example. Still another useful smoothing filter is the Gaussian filter, which smoothes the image by convolving a Gaussian function with the image (see Section 5.1.3 for definition of convolution). Figure 9.9A illustrates the Gaussian smoothing of Figure 9.7A. Notice that the smoothing procedures described here are different from those described in Section 2.5.2. In the latter the smoothing is done with many images, whereas in this case the smoothing is performed on pixels within a neighborhood of an image.

The deblurring procedure described earlier in Eq. (9.10) is a linear filtering technique used to sharpen an image. The difference $\bar{f} - \bar{f}_{av}$ represents the sharper edges in the image, which are emphasized and added back to the original image $\bar{f}$. The image f appears to be sharper than $\bar{f}$.

Frequency Domain

Filtering in the frequency domain is performed as follows. The image is first transformed to the frequency domain, and the amplitude of each frequency component of the image is modified (or filtered). The modulated image is transformed back to the spatial domain as the filtered image. Depending on how each frequency component is manipulated, the filtered image is either smoother or sharper than the original image.

The Fourier transform described in Section 2.4 is a common method used to perform the image transform. Recall from Eq. (2.5) that after $f(x,y)$ has been transformed, the real and imaginary components $Re(u,v)$ and $Im(u,v)$ of $F(u,v)$

$$F(u,v) = \frac{1}{N} \sum_{x=0}^{N-1} \sum_{y=0}^{N-1} f(x,y) \exp\left[\frac{-i2\pi(ux + vy)}{N}\right] \tag{2.5}$$
$$= Re(u,v) + iIm(u,v)$$

can be modified for each frequency (u,v). In the process called low pass filtering, we write

$$Re(u,v) = 0 \quad \text{and} \quad Im(u,v) = 0 \quad \text{for} \quad (u^2 + v^2)^{1/2} \geq r \tag{9.13}$$

where r is some constant. That is, all frequency components with a radius greater than and equal to r are deleted, and only low frequency components remain. In high pass filtering, we have

$$Re(u,v) = 0 \quad \text{and} \quad Im(u,v) = 0 \quad \text{for} \quad (u^2 + v^2)^{1/2} < r \tag{9.14}$$

Here all frequency components with a radius less than r are deleted, and only high frequency components remain in the inverse transformed image. Figure 9.11 shows results applying high pass and low pass filters on a chest radiograph for different values of u and v.

When $Re(u,v)$ and $Im(u,v)$ are modified for a given (u,v), the process is called a frequency emphasis. The inverse transformed image will emphasize the change of the particular frequency component (u,v).

9.3.2 Image Display and Measurement Functions

Although display workstations should have the image processing functions described in Section 9.3.1, it is not advisable to introduce these advanced image processing features into the clinical environment until the users thoroughly understand the consequences of such operations. Advanced features that are not well understood only cause confusion in the analysis of images. For these reasons, advanced image processing functions should be an option in the image workstation. On the other hand, a set of easy-to-use image display and measurement functions should be included in the image workstation to assist users in diagnostic work. Sections 9.3.2.1–9.3.2.5 describe some of these functions.

9.3.2.1 Zoom and Scroll

Zooming and scrolling is an interactive command manipulated via a trackball or a mouse. The operator first uses the trackball to scroll about the image, centering the region of interest on the screen. The ROI can then be magnified by pressing a designated button to perform the zoom. The image becomes more blocky as the zoom factor increases, reflecting the greater number of times each pixel is replicated.

Although it is useful to be able to magnify and scroll the image on the screen, the field of view decreases in proportion to the square of the magnification factor. Magnification is commonly performed via pixel replication or interpolation. In the former, one pixel value repeats itself several times in both the horizontal and vertical directions, and in the latter, the pixel value is replaced by interpolation of its neighbors. For example, to magnify the image by 2 by replication is to replicate the image 2×2 times.

9.3.2.2 Window and Level

The window and level feature allows the user to control the interval of gray levels to be displayed on the monitor. The center of this interval is called the *level value* and the range is called the *window value* (see also Section 7.6.1.4). The selected gray level range will be distributed over the entire dynamic range of the display monitor, and thus, using a smaller window value will cause the contrast in the resulting video image to increase. Gray levels present in the image outside the defined interval are clipped to black or white (or both), depending on which side of the interval they are positioned. This function is also controlled by the user via a trackball or mouse. For example, moving the trackball in the vertical direction typically controls the window value, while the horizontal direction controls the level of which gray levels are displayed on the video monitor. Window and level operations can be performed in real time using an image processor with a fast access memory called a lookup table (LUT). A 256 -value LUT inputs an 8-bit address whose memory location contains the value of the desired gray level transformation (linear scaling with clipping). The memory address for LUT is provided by the original data.

Figure 9.12 illustrates the concept of the LUT. Thus, for example, if one fixes a window value to 1 and changes the level value with the trackball one gray level at a time, the monitor will effectively display all 256 values of the image with one gray level at a time.

9.3.2.3 Histogram Modification

Another function that is useful for enhancing the display image is histogram modification. A histogram of the original image is first obtained, then modified by rescaling each pixel value in the original image. The new enhanced image that is formed will show the desired modification.

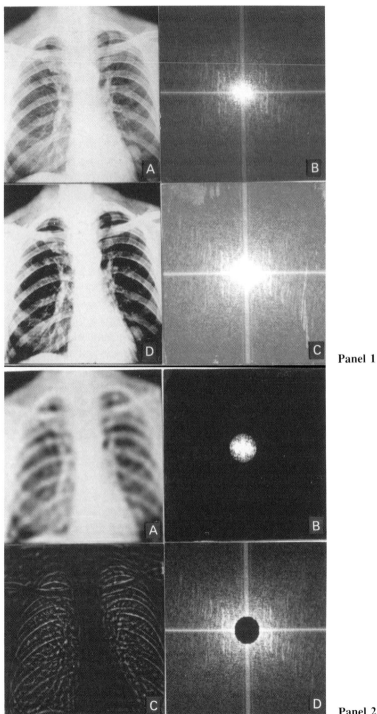

Panel 1

Panel 2

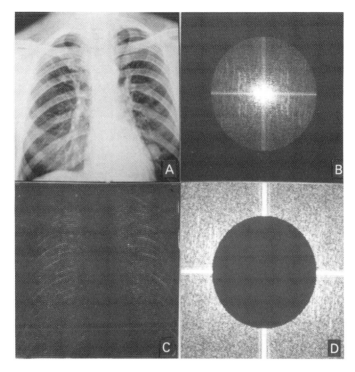

Panel 3

Figure 9.11 *Panel 1:* (A) Digitized chest X-ray. (B) Its Fourier transform, $N = 256$; the origin (0,0) of the display is at the center of the image, and the coordinates of the edges are ± 128. (C) The Fourier transform is modulated by an exponential filter for contrast enhancement. (D) The inverse modulated Fourier transform shows that it is higher contrast than (A). *Panel 2, upper row:* Results from a low-pass filter, Eq. (9.13), $r = (u^2 + v^2)^{1/2} \geq 20$ in the display coordinate system: (B) is the filtered transform image; (A), the inverse filtered transform image, has lost its sharpness. *Lower row:* Results from a high pass filter, Eq. (9.14), $(u^2 + v^2)^{1/2} < 20$: (D) is the filtered transform image; (C) is the inverse filtered transform image, (only the edges remain). By adding (A) and (C) together, we would have the original image (A, panel 1). *Panel 3:* Same as panel 2 except $r = 80$.

An example of histogram modification is histogram equalization, in which the shape of the modified histogram is adjusted to be as uniform as possible for all gray levels. The rescaling factor (or the histogram equalization transfer function) is given by:

$$g = (g_{max} - g_{min})P(f) + g_{min} \tag{9.15}$$

where g is the output (modified) gray level, g_{max} and g_{min} are the maximum and minimum gray level of the modified image, f is the input (original) gray level, and $P(f)$ is the cumulative distribution function (or integrated histogram) of f.

Figure 9.13 shows the concept of histogram equalization and an example of modifying an overexposed (too dark) chest image using the histogram equalization

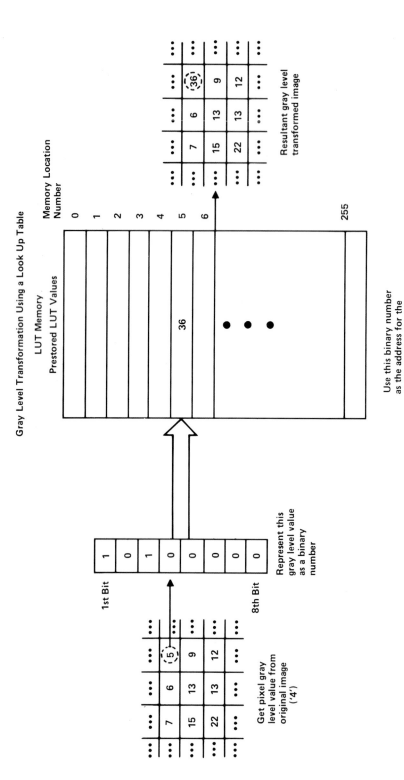

Figure 9.12 Concept of a lookup table (LUT). In this case, the pixel value 5 is mapped to 36 through a preset lookup table.

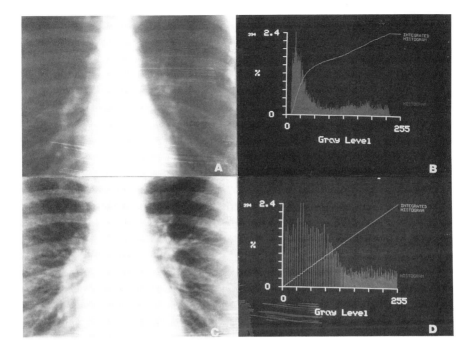

Figure 9.13   Concept of histogram equalization. (A) Chest X-ray with lung region over-exposed, showing relatively low contrast. (B) Histogram of the chest image. (C) Lung region in the image enhanced using histogram equalization. (D) The modified histogram.

method. In this example, the frequency of occurrence of some lower gray level values in the modified histogram has been changed to zero to enforce uniformity.

9.3.2.4 Image Reverse

A look-up table can be used to reverse the dark and light pixels of an image. In this function, the LUT is loaded with a reverse ramp such that for an 8-bit image, the value 255 becomes 0, and 0 becomes 255. Image reverse is used to locate external objects—for example, intrathoracic tubes in ICU X-ray examinations.

9.3.2.5 Distance, Area, and Average Gray Level Measurements

Three simple measurement functions are important for immediate quantitative assessment, because they allow the user to perform physical measurement with the image displayed on the video monitor by calibrating the dimensions of each pixel to some physical units or the gray level value to the optical density.

The *distance calibration* procedure is performed by moving a cursor over the image to define the physical distance between two pixels. Best results are obtained when the image contains a calibration ring or other object of known size. To perform *optical density calibration,* the user moves a cursor over many different gray levels and makes queries from a menu to determine the corresponding optical densities.

Finally, an interactive procedure allows the user to trace a region of interest from which the *area and average gray level* can be obtained.

9.3.3 Montage

9.3.3 Overview

A montage represents a selected set of individual images from a CT, MR, US or any other multi-image modality series. Such groupings are necessary because only a few images from most series show the particular pathology or features of interest to the referring physicians or radiologists. For an average case, such as MR, where a half-dozen sequences* may be done, averaging 30 images per sequence, there are typically 180 images in a given study on a patient. A typical montage would contain 20 images, representing the significant features that from the physicians' point of view are necessary to read the case. So, typically, then, only 10% of the images taken in an examination are essential, the rest are supplemental. Since it is difficult for the technologist at the time of the scanning to know what images will be the significant ones, a standard series is generally made covering the entire body region of interest. It is up to the radiologist/physician to select the images of interest.

In the PACS display workstation, the montage feature allows the user to select and maintain in one file images of interest from all series. This montage file is then saved for future reference, and most subsequent reviews of prior studies can be done by simply referring to the montage file, which contains only the significant images, rather than retrieving all series that were done on a given examination.

9.3.3.2 Generic Montage Design

The following features are desirable in the design of a montage function:

1. The montage should be simple to use. The end users are radiologists/physicians who have little time to learn complex tools to perform functions they already do efficiently in a film-based operation system.
2. The function should be available on all image workstations currently used to view studies.
3. It should use selection methods similar to those familiar from the image workstation–user interface.
4. If the user elects not to impose a montage file name, the system should default to a standard name (e.g., patient name/date of exam/modality).
5. When a montage is displayed, each slice should be displayed with its own correct window/level.
6. The user should be able to use the workstation features (window/level, cine, zoom/scroll, etc.) to view the displayed montage.

---

* In MR, a sequence contains a series of images.

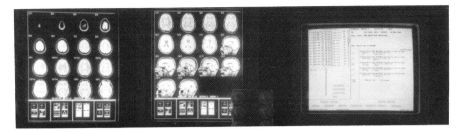

Figure 9.14 Example of a montage file: *right,* text monitor shows the montage file at the left of the screen; *middle,* right-hand 2K display monitor shows the montage images selected from different MR sequences mixing transverse and sagittal sectional images; *left,* left-hand 2K monitor shows a standard transverse sectional study without the montage. (Cf. Fig. 9.2.)

One major issue regarding the internal aspects of montage designs must be resolved: Should the actual image pixel data be stored in the montage file, or should the function simply use a pointer to the image data? The tradeoff is between storage space and immediate access to images.

Storing the image data in the montage file has the advantage of being the most efficient way to retrieve and display the images, since the data lies in one contiguous space, just as they will be loaded into the display workstation. The images will be duplicated in the database, however. Another disadvantage is that storing images in a contiguous file makes editing the montage more difficult: deleting and inserting chunks of image data is a much more CPU-intensive task than moving pointers around.

Storing pointers to image data requires the least amount of additional storage space and has the advantage of ease of editing. Since, however, the actual image data are scattered throughout the PACS, recent image data will be in the display station local storage and older studies will be in the archive. To access montages stored in this fashion, each series containing a slice in the montage must be retrieved from the archive to local storage before the images can be loaded. In the worst case, 20 such retrievals may be necessary, meaning a delay of 10–20 minutes before a montage can be displayed.

Figure 9.14 shows a montage text file on a text monitor in a 2K workstation (see also Figure 9.2) along with the MR montage images shown on the image display monitor. The montage images are selected from different MR sequences.

9.3.4 Basic Functions for a Display Workstation

Some of the basic software functions described in Sections 9.3.2 and 9.3.3 are needed in a display workstation to facilitate its operation. These functions should be easily used with a single click of the mouse, a turn of the dial knob, or a roll with the trackball through the patient's directory, study list, and image processing icons on the various monitors. The keyboard is used only for retrieving information not stored on the workstation's local disks. In this case, the user must input either the

Table 9.3 Software Functions for a Display Workstation

Function	Description
Directory	
Patient directory	Name, ID, age, sex; date of current exam
Study list	Type of exam, anatomical area; date of studies
Display	
Screen reconfiguration	Reconfigure each screen for the convenience of image display
Monitor selection	Left, right
Display	Display images according to screen configuration and monitor selected
Image manipulation	
Dials	Brightness; contrast; zoom and scroll
LUT	Predefined lookup talbes (bone, soft tissue, brain, etc.)
Cine	Single or multiple cine on multimonitors for CT, MR, and US images
Rotation	Rotate an image
Negative	Reverse gray scale
Utilities	
Montage	Select images to form a montage file
Image discharge	Delete images of discharged patients (a privileged operation)
Library search	Retrieve historical examinations (requires keyboard operation)
Report	Retrieve reports from RIS
Measurements	Linear and region of interest

patient's name or ID, or a disease category, as the key for searching the long-term archive. Table 9.3 shows some basic software functions required for a display workstation.

9.4 The Laser Film Imager

Hard copy display is sometimes needed for sending a copy of the images to a remote site where a soft copy display system is not available. For good quality hard copy, a laser film printer (imager) is used. The laser film imager uses a fine laser spot to write a digital image onto a red-sensitive film (8 in. × 10 in. or 14 in. × 17 in.). The spot moves from left to right and the film advances to the next line after a complete line has been written. The intensity of the laser spot is modulated according to the gray level value of each pixel which, in turn, determines the optical density of the pixel on the film . For convenience of discussion, consider the schematic illustration of a laser imager shown in Figure 9.15. This system can write up to 2384 × 3050 × 8 bits smaller film (8 in. × 10 in.) or 4288 × 5275 × 8 bits on a larger film (14 in. × 17 in.); each pixel corresponds to an area of 8 μm^2. The film advance speed is 16 mm/s. Table 9.4 lists the specifications of a laser imager.

9.4.1 The Block Diagram

To start, digital image data supplied by the host computer reach the imager's formatter module through a dedicated interface board. The data are sent through a programmable lookup table in the printer, which corrects for nonlinearities in the laser production of film density.

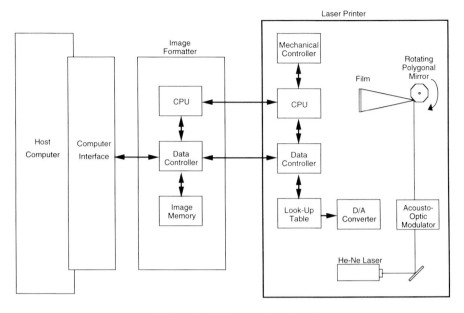

Figure 9.15   Block diagram for a laser imager.

The lookup table is calibrated with the optical density–gray level transfer characteristics of the imager. The output signal from the lookup table is used to modulate the intensity of a 5 mW helium–neon laser beam using a lead molybdate ($PbMoO_4$) acousto-optic modulator such that the input data will be linearly mapped onto a range of optical densities on film. A conventional X-ray film processor is used to develop the exposed film. However, the red-sensitive film requires a green safe light in the darkroom.

9.4.2   Evaluation of the Performance Characteristics of a Laser Film Imager

Several parameters are important in determining the performance characteristics of a laser film imager: the transfer characteristics between the optical density and the gray level, and characteristics of the laser spot, including uniformity, spatial resolu-

Table 9.4   Specifications of a Laser Imager

Pixel size	80 μm × 80 μm
Density resolution	8 bits
Film size and corresponding matrix size	8 in. × 10 in. (2348 × 3050)
	14 in. × 17 in. (4288 × 5275)
Scan speed	16 mm/s
Magnification	× 0.5, 1, 2, 3, . . . , 16
Image format	Up to 16 images/film
Laser power	5 mW

tion, and spatial linearity. Sections 9.4.2.1–9.4.2.5 discuss materials and methods used to measure these parameters. The measurements can be verified by densitometers—for example, the Sakura PDM-5 scanning microdensitometer, with a resolution of 10.0 μm, and the Macbeth TD502LD densitometer, with an aperture size of 1.0 mm.

9.4.2.1 Optical Density Versus Gray Level

The gray level–optical density transfer characteristics of the imager can be investigated by writing a computer-generated gray level step wedge with 256 levels onto a film and measuring the corresponding optical densities of the film with the Macbeth densitometer. Figure 9.16 plots optical density (OD) versus gray level using this method. The relationship between input gray level and output optical density is quite linear for gray levels between 4 and 235, corresponding to optical densities 0.16 and 3.06. The slope of the linear portion of the curve is 0.0126 OD/gray level. Beyond a gray level of 235, the H-D curve characteristics of the film (see Section 3.1.2.1, Fig. 3.3) cause the film density to saturate at 3.06 OD. The slope of film density versus gray level curve can be changed via the software lookup table, however, and thus it is possible to manipulate the contrast of the original digital data directly at the time of printing. This very important feature of a laser imager allows the printer to move away from the toe and shoulder regions of the H-D curve, thus preventing the printed image from being too bright or too dark.

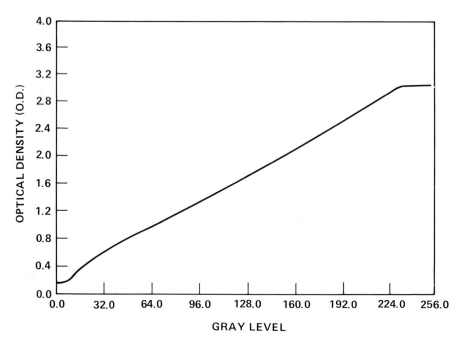

Figure 9.16 Relationship between the computer-generated digital gray level (input) and the film optical density (output) of a laser imager.

9.4.2.2 Spot Analysis of the Printer

The laser spot characteristic provides the system's flat field response and spatial resolution capability. A laser spot, as defined here, is the two-dimensional analog optical density distribution on the film resulting from a digital impulse input to the laser imager. The smaller the spot size, the higher will be the spatial resolution of the system. Even with a uniform impulse, the spot will vary slightly in amplitude depending on its position on the film. The spot will be larger at the periphery of the scanning field than at the center, as a result of the oblique angle between the beam and the film.

To study the effect of a laser spot on the image quality, measurements should be taken from the periphery of the film, which represents the worst possible case. The film with the spot can be analyzed using a high resolution light microscope connected to a vidicon camera (see Section 3.2.1.1). Figure 9.17, which shows the

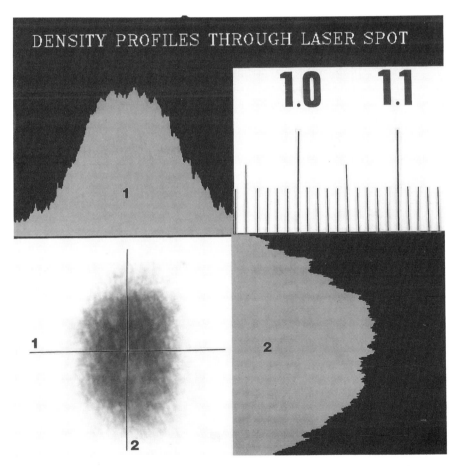

Figure 9.17 *Lower left:* Magnified view of laser spot profiles taken at the center of the spot (1) parallel and (2) perpendicular to the scan direction. *Upper right:* Scale indicating distance (from 1.0 to 1.1 is 100 μm).

optical density profiles at the center of a spot taken parallel and perpendicular to the beam transversal direction, respectively, reveals that the spot is not circularly symmetric but is elliptical, with an approximately Gaussian distribution.

Often, because of differences in motion of the spot in directions parallel and perpendicular to the scan direction, the optimum spot shape in laser writing systems is not circular. In the parallel direction, spot motion is continuous, and resolution is determined from the spot size and shape, and the response time of the acousto-optic modulator. In the perpendicular direction, spot motion is discrete and resolution is determined by line spacing distance and the spot size and shape. The display aperture in the perpendicular direction must be large enough to avoid any aliasing artifacts, and it also needs to be large enough to avoid banding artifacts, created when the beam is mispositioned from one line to the adjacent line. This laser utilizes a spot with full width at half-maximum (FWHM) dimensions of 83.6 and 126.3 μm in the parallel and perpendicular to the scan directions, respectively. The sampling distance in both directions is 80 μm.

9.4.2.3 Uniformity

The uniformity of the imager can be measured by printing a uniform digital image and using a Macbeth densitometer to analyze the output film. Analyses should be performed over the entire writing field (flat field response) as well as over local regions of interest (noise). The flat field response can be determined by measuring the optical densities of 100 random samples along the entire film and computing their standard deviations. The deviation over the entire film in this imager does not exceed 0.04 OD (Fig. 9.18A).

Noise values for the imager can be obtained by taking the optical densities of 100 samples within a 2.0 cm^2 area of the printed film and computing the mean and standard deviations of these measurements. Figure 9.18B plots the results of the noise measurements for the laser imager.

Note that variations parallel to the scan direction arise mainly from fluctuations in the laser output intensity, as well as from instabilities in the acousto-optic modulator. Variations perpendicular to the scan direction are due mainly to positional errors when the film moves to the adjacent line, which results in improper overlapping of adjacent spot distributions.

9.4.2.4 Spatial Resolution

The spatial resolution of the laser imager can be determined by two methods. In the first method, the modulation transfer function (MTF) parallel to the scan direction (Fig. 9.19) is measured by fitting the central parallel density profile of the spot (optical density distribution through the center of the spot of the direction parallel to the scanning beam) to a Gaussian function and computing its Fourier transform under the assumption that the system is linear. In this case, the frequency corresponding to an MTF of 0.5 is 4.6 cycles/mm.

The second method is the contrast frequency response (CFR), in which the

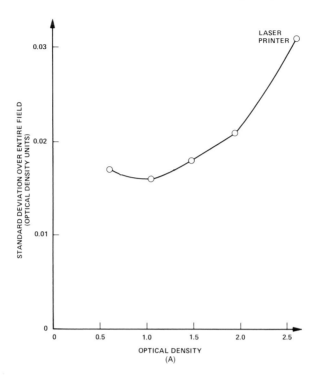

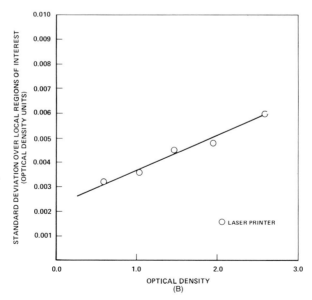

Figure 9.18 Standard deviations of optical density over the total range of the laser imager. (A) Flat field response: data are accumulated over the entire imaging field (global variations). (B) Noise: data are accumulated over small regions of interest (local variations).

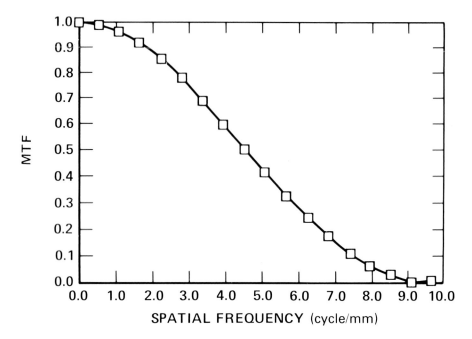

Figure 9.19 The modulation transfer function (MTF) of a laser film imager in the direction parallel to the scan.

spatial resolution can be determined by printing a computer-generated line pair image on film and using a high resolution scanning microdensitometer (Sakura PDM-5) to measure the densities across the line pair pattern on the printed film. For this line pair image, the optical densities of the spaces and lines are 0.16 and 2.3, respectively.

Figure 9.20 plots the results of the contrast frequency response parallel and perpendicular to the scan of the laser imager obtained using the CFR method (see Section 3.3.1.3). The response at 3.0 cycle/mm is 0.89 in the parallel direction and 0.75 in the perpendicular direction. Note that in the perpendicular direction, the writing is discrete, while in the parallel direction it is continuous. Three line pairs per millimeter are easily resolvable on the processed film in both parallel and perpendicular directions.

9.4.2.5 Spatial Linearity

To investigate spatial linearity parallel to the scan direction of a laser film imager, one can print an ideal computer-generated image consisting of parallel and equally spaced lines and observe the deviation of the lines on the resultant film from the ideal image. This can be accomplished by performing a digital subtraction of

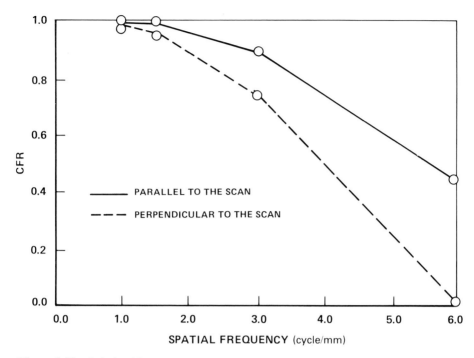

Figure 9.20   Relationship between spatial frequency and contrast frequency response (CFR) parallel and perpendicular to the scan direction of a laser film imager.

the resulting film with a 180° rotation about the normal axis of the same film. The resultant subtracted image provides the visualization of vertical distortions of the lines parallel to the scan direction.

Similarly, a subtraction of a film with vertical lines from a 180° rotation about the axis parallel to the scan direction of the same film results in the visualization of distortions parallel to the scan direction. The digital subtraction can be performed using a vidicon camera connected to an image processor that digitizes the film to $512 \times 512 \times 8$ bits as described in Section 3.2.1.4.

The distortion due to the vidicon camera used instead of the laser imager in this experiment can be measured by digitizing a test image with known linearity. The subtraction of the image from its 180°-rotated image is seen to produce a highly uniform result, thus validating the assumption that vidicon camera digitizing did not cause the nonlinearity.

The results of measuring the spatial linearity indicate that there are slight distortions in the perpendicular direction (maximum deviation of 370 μm for a 20.3 cm² film) and no detectable distortions in the direction parallel to the scan. The same test performed on line patterns from a multiformat video camera (MULTI-IMAGER 7 by Matrix Instruments, an earlier generation film imager that uses vidicon scanning techniques) reveals a maximum deviation of 1490 μm for film of the same size.

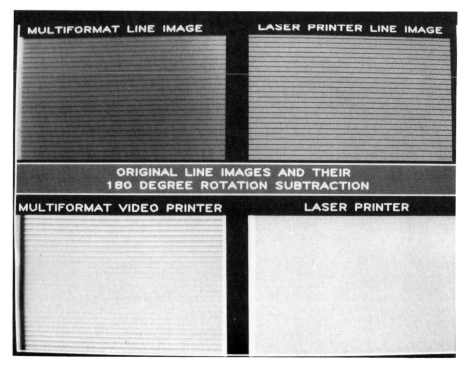

Figure 9.21 Linearity test results of a laser imager and a multiformat camera: *top,* original line images; *bottom,* subtraction images (original rotated 180° about the normal axis of the film). The laser imager (right) shows minimum perpendicular distortion (no line residues) in the subtraction image, whereas the subtraction image from the multiformat video printer (left) shows significant perpendicular distortions.

Vertical distortions correspond to deviation in line scanning speed, while horizontal distortions correspond to nonlinearities in the optics. A special lens (flat field f-theta lens) used in the laser imager corrects for most nonlinearities introduced by conventional lens.

Figure 9.21 compares linearity test results of the laser imager with results obtained using the multiformat camera. The laser imager is clearly superior to the video-based imager in terms of spatial linearity.

The principle of the laser imager system discussed here is identical to that of the film recorder in the computed radiography system discussed in section 4.1. Not only do both systems write a digital image onto a single emulsion film, but in both cases the image recorded has an almost linear relationship of gray level to optical density, a uniform flat field response, a high spatial resolution, and an excellent spatial linearity. Results from these measurements indicate that the laser imager is a very good hard copy recorder for digital radiologic images. The trend in diagnostic radiology is to use the laser imager to record hard copy from digitally generated images.

9.5. Information Retrieval and Display

In Section 8.5.3 we discussed the PACS system software, for image receiving, stacking, routing, archiving, studies grouping, platter management, and RIS and HIS interfacing. These software functions are needed for optimal image and information retrieval at the display workstation. Now we turn to methods and essentials of grouping patients' image and data effectively based on the patient folder manager concept introduced by Arenson (see Arenson et al., 1994).

9.5.1 Patient Folder Manager Concept: Preliminary

Folder Manager (FM) is a software package that drives a picture archiving and communication system (PACS) by means of event trigger mechanisms. The concept emphasizes standardization, modularity, and portability.

The preliminary task of FM is to establish an FM infrastructure, which includes:

- HIS–RIS–PACS interface
- image routing
- image selection
- online radiology reports
- patient folder management

The first three functions were described in Section 8.5.3. We briefly discuss the online reports and folder management here.

9.5.1.1 Online Radiology Reports

The PACS receives radiology reports and impressions from RIS via the RIS–PACS interface and stores these text information files in the PACS database. These reports and impressions can be displayed instantaneously at a PACS display station along with the associated images from a given examination. The PACS also supports online queries of reports and impressions from a display station.

9.5.1.2 Patient Folder Management

The PACS manages patient studies in folders. Each folder consists of a given patient's demographics, examination descriptions, images from current examinations, selected images from previous examinations, and relevant reports and impressions. A patient's folder will remain online at a specific display workstation during the patient's entire hospital stay or visit. Upon discharge or transfer of the patient, it is automatically deleted from the display station.

9.5.2 Patient Folder Manager: Modules

Three software modules are in the patient folder manager:

- Archive Management

Table 9.5 Summary of Patient Folder Manager
Software Modules

Module	Submodules	Essential Level*
1: Archive Manager	Image Archiving	1
	Image Retrieving	1
	HL7 Message Parsing	2
	Event Triggering	2
	Image Prefetching	2
	Platter Management	3
2: Network Manager	Image Sending	1
	Image Receiving	1
	Image Routing	1
	Job Prioritizing and Recover Mechanism	1
3. Display/Server Manager	Image Selection	2
	Image Sequencing	3
	Window/Level Preset	2
	Report/Impression Display	1

* Essential Level (1, highest; 3, lowest): 1, minimum requirements to run the PACS; 2, requirements for an efficient PACS; 3, advanced features.

- Network Management
- Display/Server Management

Table 9.5 describes these three modules and associated submodules and gives their essential level for PACS.

9.5.2.1 Archive Management

The Archive Manager module provides the following functionalities:

- manages distribution of images on multiple storage media
- optimizes archiving and retrieving operations for PACS
- prefetch historical studies to display stations

Mechanisms supporting these functions include event triggering, image prefetching, job prioritization, and platter management.

Event Triggering

Event triggering can be achieved by means of the following algorithm.

ALGORITHM NAME: EVENT TRIGGERING
DESCRIPTION

Events occurring in RIS are sent to the PACS in HL7 format over TCP/IP, which then triggers the PACS controller to carry out specific tasks such as image retrieval and prefetching, PACS database update, platter management, and patient folder cleanup. Events sent from RIS include patient admission, discharge, and transfer (ADT), patient arrival, examination scheduling, cancellation, completion, and report approval.

SOFTWARE CODING

ESSENTIALS

HIS/RIS/PACS interface

HL7 message parsing

Image prefetching

PACS database update

Patient folder management

Platter management

PSEUDOCODE

Wait for HL7 message from the RIS

receive HL7 message

parse HL7 message

case of ⟨message type⟩:

patient transfer or discharge:

group patient images from magneto-optical disks and copy to write once, read many disk(s)

delete patient image folder form display server

examination scheduling:

perform prefetch table lookup

select previous examinations from PACS database

schedule retrieval of patient images

schedule retrieval of patient textual data

examination cancellation:

remove scheduled retrieval jobs

patient arrival:

check existence of patient images in display server

retrieve patient's selected images from optical archive

retrieve patient text data from PACS database

generate or update patient image folder

patient demographics, examination description, or radiology reports:

update PACS database

loop back

Image Prefetching

The prefetch mechanism initiates as soon as the PACS controller detects the arrival of a patient by means of the ADT message from the RIS. Selected historical images, patient demographics, and relevant radiology reports are retrieved from the optical archive and the PACS database. These data are distributed to the destination display station(s) before completion of the patient's current examination.

The prefetch algorithm is based on predefined parameters such as examination type, section code, radiologist, referring physician, location of display station, and

Current Exam Type, n / Section	Pediatrics		Neuroradiology	Chest	Bone	· · ·	Default
	Radiol	Ref Phys					
1-View Chest				2			
2-View Chest				1			
CT-Head				0			
CT-Body				2			
Angio				0			
Conventional Radiography				·			
MR				·			
US				·			
Fluoro							

(Back axes: Disease Category, Standard Rule, Disease 1, Disease 2, · · ·)

Figure 9.22 Four-dimensional prefetching table for examination type, disease category, section radiologist, and referring physician.

number and age of the patient's archived images. These parameters determine which historical images should be retrieved. Figure 9.22 shows a four-dimensional prefetching table that focuses on examination type, disease category, section radiologist, and referring physician. This table determines which historical images should be retrieved from the central archive system. For example, for a patient scheduled for chest examination, the n-tuple entries in the chest column $(2, 1, 0, 2, 0, \ldots)$ represent an image folder consisting of two single-view chest images, one two-view chest image, no CT head scan, two CT body scans, no angio image, and so on.

In addition to this lookup table, the prefetch mechanism utilizes patient origin, referring physician, location of display station, number of archived images for this patient, and age of these individual archived images in determining the number of images from each examination type to be retrieved.

The Prefetch Algorithm

The prefetch mechanism is carried out by several processes within the archive server (see Section 8.5.3.4). Each process runs independently and communicates simultaneously with other processes utilizing client–server programming, queuing control mechanisms, and job prioritizing mechanisms. The prefetch algorithm can be described in the following pseudocode.

ALGORITHM NAME: IMAGE PREFETCHING
DESCRIPTION

> The prefetching mechanism is triggered when the examination scheduled, examination canceled, and patient arrived events occur in the RIS. Selected historical images, patient demographics, and relevant radiology reports are retrieved from the optical archive and the PACS database. These data are distributed to the destination display station(s) before completion of the patient's current examination.

> The prefetch algorithm is based on predefined parameters including examination type, section code, radiologist, referring physician, location of display station, and the number and age of the patient's archived images.

SOFTWARE CODING

> *ESSENTIALS*
> RIS–PACS interface
> Event triggering
> Prefetch table lookup
> Image retrieval
> Database query

> *PSEUDOCODE*
> *Wait for event from the RIS*
> *receive event (HL7 message)*

case of ⟨event type⟩
> *examination scheduled:*
> *perform prefetch table lookup*
> *select previous examinations from PACS database*
> *schedule retrieval of historical images*
> *schedule retrieval of patient demographics and radiology reports*
> *examination canceled:*
> *remove scheduled retrieval jobs*
> *patient arrived:*
> *retrieve patient's selected images from optical archive*
> *retrieve patient demographics and radiology reports from PACS database*
> *generate or update patient folder*
> *loop back*

RULES

Parameters used in the prefetch table lookup process include:

Examination type

Radiologist

Referring physicians

Section code

Display station site

Age of archived image

Number of historical images in the archive

- Current examination type determines number of images from same type or similar type of previous examinations to be prefetched.
- Radiologists and referring physicians may have individual preferred entries.
- Section code and display station site may alter the maximum number of images to be prefetched by changing the 4-D prefetching table. For example, an ICU station would require fewer historical CR images to be prefetched than a chest station.
- Age and number of a patient's archived images may limit the maximum number of images to be prefetched.

Job Prioritization

The PACS controller manages its processes by prioritizing job control to optimize the archiving and retrieving activities. For example, a request from a display station to retrieve an image from an optical disk will have the highest priority and be processed immediately. And, upon completion of the retrieval, the image will be queued for transmission with a priority higher than other images that have just arrived from the image acquisition nodes and are waiting for transmission. By the same token, an archive process must be compromised if there is any retrieval job executing or pending.

The use of job prioritizing and compromising between the PACS processes will result in dramatic decreases in delays in servicing radiologists and referring physicians in the clinic.

Platter Management

During a hospital stay or visit, a patient's current images from different examinations are copied to magneto-optical disks (MODs) for long-term storage. Upon discharge or transfer of the patient, these images are then be grouped from the erasable MODs and copied contiguously to a single write once, read many optical disk or to consecutive WORM disks for permanent storage (see Section 8.5.3.5).

9.5.2.2 Network Management

The network manager handles the distribution of images and text data from the PACS controller. This module, which controls the image traffic across the entire

PACS network, is a routing mechanism based on some predefined parameters (see Section 8.5.3). It includes a routing table composed of the predefined parameters and a routing algorithm that is completely driven by the routing table. The routing table should be designed to facilitate updating as needed. Any change of the routing table should be possible without modification of the routing algorithm.

In addition to routing images to their designated display stations, the network manager performs the following tasks:

- queue images in the event of network or workstation failure
- switch network circuit from ATM to Ethernet when the ATM network fails
- distribute images based on different priority levels

The image sending algorithm can be described in the following pseudocode.

ALGORITHM NAME: IMAGE SENDING

DESCRIPTION

The send process catches a ready_to_send signal from the routing manager, establishes a TCP/IP connection to the destination host, and transmits the image data to the destination host.

Upon successful transmission, the send process dequeues the current job and logs a SUCCESS status. Otherwise, it requeues the job for a later retry and logs a RETRY status.

SOFTWARE CODING

ESSENTIALS

TCP connect

dequeuing

requeuing

event logging

PSEUDOCODE

Wait for ready_to_send signal from image routing manager

catch ready_to_send signal

get next pending job from comm_out queue

open ATM TCP socket

if (TCP_OPEN_FAIL)

open Ethernet TCP socket

if (TCP_OPEN_FAIL)

log error

requeue job

go to loop back

else

go to send_data

else

go to send_data

send_data:

send data to destination host

wait for acknowledgment

```
    if (NEGATIVE_ACK)
       log error
       requeue job with RETRY status
       go to loop back
    else
       de queue job with SUCCESS status
  loop back
```

9.5.2.3 Display–Server Management

Display–server management includes the following tasks:

* image sequencing
* image selection
* window/level preset
* coordiantion with reports and impressions

Window/level preset and coordination with reports and impressions have been described in Sections 8.6.5, 9.3.2.2, and 9.5.1, respectively. Image sequencing is one of the most difficult tasks in display–server management because it involves users' habits and their subjective opinions, but does not supply universal rules to govern these preferences. Algorithm development requires a certain amount of artificial intelligence. The current thought is that this module will be application specific and will require heavy customization. Image selection can be handled by the display–server management using basic rules through user interaction by the following algorithm.

ALGORITHM NAME: IMAGE SELECTION
DESCRIPTION

The image selection process allows a user to select a subset of images from a given image sequence (as in an MR or CT study; see Section 9.3.3) on the display monitor(s). These selected images are then extracted from the original sequence and grouped into a new sequence for future display.

SOFTWARE CODING

ESSENTIALS

Image display
Montage function
PACS database update

PSEUDOCODE

Display complete sequence of images
wait for user to select images through the montage function
accept selection from user
while (SELECT_NOT_DONE)
   read index from selected image
group indexes
insert indexes into PACS global database

RULES
- Indexes stored in PACS database are global (i.e., are accessible from any PACS display stations).
- Individual radiologists and referring physicians may select image subsets and save indexes using the montage function in separate index tables under user's preferred image file names.

9.6 Physician's Desktop Retrieval

9.6.1 Distributed Image File Server

PACS was first developed to meet the needs of image management in the radiology department. As the PACS concept evolved, the need for applications of PACS to cross borders to other health care disciplines increased. For this reason, second-generation or hospital-integrated PACS design should include a distributed image file server to provide integrated image and textual data for other departments in the medical center.

The PACS components and data flow diagrammed in Figure 7.1 represent an open architecture design: the display component can accommodate many types of display workstation as descried in Section 9.1.4. When the number of display workstations (e.g., physician desktop workstations) increases, each with its own special applications and communication protocols, however, the numerous queries generated by the more active system may affect the performance of the PACS controller (see Section 9.1.4). Under such circumstances a distributed image file server(s) linked to the PACS controller should be designed. Figure 9.23, an extension of Figure 7.1, shows such a design for a Macintosh user cluster.

9.6.1.1 Design Criteria

Consider a radiology department in which an existing departmental Ethernet network is supporting over 100 Macintosh users. In this network, the users have access to a variety of output devices such as laser printers and slide makers, and a Quick-Mail (CE Software, West Des Moines, IA) server for electronic mail. Based on this working environment, let us design a departmental image file server that will permit these Macintosh users to access images and data from the hospital-integrated PACS via the PACS controller.

9.6.1.2 The Distributed Image File Server (DIFS) and the Clients

The DIFS should consist of a relatively powerful server—for example, a Sun SPARC20 with a large disk capacity for storing images and related data, an ATM connection with an Ethernet backup to the PACS controller, and a powerful relational database for client–server queries. In each Macintosh client machine, a C-lan-

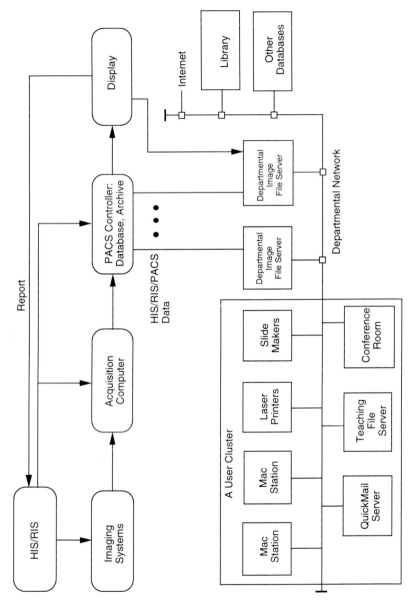

Figure 9.23 Distributed image file servers connected to the PACS controller. Each server provides specific applications for a given cluster of users.

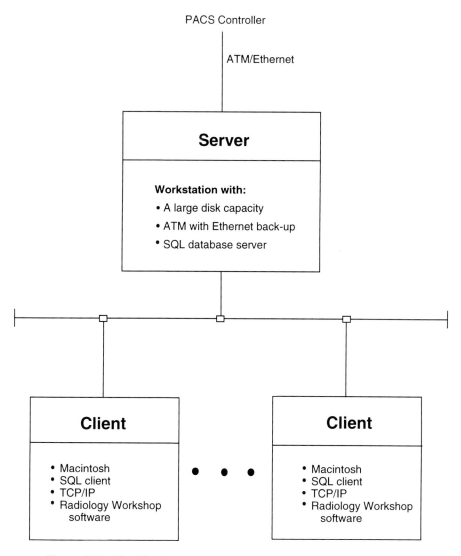

Figure 9.24 Specifications of and connections between server and clients.

guage software package (e.g., Radiology Workshop, developed at UCSF) enables the computer to establish a network communication link with the PACS controller and other databases connected to the departmental network through the use of a variety of TCP/IP based messages. Figure 9.24 shows the specifications and the connections between the server and clients.

Let us use the Radiology Workshop software package in the sample client–server queries that follow.

A. Text Request

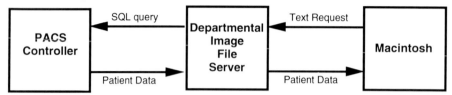

B. Thumbnail Request

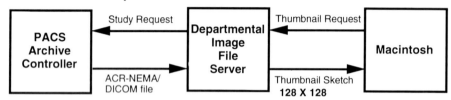

C. Full-Resolution Request

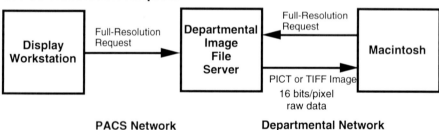

PACS Network   **Departmental Network**

Figure 9.25 Communication between the departmental image file server and the PACS controller and display in response to requests of three types: (A) text requests, (B) thumbnail requests, and (C) full-resolution requests. SQL, structured query language; PICT, Macintosh picture format; TIFF, tagged image file format.

9.6.1.3 Three Types of Query

Text Requests

The Macintosh user may request a patient's demographic and examination information and study reports (Fig. 9.25A) based on the patient's name, the patient's ID, or a variety of search parameters (Table 9.6). The DIFS converts these requests into Structured Query Language queries and transmits them to the PACS controller. Any resulting text information is then passed back to the requesting Macintosh.

Table 9.6 Functionality Provided by the Radiology Workshop Software

Functions	Items
Ability to search for information on the basis of several criteria	Patient's identification number and name
Access to image information	Patient's demographics
	Examination information
	Diagnostic reports
Access to image information	Study thumbnails (128 × 128 resolution thumbnails of each image in a given study)
	Full-resolution study images (of key images) available in one of three forms:
	8-bit Macintosh picture format
	8-bit tagged image file format
	16-bit raw data file
Ability to receive key full-resolution images selected at remote viewing workstations	
Access to radiology information system, hospital information system, and library information system through initiation of online session	

Thumbnail Requests

After acquiring the text information concerning a particular study, the user may request a "thumbnail sketch" of the entire study (Fig. 9.25B). The DIFS requests the particular study from the PACS controller in the ACR-NEMA or DICOM format, generates a "thumbnail sketch" consisting of 128 × 128 resolution image subsamples, and delivers the entire thumbnail sketch to the requesting Macintosh. After the DIFS has sent this thumbnail sketch to the Macintosh, it discards its own copy. The original ACR-NEMA image file, however, can be kept in the DIFS for a certain period of time, perhaps a week, to satisfy any subsequent full-resolution requests. Aside from this temporary storage, no images are archived on the DIFS—it is meant only to act as a gateway into the PACS for radiologists' personal computers. Figure 9.26 shows two thumbnail sketches, as well as the screen output of a patient study list, detailed study information, and a diagnostic report.

Full-Resolution Requests

After viewing a thumbnail sketch, the user may select key images to be retrieved from the DIFS at full resolution using the route outlined in Fig. 9.25C. The DIFS converts these images from the ACR-NEMA format to a standard Macintosh format, such as the Macintosh picture (PICT) format or the tagged image file format (TIFF), in full resolution 8 or 12 bits/pixel, and transfers to the Macintosh's hard drive with the user's specific file name(s), where they may be viewed or manipulated by any standard Macintosh application. Information describing the particular patient and study is inserted into an image header before being transferred

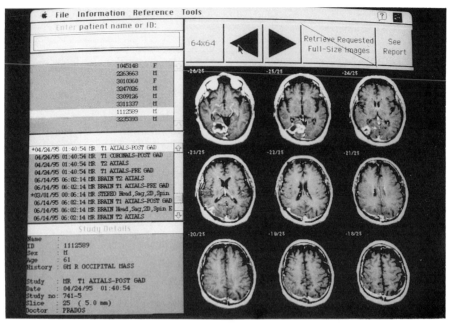

A

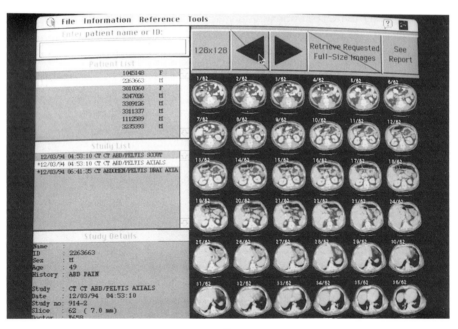

B

Figure 9.26 (A) Macintosh-based physician's desk workstation used for multimedia display: Upper left, patient list; middle left, study list; lower left, patient information; middle and right side, thumbnail screen with a set of MR T1 images subsampled to 128 × 128.

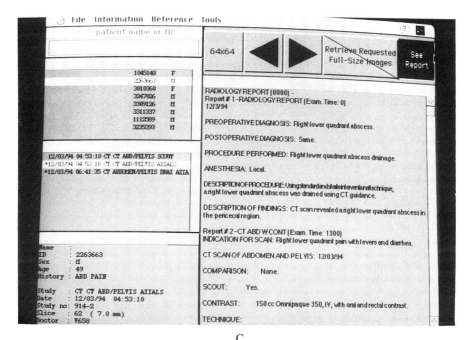

C

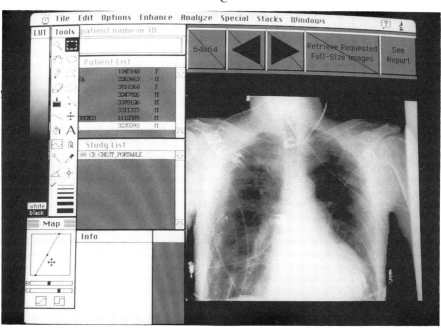

D

(B) Thumbnail screen with a set of CT abdominal images subsampled to 64 × 64. (C) Screen showing the diagnostic report describing the images presented in (B). (D) Screen with a CR image subsampled to 256 × 256 and enhanced with the NIH IMAGE software.

to the Macintosh. The option of letting users create specific file name(s) helps users to keep track of their own large collections of images. In addition, interfaces that allow key images to be selected during image interpretation at the display workstation should have been established (see Fig. 9.23: directional arrow from Display to the DIFS). These selected images and related data can be stored and tagged with the DIFS and later forwarded to the Macintosh by a user's query there.

9.6.1.4 Radiology Workshop Software Package

Radiology Workshop is a C-language software package that allows the user to formulate text, thumbnail, and full-resolution requests to the DIFS and displays any resulting information. Its easy-to-use interface consists of graphic icons and is driven by mouse and keyboard input. The hardware requirements to use this software are minimal—a Macintosh II or better with at least 4 Mbytes of random access memory, a hard drive, and a network connection to the departmental network (either directly or through the Internet). Figure 9.26 shows various types of images and patient information retrieved from PACS through Radiology Workshop. Figure 9.26D shows a full-resolution CR image displayed by a public domain software package, NIH IMAGE, all within the Radiology Workshop domain.

9.6.2 Some Issues Related to Image and Information Retrieval

The distributed image file server (DIFS) allows users with a minimum desktop computer resource to access a wealth of hospital-integrated PACS data effectively. Since the hospital-integrated PACS is open to every potential user in the medical center community, several issues arise, related to system usage, system performance, communication bandwidth, access priority, and data security.

9.6.2.1 System Usage

The images and data retrieved from DIFS are best used in two major applications: the acquisition of Macintosh picture images for slide making and the acquisition of raw image data for image processing. Typically, the user has seen an interesting case during readout and wants to use the system to transfer a few full-resolution key images to his or her Macintosh for storage in a personal teaching file and for slide production. Because of the large amounts of storage required by these images (8-bit MR and CT images need about 64 and 200 Kbyte per slice, respectively), it may be necessary to install other peripheral storage devices, such as the small optical disk drive, to increase the storage capacity for the user. As for slide production, the quality of slides varies greatly from user to user, necessitating the identification of a consistent method of producing good quality slides from computer slide printers.

9.6.2.2 System Performance

The system's response to queries of the PACS controller should be timely. For example, queries of text information should be completed within seconds. The time to acquire a thumbnail sketch of a study is quite variable and is generally deemed to be slow, but it depends primarily on the age of the requested study. While a patient is within the hospital, his or her studies are stored temporarily on high speed magnetic storage. After discharge, this study information is moved to long-term storage in the much slower optical disk library. Thumbnail sketches of these recent studies should be ready within one minute, whereas older studies require several minutes (depending on the size of the study). Because 90% of the retrieval time is spent reading the image from disk, this time is unlikely to be reduced and the delay must be tolerated by the users. However, the user should consider that this image retrieval has a lower priority than the image retrieval from the clinical viewing stations.

With the PACS and DIFS infrastructure in place, widespread installation of this system for use by students and staff outside the department of radiology will result. However, three fundamental issues must be considered before the PACS administration can provide such unparalleled access to patients' text and image data.

Traffic on the Departmental Network

Although the Macintosh interface is designed for selection of only a few key images from a study, the PACS controller always delivers an entire image file through the faster PACS network to the DIFS because of its standard ACR-NEMA or DICOM data format. The DIFS accepts this large image file and extracts only the requested images for delivery to the Macintosh through the slower departmental network. Through a combination of this extraction and the aforementioned data conversion (which typically reduces the number of bytes in an image), the traffic that must be carried on the departmental network is reduced. This leaves bandwidth available for the other major uses of the network, including electronic mail, printing, file transfer, and Telnet.

Priority of Clinical Activities

A priority index must be determined among diagnostic workstations, review stations, and the DIFS clients. The current thought is that the former two should have higher priority. It is likely that requests from DIFS will have to be handled by the PACS controller at a lower priority than clinical requests.

However, the forwarding of key image requests from the workstations to the DIFS relieves the workstations of the significant amount of work involved in transmitting full-resolution images to the user's Macintosh. Thus, key image selection is allowed to take place with little or no slowing of clinical interpretation. The DIFS also relieves the PACS controller of a significant workload by performing the data format conversion (such as ACR-NEMA or DICOM to PICT) that must precede the transmission of these full-resolution images to a Macintosh.

Data Access Rights and Security

Because Radiology Workshop operates through the use of standard TCP/IP protocols, anyone using this software can access the data stored in the PACS archive from anywhere in the world (through the Internet). Therefore, the topic of data security is of paramount importance.

In particular, the issues of data access rights and security give rise to two distinct sets of problems. First of all, data within the PACS must be secure from accidental corruption and tampering, and must be accessible to authorized users only. By limiting access to the PACS to a small number of well-defined read-only requests, the DIFS protects the integrity of the data stored in the PACS. In addition, to access the DIFS, it is necessary for users to obtain a password and register their computers with the department. Only requests from authorized machines with valid user passwords will be accepted.

Second, patients' confidentiality must be strictly maintained. One method is the removal of any identifying data from information transmitted to a user's Macintosh. However, without some type of link to this information, valid clinical research would be significantly inhibited. Policies need to be developed by each institution, based on past experience and clinical requirements, to address these patient confidentiality issues and to identify guidelines specifying who may have access to the data and how the material legitimately may be used.

10

Picture Archiving and Communication System (PACS) IV: System Integration and Implementation Strategies

10.1 System Implementation Strategies

10.1.1 Background

A picture archiving and communication system serves to integrate many components that are related in clinical practice. As we discussed in Chapter 8, depending on the application, a PACS can be simple, consisting of just a few components, or it can be a complex hospital-integrated system. For example, a PACS for an intensive care unit may comprise no more than a scanner near the film developer for digitization of radiographs, a base band communication system to transmit the images, and a video monitor to receive and display images in the ICU itself. On the other hand, the establishment of a comprehensive hospital-integrated PACS is a major undertaking that requires careful planning and millions of dollars of investment.

During the past 10 years, many hospitals and manufacturers in the United States and abroad have researched and developed PACS of varying complexity. Some of these systems are in clinical trial and use. These systems can be loosely categorized into two groups according to methods of implementation. The first category is the homegrown system, developed within the department or hospital because of clinical needs. The second category is market driven. That is, manufacturers see potential profit in developing a turnkey PACS, as a new product component for a special application to enhance the sales of other product lines.

In the late 1980s, the surgeon general of the U.S. military services initiated the Medical Diagnostic Imaging Support (MDIS) system concept. The MDIS adopted military procurement procedures in acquiring PACS for military hospitals and clin-

ics. This approach created a third category of implementing PACS. Section 10.1.2–
10.1.5 discuss these approaches and provide examples for each.

10.1.2 Three Methods of PACS Implementation

Most PACS implementation efforts are initiated by university hospitals and academic departments and by research laboratories of major imaging manufacturers of
imaging equipment. There are generally three methods of approach. In the first
approach, *systems integration,* a multidisciplinary team with technical know-how is
assembled by the radiology department or the hospital. The team becomes a system
integrator, selecting PACS components from various manufacturers. Its members
develop system interfaces and write the PACS software according to the clinical
requirements of the institution. In the second approach, *requirements specification
and contracting,* a team of experts, from both outside and inside the hospital, is
assembled to write detailed specifications for the PACS for a certain clinical environment. A manufacturer is contracted to implement the system. In the third, or
turnkey approach, the manufacturer develops a PACS and installs it in a department
for clinical use.

Each approach has advantages and disadvantages. The systems integration approach, for example, allows the research team to continuously upgrade the system
with state-of-the art components. A system so designed is tailored to the clinical
environment and can be upgraded without depending on the schedule of the manufacturer; it will not become obsolete. On the other hand, a substantial commitment is
required of the hospital to assemble a multidisciplinary team. In addition, since the
system developed will be one of a kind, consisting of components from different
manufacturers, service and maintenance will be difficult.

The primary advantage of the second approach (requirements specification and
contracting) is that the PACS specifications are tailored to a certain clinical environment, yet the responsibility for implementation is delegated to the manufacturer.
The department acts as a purchasing agent and does not have to be concerned with
the installation. The specifications tend to be overambitious, however, because of
the potential for experts, not familiar with the clinical environment, to underestimate
the technical and operational difficulty of certain functions. The designated manufacturer, who may lack experience with some components in a clinical environment,
may in turn overestimate the performance of each component. As a result, the
completed PACS may not meet the overall specifications. The cost of contracting
with a manufacturer to develop a specified PACS is also high because when only
one system is built, the narrow profit margin will not always permit the realization
of economies of scale.

The advantage of the third or turnkey approach is that in a generalized production
system, the cost tends to be lower. In this approach, the manufacturer needs a couple
years to complete the production cycle. By the time system is commercially available, however, some components from the fast moving computer and communication fields may have become obsolete. Also, it is doubtful whether a generalized

Table 10.1 Advantages and Disadvantages of Three Methods
of PACS Implementation

Method	Advantages	Disadvantages
1. Systems integration	Built to specifications State-of-the art technology Continuously upgraded Not dependent on a single manufacturer	Difficult to assemble a team One-of-a-kind system Difficult to service and maintain
2. Requirements specification and contracting	Specifications written for a certain clinical environment Implementation delegated to the manufacturer	Specifications may be over ambitious Technical and operational difficulty may be underestimated Manufacturer may lack clinical experience Expensive
3. Turnkey	Lower cost Easier maintenance	Too general Not state-of-the-art technology

PACS can be used for every specialty in a single department and for every radiology department.

Most likely, all three approaches will gradually merge as additional clinical data regarding PACS become available. Table 10.1 summarizes the advantages and disadvantages of these approaches.

Because of various operating conditions, the emphasis in PACS research and development is different in North America, Europe, Japan, and South Korea. In the United States, PACS research and development is mostly supported by government agencies and manufacturers. In the European countries, it is supported through either multinational consortia or country or regional resources. European research teams tend to work with a single major manufacturer, and most PACS components, which are developed in the United States and Japan, are not as readily available in Europe. European research teams emphasize PACS modeling and simulation, as well as investigation of the image processing component of PACS.

In Japan, PACS research and development is a national project, with the country's resources distributed among various manufacturers and university hospitals. A Japanese manufacturer integrates a PACS system and installs it in a hospital for clinical evaluation, but the manufacturer's PACS specifications tend to be rigid, leaving little room for the hospital research team to modify the technical specifications.

South Korea, a recently emerging force in PACS installations, receives support from large private manufacturers.

10.1.3 Method 1: Systems Integration

For the method 1 approach, we give two examples at the University of California: Los Angeles (UCLA) and UC San Francisco. The UCLA approach, which began in

1984, has three phases. Phase 1, from 1984 to 1990, encompassed demonstration of the concept of PACS and the design of the PACS infrastructure. Phase 2, from 1990 to 1991, comprised clinical implementation of several PACS modules. Phase 3, which began in 1992, includes systems refinement, maintenance, and applications.

10.1.3.1 The UCLA Approach

Phase 1: Demonstration of Concept and Design of PACS Infrastructure

To demonstrate the concept of PACS to physicians, in 1987 UCLA implemented two PACS modules, one in the pediatric radiology section (within the department) and the other in the coronary care unit. The pediatric radiology section was selected because it operates independently and resembles a miniradiology department. It is an excellent model with which to study the implementation of a complete PACS within a radiology department. In this module, images are displayed on two 2048-line monitors. The module is used for daily conferences and case reviews. The coronary care unit was chosen for the second PACS module because a viewing station in this unit is convenient for clinicians who need to stay near their patients. It is a model of a PACS outside the radiology department. In this module, images are displayed on three 1024-line monitors. Both modules are in clinical operation 24 hours a day, 7 days a week. Radiologists and clinicians alike had very positive reactions to their experiences with these two systems.

From 1988 to 1990, the UCLA team concentrated on the design of the PACS infrastructure. The critical components in the infrastructure, which supports a digital-based radiology operation, are the communication system, PACS controllers, database, fault-tolerance design, and system integration software.

The infrastructure was implemented from 1990 to 1991. There are 64 multimode and 48 single-mode fiber-optic cables connecting the three buildings (Center for the Health Sciences, Medical Plaza, and Taper Building) housing the radiology department. There are two PACS controllers, one at the Center for the Health Sciences and one at the Medical Plaza. The infrastructure has been online since the beginning of 1991.

Communication System. UCLA designed a three-tiered fiber-optic communication system with Ethernet, FDDI (fiber-distributed data interface), and Ultranet. The Ethernet is used to transmit images from acquisition devices to the acquisition computer. Since the acquisition device is slow in generating images, transmission speed between these two nodes is not crucial. Images are reformatted at the acquisition computer and sent to the cluster controller by means of FDDI. Images are archived onto optical disks and distributed to the image display stations with the 1.0 Gbit/s Ultranet. The three communication networks are coexistent in the infrastructure and serve as backups for each other.

PACS Controllers. There are two PACS controllers in the infrastructure. Each controller is composed of a SPARC 4/490 image server (Sun Microsystems, Mountain View, CA) with a 4- Gbyte magnetic disk storage, a 1- Tbyte optical disk library for archiving images, and a Sun SPARC 4/490 server running the database (Sybase; Emeryville, CA) for patient directory and text information. The controllers are identical in architecture and can be used as mutual backup. PACS controllers are connected with the Ultranet. Images can be transmitted between PACS controllers at 4–8 Mbyt/s. An identical Sybase database in each PACS controller serves as the mirrored system. Current patient image information is updated continuously on the database of every controller.

Fault-Tolerance Design.   In the infrastructure, every component has a backup. The database exists in multiple copies, one in each cluster controller. Each PACS controller is located in a separate room to diminish the potential for disaster. The three communication networks back up each other, and all active fiber-optic cables have a duplicate. Each cluster controller is powered by an uninterruptable power supply (UPS) with up to 20 minutes of back-up power.

Systems Integration Software.   The communication system, PACS controllers, database, and backups are integrated as the PACS infrastructure by means of an elaborate system software. The system software was written in C programming language and runs under the UNIX operating system.

Phase 2: Implementation of PACS Modules

Two tasks are required to implement PACS modules in a clinical environment. The first task is to connect image acquisition devices to the PACS controller through the infrastructure. The second is to design and implement display stations in the department and in the clinics. With respect to image acquisition, three computed tomographic (CT) and three magnetic resonance (MR) scanners with direct digital interface to acquisition computers and to two PACS controllers were connected to the infrastructure. Also, three computed radiography units and three film digitizers were connected. The establishment of the infrastructure made these connections possible.

Phase 3: Systems Refinement, Training, Maintenance, and Applications

Phase 3 comprises three stages. Stage 1 is the continuing development of display stations and their clinical implementation. Stage 2 consists of refining the system, upgrading the display station software, and establishing protocols for training, maintenance, and service. Stage 3 consists of researching PACS applications.

Stage 1: Display Stations and Clinical Implementation.   Five stations, each with two 2048-line monitors, were implemented in the pediatric radiology (two stations), neuroradiology, chest radiology, and bone radiology sections. One printing station was installed as a hard copy device. In addition, two three-monitor 1K stations were installed in the coronary care unit and in the pediatric ICU. Figure 10.1 shows the UCLA PACS infrastructure and image acquisition and display stations.

Stage 2: Systems Refinement and Training, Maintenance, and Service.   During clinical implementation, procedures were set up for training, systems maintenance,

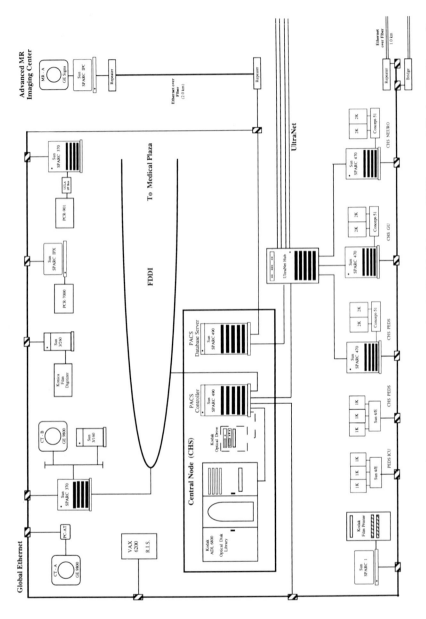

Figure 10.1 The UCLA PACS network at the Center for the Health Sciences (CHS) remote MR site: GenUn, genitourinary radiology; PCR, Philips computed radiography; Peds, pediatric radiology; RIS, radiology information system.

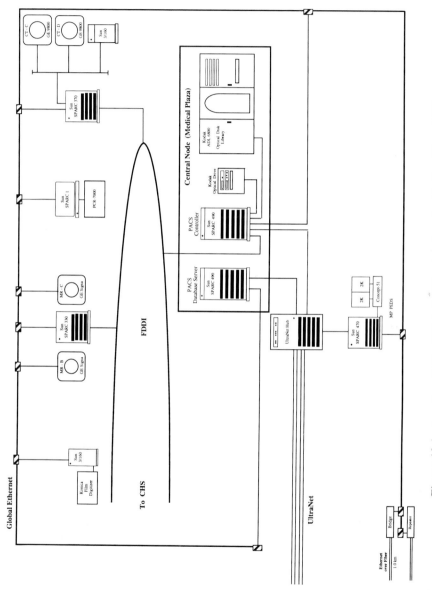

Figure 10.1 (*continued*) The UCLA PACS network at the Medical Plaza (MP).

419

and service. Three groups of personnel must be trained. First, radiologists and clinicians must learn to use the display stations. The second group, which includes the PACS coordinator, technologists, and clerical personnel, requires extensive training that covers image quality assurance, updating the patient directory, and first-line troubleshooting. Members of the third group, the PACS engineers, need to become familiar with all operational aspects of the PACS; hence their training is the most extensive.

10.1.3.2 The UCSF Approach and Other Examples

The core team that developed the UCLA PACS relocated to UCSF in October 1992 with the goal of developing in northern California a system based on a similar philosophy. In addition, the UCSF team believes that a PACS is more than a management tool; it is in fact a vehicle for future medical practice and research. For this reason, the UCSF PACS infrastructure design provides the framework for future PACS research (see Fig. 8.17 and Fig. 11.4). The first research area is image quantification, which includes the conventional image measurement methods, image reformatting, registration, fusion, and image content extraction and indexing. The purpose of this research is to extend medical diagnoses from qualitative to quantitative. The second area of research is interactive teaching. Traditional medical teaching is passive in the sense that knowledge is transmitted by the teacher and the textbook to the learner. The PACS can be used as an interactive teaching tool for diagnostic radiology through the rich PACS database (see Section 9.6). The third area of research is the development of a digital imaging database management system. Information science provides the methodology to derive knowledge from databases. Thus far, however, traditional databases have been limited to text information because no large medical digital image database has ever existed. The PACS database, including both images and textual information, is a hidden treasure that awaits probing by the researchers to develop new research and diagnostic tools. It is anticipated that this rich PACS database will open a new horizon in medical research. Section 11.2 will discuss the PACS future research directions in more detail.

Examples of other medical centers following the method 1 approach are the Geneva University Hospital in Switzerland, and ASAN Medical Center (AMC) in Seoul, South Korea. The developers of AMC adopted the UCSF approach and worked with Hyundai Electronic, Ltd. for implementation starting in February 1995. The project is to develop the PACS at AMC in Seoul first and then extend it by connecting other Hyundai-related hospitals in South Korea with wide area networks.

10.1.4 Method 2: Requirements Specification and Contracting

Sections 10.1.4.1–10.1.4.4 present examples of how some PACS were implemented with method 2 by medical centers all over the world. The Hokkaido University Medical Information System Project in Japan was founded by the late Professor Goro Irie. The second Social and Medical Center East project in Vienna, known by its acronym SMZO, is directed by Professor W. Hruby. The third example, the

MDIS for the U.S. Military Medicine Project, is by far the largest PACS installation with multiple sites. Finally, we have the Hammersmith Hospital project in London, which is based on the MDIS architecture.

10.1.4.1 The Hokkaido University Medical Information System Project

The Hokkaido University PACS project was probably one of the earliest and largest projects in medical information systems. It integrates PACS, hospital information systems, and medical records. There are three networks, one for each system. The project, started in 1989, adopts a top-down approach and is a whole-hospital information system, connected through a PACS loop. The system was planned by a team of experts from Hokkaido University, Fuji Medical Systems, and Nippon Electronic Corporation (NEC). The final system was designed and implemented by NEC. The department uses computed radiography exclusively, and all these units are connected to the network.

The Japanese system uses 1024-line monitor display stations, each equipped with software providing lookup table, rotation, inverse, and zoom and scroll capabilities, as well as subtraction, edge enhancement, and linear and angular measurement functions. The system handles 30% of the computed radiography images (300/day) and 100% of the CT and MR images and digital subtraction angiograms (500/day). Images are stored on magnetic disk for a week, and older images can be retrieved from the optical disk library in 40–60 seconds. The system is continuously upgraded by NEC. The number of terminals is targeted for approximately 200.

10.1.4.2 The Vienna Social and Medical Center East (SMZO)

The SMZO in Vienna, Austria, is a 1400-bed teaching hospital with nurse training and a geriatric center. It started operation in 1991 and serves 100,000 people. The planning of a PACS for this institution started in November 1989, with a team comprising members from the staffs of the hospital and the designated manufacturer (Siemens AG, Erlangen, Germany). This PACS adopts a top-down approach, integrating PACS, RIS, and HIS. The planning is based on a two-level approach: macro and micro. The computer sciences department in the hospital and the development group from Siemens are in charge of the macroplanning, whereas the radiology department is in charge planning at the microlevel. The system architecture is based on a token ring topology with the 100 Mbit/s FDDI; its database and network adhere to the ACR-NEMA standard.

There are two optical disk libraries with online access of 2×179 Gbyte. The system has a fault-tolerant control image management system including storage and archiving. The workstations in the radiology department have from two to eight monitors, whereas inexpensive PC-based display stations were chosen for clinical use. The system data volume ran to about 9 Gbyte/day in the first 2 years of operation. The system started clinical operation in 1992 with continuing modification and fine-tuning. The project has a built-in 5-year upgrade and update program.

10.1.4.3 *Medical Diagnostic Imaging Support Systems (MDIS) for the Military Medicine Project*

The MDIS project in the United States, one of the largest PACS development efforts, has the objective of implementing filmless medical imaging systems at several military medical treatment facilities over several years. The surgeon general of the military services created the MDIS project to exploit the results of extensive imaging research efforts over the past 10 years. These filmless MDIS systems were acquired from industry (Loral, Sunnyvale, CA) through a contracting approach that (1) functionally describes subsystem and system performance for acceptable clinical operations, (2) validates proposed systems in performance evaluation, and (3) selects a system and awards a contract based on the best value to the U.S. government.

The first four sites of the MDIS project are Madigan Army Medical Center (MAMC), Washington; Brooks Air Force–Army Hospital, Texas; Wright–Patterson Air Force Hospital, Ohio; and Luke Davis–Monthan Air Force Hospital, Arizona. The targets of the first four sites are organized as follows. By the end of phase I, 6 months after the contract is awarded, basic MDIS for inpatients should be operational (40% digital). Phase II consists of a graceful MDIS transition, including the high volume outpatient examinations (65% digital). Finally, phase III is for refinement and to achieve inclusion of low volume outpatient examinations (90%). The MDIS technical specifications constitute one of the most comprehensive PACS implementation plans ever devised.

These four large-scale PACS projects have passed the hurdles of system design, fund raising, system selection, system implementation, and clinical use. The success of their clinical operation will demonstrate that a manufacturer can provide a PACS installation for a specific site. It will also provide the medical community with solid data for future PACS planning and implementation. The paragraphs that follow give a brief overview, focusing on the installation at Madigan.

The military first assembled a team of experts in 1989, and the team traveled around the country visiting different PACS research and development sites. They then wrote the technical specifications, including those pertaining to service, maintenance, and training, for the four sites. The military contracting office issued a request for proposals, inviting potential manufacturers to bid for the project. In the last quarter of 1991, the military selected Loral and Siemens Gammasonics and started the installation at Madigan.

The MAMC is the army's newest tertiary care center with over 400 inpatient beds and a large outpatient clinical facility. The PACS at this facility started clinical operation in March 1992. Its current main focus is connecting the PACS to five computed radiography (CR) systems, computed tomography (CT) and digital-spot imaging (DSI) devices. Images are stored in both hard copy and soft copy form. In the case of soft copy storage, a 10:1 lossy compression is used in the optical disk library after the image has been reviewed, and a 2.5:1 lossless compression is used in the temporary working storage unit (WSU) before the image is read.

The clinicians at the MAMC accept the system without any hesitation, whereas the radiologists are more conservative. Both groups have benefited from the PACS operation in terms of patient care. A very conservative estimate is that 1 hour per week will have been saved by the clinicians regarding image and report availability. With 400 doctors in MAMC, this translates to a savings of 20,000 physician-hours per year. The MAMC PACS is continuously evolving: an increase in the number of display workstations is planned, and connecting the PACS with the hospital information system (HIS) and radiology information system (RIS) is projected.

Since the installation of the Loral system in Madigan Army Hospital and other military hospitals, similar systems with slight modifications have been installed in non-military hospitals including the VA Medical Center in Baltimore and Samsung Medical Center in Seoul, mentioned earlier, and London's Hammersmith Hospital, which we discuss next.

10.1.4.4 Hammersmith Hospital Project

The Hammersmith Hospital in London, England, has built a new radiology department. A committee chaired by the hospital's director of finance and information planned a top-down, whole-hospital PACS project. The hypothesis of the project is that cost savings arising from PACS will be due to increases in the efficiency in the hospital. The 453-bed Hammersmith Hospital which includes the Royal Postgraduate Medical School and the Institute of Obstetrics and Gynecology, serves 100,000 people. The specifications of the system are based on the MDIS described in Section 10.1.4.3. The project is justified by the committee on the basis of the direct and the indirect cost-saving components. The following direct cost/saving components are considered: archive material and film use, labor, maintenance, operation and supplies, space and capital equipment, and buildings. The indirect cost savings are in the areas of junior medical staff time, reductions in unnecessary investigations, (saving the time of radiologists, technologists, and clinicians) redesignation and change of use of a number of acute beds, and reduction in the length of stay. The project is in the evaluation phase.

10.1.5 Method 3: Turnkey Approach

Sometimes a medical center will order a turnkey system from a manufacturer, with some modifications made for its own specific clinical application. One example, the COMMView system developed by AT&T and Philips (Shelton, CT), is used by Georgetown University in Washington, DC, the University of Washington in Seattle (see also Section 1.3), and the Bowman Gray School of Medicine at Wake Forest University in Winston-Salem, North Carolina.

10.1.6 Current Trends

During the past years, we have witnessed many hospitals implementing PACS by merging gradually these three approaches, retaining suitable but discarding some irrelevant features based on their clinical requirements. This phenomenon is especially pronounced in the merging of methods 2 and 3 in several recent installations. An example is the turnkey system by Loral which was originally developed for U.S. military medical centers from the method 2 approach. Since then, Loral has modified the MDIS specified system to turnkey systems and installed them worldwide: in the Veterans Administration Medical Center in Baltimore, in Hammersmith Hospital in London, and in Samsung Medical Center in South Korea. The merging between method 1 and method 2 can be exemplified by the AMC, Seoul, project in which AMC adopted an open architecture approach and contracted with Hyundai Electronic, Ltd. for the installation. Methods 2 and 3 approaches are necessary for large scale implementation whereas method 1 remains as the driving force to stimulate methods 2 and 3 in adopting standardization, open architecture, and the utilization of state-of-the art technologies. While more PACS are being implemented, the importance of standardization, open architecture, reliability, and security must not be ignored by the medical centers and manufacturers.

10.2 Planning to Install a PACS

10.2.1 Film-Based Operation

The first step in planning a PACS is to understand the existing film-based operation. In most radiology departments, the film-based operation procedure is as follows.

Conventional diagnostic images obtained from either X-ray or other energy sources are recorded on films, which are viewed from alternators (light boxes) and archived in the film library. Images obtained from digital acquisition systems—for example, nuclear medicine, ultrasound, transmission and emission computed tomography, computed radiography, and magnetic resonance imaging—are displayed on the acquisition device's monitor for immediate viewing, then recorded on magnetic tapes or disks for digital archiving. In addition, they are recorded on films for viewing as well as for archival purposes. Since films are convenient to use in a clinical setting, clinicians prefer to view digital images on films even though this method reduces image quality. As a result, most departments still use films as a means of diagnosis and as a storage medium regardless of image origin. In general, films obtained within 6 months are stored in the departmental film library and older films are stored remote from the hospital. To retrieve older films requires from 0.5–2 hours.

Most radiology departments arrange operations in an organ base with exceptions in nuclear medicine, ultrasound, and sometimes MRI and CT. Some hospitals group MRI and CT into neuro and body imaging sections. It is advantageous during planning to understand the cost of the film-based operation. The sample tables that follow are useful for collecting statistics in the planning stage. Table 10.2, an example of the tabulation of number of procedures, film used, and film cost, provides an overall view of data from each specialty. This information can be used to design the PACS controller routing mechanisms, to determine the number of display workstations required, and to arrive at the local storage capacity needed for each

Table 10.2   Record on Number of Procedures, Film Used, and Film Cost

Section (Specialty)	Number of Procedures, Year 1, . . . , Year N	Film Used (sheets) Year 1, . . . , Year N	Film Cost (dollars)* Year 1, . . . , Year N
Nuclear Medicine			
Ultrasound			
CT/MRI			
Pediatrics			
Genitourinary and gastrointestinal (abdominal)			
Neuroradiology			
Cardiovascular			
Interventional			
General outpatient[†]			
General inpatient[†]			
Mammography			
Emergency			
ICUs[‡]			
Total			

*   Film cost is for X-ray film purchase only; film-related costs are not included.
†   Include chest and musculoskeletal examinations.
‡   Inlcude all portable examinations.

display workstation. The film cost can be used to estimate the film-based operation cost compared with the digital-based or PACS operation cost.

Table 10.2 also can be used to generate a film-based operation cost estimate as shown in Table 10.3. Direct and indirect film library expenses included under item 1 in Table 10.3 are X-ray film jackets, mailing envelopes, insert envelopes, negative preservers, rental on film storage both inside and outside the department, and fleet services for film deliver; direct and indirect film processor expenses (item 2) are

Table 10.3   Multiple-Year Estimation of Film and Film-Related Costs*

	Year 1	. . .	Year N
1. Film library	$		$
Indirect expenses	$		$
2. Film processor	$		$
Indirect expenses	$		$
3. Personnel			
Darkroom	$ (FTE)		$ (FTE)
Film library	$ (FTE)		$ (FTE)
4. Film-related costs			
Total (1 + 2 + 3)	$		$
5. Film cost	$		$
(from Table 10.2)			
Total costs	$		$

*   FTE, full-time equivalent.

Table 10.4   Percentage Distribution
                of Conventional Projection
                X-Ray Procedures Performed
                and Effort Required According
                to Body Region

Procedure	Percentage	Effort Required*
Chest	40	18%
Skeletal	39	25%
Gastrointestinal	9	22%
Genitorurinary	1	8%
Neuroradiology	1	9%
Others	7	15%

*   Effort required means that it takes 18% effort to perform all chest
x-ray examinations which amounts to 40% of all departmental examinations, and so forth.

equipment purchases, developing solutions, replacement parts, facilities repairs and installations, and other miscellaneous supplies. In a typical film-based operation in a large teaching hospital, 70% of the film-based operation budget is allocated to the film library (item 3). The film cost (item 5) should be derived based on the number of procedures performed and films used per year given in Table 10.2. The film operation (not including film viewing) requires a large amount of premium space within the department, which should be translated to overhead cost in the estimate.

Table 10.3 is necessary in the estimation of the cost of the film-based operation in a radiology department. Using this table and the PACS checklist (Section 10.2.2.2) will allow a comparison of the PACS installation and operation costs with that of the film-based operation. Tables 10.2 and 10.3 give an overview of the film-based operation and its cost. Tables 10.4 and 10.5 provide comparative statistics, as well.

Table 10.4 is an estimated breakdown of the percentage distribution of procedures performed and efforts required in conventional projection X-ray examinations according to body region in a large urban hospital in the northeastern United States. A similar table can be generated for digital sectional images including CT, MR, and US. The effort required is a measure of time and labor required to perform the procedure. Table 10.5 gives estimated annual percentage volumes of procedures from three civilian and three military hospitals. MR head procedures are not entered as an item in either table because there is considerable deviation among hospitals in both number of procedures and number of images generated per procedure. A hospital or a department planning to install a PACS should generate such a table to allow comparison with hospitals listed in these tables and make a judgment accordingly.

There are several two-phase cost analysis models available in the market to help a hospital to analyze the cost impact of PACS. The first phase is to assess the present film-based operation cost. In this phase, the user completes data forms similar to

Table 10.5 Estimated Annual Percentage Volume of Procedures:
Comparing a Site Planning for PACS with Six Other Hospitals

	Hospital X, Planning a PACS	Civilian Hospitals, % (images/procedure)			Military Hospitals, % (images/procedure)		
		A	B	C	D	E	F
Chest		30 (2)	20 (2)	17 (2)	33 (2)	41 (2)	23 (2)
Extremities		12 (2.5)	10 (2.5)	22 (3)	17 (2.5)	16 (3)	20 (3)
Spine, rib		4 (3)	4 (4)	7 (2)	5 (3)	7 (2)	7 (3)
CT*		4 (12)	8 (20)	7 (12)	5 (/)	4 (/)	6 (/)
Other (MR, US, CT body, etc.)		50	58	47	40	32	44
Total %		100%	100%	100%	100%	100%	100%
Total number of procedures		160,000	98,000	66,000	106,000	79,000	101,000

* Head only.

Tables 10.2 and 10.3, and the model will present a detailed costing of the film-based operation. In the second phase, the user evaluates how these costs might differ upon implementation of the PACS. A model like this will allow the hospital to have an overview of the financial impact on the current film-based operation of a PACS implementation.

10.2.2 Digital-Based Operation

10.2.2.1 Planning a Digital-Based Operation

Interfacing to Imaging Modalities and Display Workstation Usage

In a digital-based operation, two components (see Fig. 7.1) are not under the absolute control of the PACS developer/engineer: namely, interfacing to imaging modalities and the use of display workstations. In the former, the PACS installation must coordinate with imaging modality manufacturers to work out the interface details. In the latter, radiologists and clinicians are the ultimate users to approve the system. For these reasons, human interface and communication play important roles in planning the installation. When a new piece of equipment is purchased, it is important to negotiate with the manufacturer on the method of interfacing the imaging modality to the PACS controller. It is necessary to include the ACR-NEMA or DICOM standard in the equipment specification for image communication purposes.

In designing the display workstation and its environment, user input is mandatory, and several revisions are necessary to assure user satisfaction.

Cabling

We described cabling and the hub room concept in Section 8.2. This section discusses the overall cable plan. Proper cabling for the communication of images and patient text information within the department and within the hospital is very crucial for the success of a digital-based operation. The traditional method of cabling for computer terminals is not recommended because as the magnitude of the digital-based operation grows, the web of connecting wires very quickly becomes unmanageable.

Cabling is much simpler if the entire department is on the same floor. Greater complications ensue when the communication cable must traverse the whole hospital, which may occupy many floors or even many building complexes.

The plan of laying out cables to support the digital-based operation should be very carefully thought through. Fiber-optic video broadband communication systems seem to be a good plan, since only two cables (one for backup) will suffice for up to twenty-five 512-line video channels for real-time telemanagement (see Section 8.3.2.1). When cables become long, signal amplification must be provided at certain strategic points in the network, to retain the integrity of the signal.

In the case of a digital network, ATM with an Ethernet backup is the preferred choice; details were described in Section 8.1.3.

Air Conditioning

Most digital equipment in a digital-based operation requires additional air conditioning. If a new radiology department is planned, adequate air conditioning should be supplied to the central computing, server, and image processing facility. Normally, display stations do not require special air conditioning, but certain room temperature requirements are still necessary.

Because a hospital is always limited in space, it may be difficult to find additional central air conditioning for the large area housing the PACS central facility. Sometimes individual, smaller air-conditioning units must be installed. The individual air conditioner can be a stand-alone floor unit or a ceiling-mounted unit.

Each time another air-conditioning unit is installed, additional cool water from the hospital is required. Thus the hospital's capacity for cooling water should be considered. Also, as noted earlier, additional air-conditioning units will create a lot of noise in the room. To ensure that the room housing the display workstations is suitable for viewing images, adequate soundproofing should be used to insulate these areas from the extra noise created by the air-conditioning and cooling system.

Staffing

The hospital or department should allocate special technical staff to support the digital-based operation. In particular, categories in system programming, digital engineering, and quality assurance personnel are necessary to make a digital-based operation run smoothly and efficiently. These new full-time equivalents (FTEs) can be allocated from switching some FTEs in the film-based operation. Even with the manufacturer installing a digital-based operation for the department and providing support and maintenance, the department retains the responsibility for supplying the personnel to oversee the operation. In general, the staff requirements consist of one hardware engineer, one system/software engineer, and a quality assurance technologist, all under the supervision of a PACS manager.

Training

The department or hospital should provide four categories of training to the staff.

Continuing Education for the Radiologists/Clinicians.   Adequate training by the department should be provided to staff radiologists/clinicians on the concept of a digital-based operation as well as the use of the display workstation. This training should be periodic, and updates should be offered as new equipment or display workstations are implemented.

Residents' Training.   The training for radiology and other specialty residents should be more basic: the four- or three-year residency program should include training in a digital-based operation. A one-month elective in PACS would be advantageous to radiology residents, for example. In this period, one or two residents would rotate through the PACS unit and obtain basic training in computer hardware architecture, software overview, architecture of the image processor, communication protocols, and the concept of the display workstations.

The residents also can learn all the basic image processing functions that are useful for image manipulation, as described in Section 9.3. The training schedule should be in the first or second year of residency to allow the physicians to understand the concept and the complete procedure involved in a digital-based operation early in their training. This will facilitate future digital-based operations for the department and the hospital. In addition, a quick refresher course every year in July, when new house staff starts in radiology and other specialities, will minimize the downtime of the display workstations.

Training of Technologists.   Some retraining of the technologists in the department must precede the changeover to a digital-based operation. Digitization of images using the laser scanner on X-ray films, and the use of a computed radiographic system with imaging plates, are quite different from the screen–film procedure familiar to technologists. Also, the integration of image workstations for diagnosis and computer terminals for logging in information of the patients in RIS is a new concept that requires additional training. The department should provide regular training classes, emphasizing hands-on experience with existing equipment.

Training of Clerical Staff.   Past experience in training secretarial staff to use word processors rather than typewriters has proven that the switch to digital operations at the clerical level is not difficult. The training should emphasize efficiency and accuracy. Ultimately, the move to digital-based operation will reduce the number of FTEs in the department.

10.2.2.2 Checklist for Implementation of a PACS

This section provides a checklist for implementation of a hospital-integrated PACS. Implementation cost and operational cost can be estimated by multiplying the component price by the number of units and adding the subtotals. Component prices can be obtained from vendors.

    I. Acquisition Computers
        (one computer for every two acquisition devices)   No. ____
        Local disk   No. ____
        ATM connection   No. ____
        Interface connections   No. ____
   II. PACS controller
        Database machine   No. _2_
        File server   No. ____
        Optical disk library   No. ____
        ATM connection   No. ____
  III. Communication Networks Cabling (contracting)
        ATM switches   No. ____
        Ethernet hub   No. ____
        Router   No. ____
        Bridge   No. ____
        Video monitoring system   No. ____

IV. Display Workstations   No. ___
    Four-monitor 2K station   No. ___
    Two-monitor 2K station   No. ___
    Four-monitor 1K station   No. ___
    Two-monitor 1K station   No. ___
    One-monitor 1K station   No. ___
V. Interface to Other Databases
    HIS   Yes ___   No ___
    RIS   Yes ___   No ___
    Other database(s)   Yes ___   No ___
VI. Software Development
    The software development cost is normally about 1 to 2 times the hardware cost.
VII. Equipment Maintenance/year
    10% of hardware + software cost
VIII. Consumable
    Optical disks/year   No. ___
IX. Supporting Personnel
    FTEs (full time equivalent)   No. ___

10.3 PACS System Evaluation

Finally, we discuss several methodologies of PACS system evaluation. The first method is to evaluate subsystem throughputs, which does not involve a comparison of film-based and digital-based operations. The second is a method of directly comparing the performance of film-based and digital-based operations. The third method is a standard ROC (receiver operating characteristic) analysis, comparing image quality of hard copy versus soft copy display. Sections 10.3.1–10.3.3 give examples of each method.

10.3.1 Subsystem Throughput Analysis

When analysts evaluate the throughput rates of individual PACS subsystems, including the acquisition, archive, display, and communication networks, the overall throughput rate of the PACS is the total of those for all these subsystems. Figure 10.2 shows a block diagram of PACS subsystems and image residence times. Table 10.6 defines acquisition, archival, retrieval, distribution, display, and network residence times.

The throughput of a PACS subsystem can be measured in terms of the average residence time of individual images in that subsystem. The residence time of an image in a PACS subsystem is defined as the total time required to process the image in order to accomplish a particular task within that subsystem. The overall throughput of a PACS can then be measured by the total residence time of an image in the various subsystems.

Each of the PACS subsystems may perform several tasks, and each task may be accomplished by several processes. An archive subsystem, for example, performs three major tasks: image archiving, image retrieval, and image routing. To perform

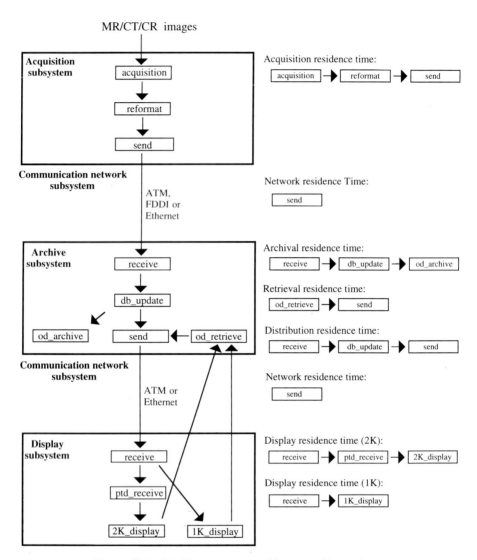

Figure 10.2   PACS subsystems and image residence times.

the image retrieval task, a server process accepts retrieve requests from the display station, a retrieve process retrieves an image file from the optical disk library, and a send process sends the image file to the destination display station. These three processes communicate with each other through a queuing mechanism and run cooperatively to accomplish the same task. In this example, the retrieval residence time of an image file in the archive subsystem can be measured by the elapsed time from the moment an archive server receives a retrieve request, then retrieves the image file from the optical disk library, to the moment the server has finished sending the image file to the destination display station.

Table 10.6 Definitions: Acquisition, Archival, Retrieval, Distribution, Display, and Network Residence Times

Image Residence Time	Subsystem Where Measurement Performed	Definition
Acquisition	Acquisition	Total time of receiving an image file from a radiologic imaging device, reformatting images, and sending the image file to the PACS controller.
Archival	Archive	Total time of receiving an image file from an acquisition computer, updating the PACS database, and archiving the image to an optical disk.
Retrieval	Archive	Total time of retrieving an image file from an optical disk and sending the image file to a display station.
Distribution	Archive	Total time of receiving an image file from an acquisition computer, updating the PACS database, and sending the image file to a display station.
Display (2K)	Display	Total time of receiving an image file from the PACS controller, transferring the image file to the disk storage array and displaying it on a 2K monitor.
Display (1K)	Display	Total time of receiving an image file from a PACS controller and displaying it on a 1K monitor
Network	Network	Total travel time of an image from one PACS component to another via a network.

10.3.1.1 Acquisition Residence Time

An acquisition subsystem performed three major tasks: (1) acquiring image data and patient demographic information from radiologic imaging devices, (2) converting image data and patient demographic information to the DICOM format, and (3) sending reformatted image file to a PACS controller. Images from various modalities are acquired via different data interface methods, described in Section 7.5.2. The current technology adopted by major manufacturers limits the transfer speed of image data from a radiologic imaging device to its acquisition computer. This constitutes the major deleterious factor that affects the overall throughput of a PACS. The real-time acquisition residence times of the MR, CT, and CR images are described in the subsections that follow. We use the GE Signa MR, the GE 9800 CT, and the Fuji CR 901 as examples.

MR and CT Image Acquisition

GE MR and CT (General Electric Medical Systems, Milwaukee, WI) transmitted images at a slow data rate (< 100 Kbyte/s) via the Ethernet, utilizing a standard file transfer protocol (see Section 7.5.2.5). The acquisition computers scanned the image directories within the scanners periodically and extracted new images from the scanners. However, since there is no information from the scanners to indicate the completion of a scan, the acquisition process knows that a scan is complete only when a slice image from a new sequence or patient scan is detected or the number of slice images remains constant over a certain period of time. Thus there is a significant delay in acquiring a complete sequence of slice images (or image file) to the PACS (all slice images from one scan are defined as a complete sequence and are packed into a PACS image file through the reformat process). Reformatting slice images from one scan into a PACS image file is done during the waiting time (i.e., before the next slice image is received), and therefore the acquisition time of an image sequence overlaps the reformat time of its individual slice images.

CR Image Acquisition

Images from the CR are acquired through a PIP (Philips Interface Processor) or DASM (data acquisition system manager) interface (see Section 7.5.2.2) and are transmitted to the acquisition computer. Figure 10.3 shows the average acquisition residence times of the MR, CT, and CR images measured from the acquisition subsystem in the UCLA PACS system. These measurements can be obtained automatically through an automatic log program in the acquisition computer.

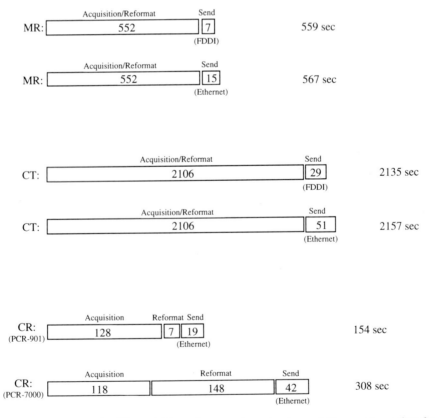

Figure 10.3 UCLA PACS acquisition subsystem throughput: acquisition residence time for three image sizes: MR, 1.96 Mbyte; CT, 13.2 Mbyte; CR, 4 (PCR-901) and 8 Mbyte (PCR-7000).

Archive Residence Time

Images in the PACS controllers are archived to the optical disk library. However, the archival residence time of an image was found to be significantly affected by the job prioritizing mechanism utilized in the PACS controller. Because of its low priority compared with the retrieve and distribute processes running on the archive subsystem, an archive process is always compromised—that is, it must wait—if there is a retrieve or distribute job executing or pending. Figure 10.4A shows the archival residence time of images in the UCLA system based on 7.5 Mbyte regardless of modality. These residence times represent the required times for an image to be processed in the archive, retrieve, and distribute tasks.

Distribution Residence Time

Images are retrieved from the optical disk library to the PACS controllers. Among the three major processes carried on by the PACS controller, retrieve requests always have the highest priority. Thus images intended for study comparison are always retrieved and sent to the requested display station immediately, before archive and distribute processes are initiated. Figure 10.4B shows the retrieval residence time of images.

Distribution Residence Time

All arriving images in the PACS controller are distributed immediately to their destination display stations before being archived on the optical disk library. These images are sent to the 2K stations via a high speed network (e.g., the ATM). Figure 10.4C shows the distribution residence time of images.

Display Residence Time (2K)

A 2K display station configured with a disk storage array or parallel transfer disks may need to first transfer images from a regular magnetic disk to the parallel transfer disks. Figure 10.5A shows the display residence time of the 2K (8 Mbyte) images measured in the UCLA system.

Display Residence Time (1K)

A 1K display station stores and displays 1K images only and is not required to transfer images between a regular disk to a parallel transfer disk. Figure 10.5B shows the display residence time of the 1K (1 Mbyte) images measured in the UCLA system.

Communication Subsystem: Network Residence Time

The residence time of an image in the multiple communication networks can be measured as an overlapped residence time of the image in the acquisition, archive, and display subsystems (see preceding subsections). The ATM or other high speed communication network throughput is limited by the magnetic disk input/output rate.

Archival:

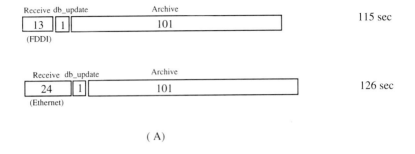

(A)

Retrieval:

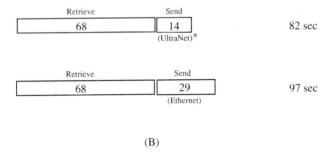

(B)

Distribution:

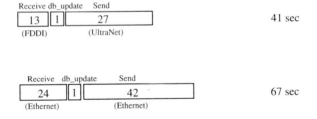

(C)

Figure 10.4 UCLA PACS archive subsystem throughput: (A) archival, (B) retrieval, and (C) distribution residence times; image size is 7.5 Mbyte regardless of image modality. Ultranet, a 1 Gbit/s proprietary network, is no longer in use at UCLA.

* Ultranet is a 1.0 gigabit/s network using TCP/IP. This technology has since been replaced by other high speed networks like the ATM.

2K station:

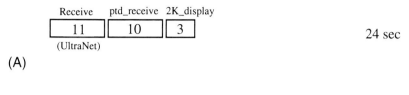

(A)

24 sec

1K station:

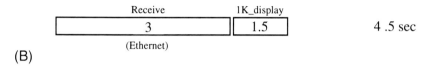

(B)

4 .5 sec

Figure 10.5 UCLA PACS display subsystem throughput: display residence time for (A) 2K station, 8 Mbytes (2048 × 2048 × 2 bytes) and (B) 1K station, 1 Mbyte (1024 × 1024 × 1 byte).

PACS Overall Throughput: Total Image Residence Time

The overall throughput of the PACS can be determined by the total residence time of an image from its original source (a radiologic imaging device) to its ultimate destination (a display station or the optical disk library). For example, the total residence time of a CT image from acquisition to display can be measured as the total of its acquisition residence time, distribution residence time, and display residence time (Table 10.7). In this example, a total of 2205.5 seconds, or 36.8 minutes, is required for a 13.2 Mbyte CT image to become available for review in a 2K display station upon completion of an examination as measured in the UCLA system. This overall throughput performance is very typical for delivering a CT examination.

10.3.1.2 *Prioritizing*

Using job prioritizing control allows urgent requests to be processed immediately. For example, a request from a display station in the archive subsystem to retrieve an image from the optical disk library has priority over any other processes running on the archive subsystem and is processed immediately. Upon completion of the retrieval, the image is queued for transmission with a priority higher than that assigned to the rest of the images that have just arrived from the acquisition nodes and are waiting for transmission. During the retrieval, the archive process must be compromised until the retrieval is complete. Suppose, for example, that the retrieval of a 20 Mbyte image file from an optical disk library takes 54 seconds; if this image file is retrieved while another large image file is being archived to the same library,

Table 10.7 PACS overall Throughput:
Required Processing Time for a 13.2 Mbyte
CT Image File from Acquisition to Display

PACS Subsystem	PACS Process	Required Processing Time (s)
Acquisition	*acquisition/reformat*	2106*
	send (over FDDI)	29*
Archive	*receive*	
	db_update	1
	send (over Ultranet network)	48†
Display	*receive*	
	ptd_receive	16.5†
	2K_idisplay	5†
Total processing time		2205.5
		(or 36.8 min)

* This time is modality dependent.
† Based on the following required processing times: send (7.5 Mbyte): 27 seconds (Fig 10.4C); *ptd_receive* (8 Mbyte): 10 seconds (Fig 10.5A); and *2K_display* (8 Mbyte): 3 seconds (Fig 10.5A). These averages are then extrapolated to the 13.2 Mbyte data stream.

however, the retrieval time for the former image will be 96 seconds. In other words, the time delay of the retrieval without job prioritizing is 42 seconds.

The bottleneck in PACS performance is the low speed data interface implemented by the major manufacturers in their radiologic imaging and archive devices. For example, current system design of MR and CT scanners has made it difficult for PACS developers to provide prompt, online clinical service.

10.3.2 System Efficiency Analysis

We can use image delivery performance, system availability, and user acceptance as means of measuring system efficiency.

10.3.2.1 *Image Delivery Performance*

One method of evaluating PACS system efficiency is to compare image delivery performance from the film management system and from the PACS. For example, consider the neuroradiology PACS component—in particular, the delivery of CT and MR images. We can decompose both the film and digital operating systems into four comparable stages. In the case of the film management system, the four stages are as follows:

1. At each CT and MR scanner, technologists create films by windowing images, printing images, and developing films.
2. Film librarians deliver the developed films to the neuroradiology administration office.

3. Neuroradiology clerks retrieve the patient's historical films and combine them with the current examination films.
4. Radiology residents or film library personnel pick up the prepared films and deliver them to a readout area (or neuroradiology reading room).

Similarly, the four stages in the PACS are as follows:

1. The period during which the capture computer receives images from the scanner systems and formats images into the DICOM standard image file.
2. The elapsed time of transferring image files from the acquisition computer to the data management host computer (PACS controller).
3. The processing time for managing and retrieving image files at the data management host computer.
4. The time needed to distribute image files from the data management computer to the display workstation.

The time spent in each film management stage can be recorded and estimated by technologists, film clerks, and personnel who have many years of professional experience. Circumstances that should be excluded from the calculation because their performance variances are too large to be valid include retrieving a patient's historical films from a remote film library and the lag time between pickup and delivery of films to and from the various stages in the film management system. These exclusions apparently make the performance of a film-based management system more competitive with that of a PACS module.

The performance of the PACS data management subsystem can be automatically recorded in database files and log files by software modules. The data included in these files are (1) date, time, and duration of each modularized process and (2) size of image file acquired.

The total elapsed time from creation of an image file at a scanner to availability of the image file at a display workstation is defined as the image delivery performance of a PACS system (which is similar to the residence time defined in Section 10.3.1). As an example, Table 10.8 shows the results of average image delivery

Table 10.8 Analysis of Image File Delivery Performance, in Minutes, of the Neuroradiology PACS Module

File*	Stage 1	Stage 2	Stage 3	Stage 4	Total (min)
CT					
Current	40.0	0.50	0.15	1.15	41.80
Previous	0	0	1.25	1.15	2.40
MR					
Current	7.00	0.15	0.17	0.47	7.79
Previous	0	0	0.57	0.47	1.04

* Current, image file newly acquired from the imaging scanner; previous, image file previously acquired and archived to an optical disk library.

Table 10.9 Comparison of Image Delivery Performance,
in Minutes, Between the Film Management System
and the PACS Module in a Neuroradiology Section

System	Demand on System	Stage 1	Stage 2	Stage 3	Stage 4	Total (min)
Film-based	Optimal situation*	25.0	1.0	2.0	0.0	28.0
	Regular situation	50.0	25.0	15.0	3.0	93.0
PACS	CT†	80.0	1.0	2.9	4.6	88.5
	MR‡	35.0	0.75	3.75	4.7	44.2

* The patient has no previous radiographs, the patient is scanned with a few images, and the patient's images are reviewed at a film reading room near the scanner and the film administration office.
† Two newly acquired and two previous CT image files are used to calculate the total.
‡ Five newly acquired and five previous MR image files are used to calculate the total.

performance for one currently acquired image file from the scanner and one archived image file from the optical disk library in a neuroradiology PACS module. CT and MR image files are quite different in size. On average, a CT file is approximately five times larger than an MR file. Because the image file size is one of the fundamental factors affecting the delivery performance, CT and MR image files should be recorded separately.

Table 10.9 compares the image delivery performance of a film management system and a neuroradiology PACS module. Since a consistent comparison baseline is difficult to achieve for both systems, the performance (time to complete tasks in each stage) should be redefined. For example, the images may be based on a patient's film jacket in the film-based management system and on the patient's two examinations in the PACS system. On average, approximately two image files (studies) are created for each CT examination and five image files are generated in an MR examination. The two CT image files are either contrast and noncontrast studies, or one of them is a scout view image. The five MR files are various pulse sequence studies. Therefore, in this comparison study, it is reasonable to use two newly acquired and two older CT image files and five newly acquired and five older MR image files as a basis in the digital system. In this particular example, the average image delivery performance (88.5 min for CT and 44.2 min for MR) of the PACS system is better than the average performance (93 min) of the film-based management system. However, a patient's film jacket may contain many image examinations. If more than two examinations are used to calculate the image delivery performance with the PACS system, the comparison study may show different results. It must be noted that although all historical examinations of a patient are important, the latest previous examination is essential in a clinical comparison study (see Section 9.5.1.2). Most neuroradiologists use the current image examination and the latest previous examination to make the diagnosis and refer to older examinations only if necessary.

In the PACS system, the performance of delivering one MR examination (five image files) is twice as fast as that of delivering one CT examination (two image files). The major difference is at stage 1: capturing and formatting images takes 80 minutes for a CT examination but only 35 minutes for an MR examination. In fact, the performance bottleneck, as we discussed earlier, is not the twin processes of capturing and formatting in the PACS; rather it is the system design of the CT scanner that causes a lengthy delay. The scanner has no means of indicating to the communication protocol that the last image slice of a given study in the CT image acquisition process has been sent. Lacking this information, the image capturing program must wait until the first image slice of the next study is received before it can close the last image file. Until the system design of the CT scanner is modified, therefore, any improvements in delivering CT examinations will be limited in scope.

10.3.2.2 System Availability

PACS system availability can be examined in terms of the probability that each component will be functional during the period of evaluation. In the neuroradiology example, the components considered to affect the availability of the neuroradiology PACS include (1) the image acquisition subsystem, including all CT and MR scanners and interface devices between the scanners and the acquisition computers, (2) the PACS controller and the optical disk library, (3) the display subsystem, with its display workstation computer and display monitors, and (4) the communication network.

Calculations of the probability that each component will be functional can be based on the 24-hour daily operating time. The probability P that the total system will be functional is the product of each component's uptime probability in the subsystem, defined as follows:

$$P = \prod_{i=1}^{n} P_i \qquad (10.1)$$

where P_i is the uptime probability of each component and n is the total number of components in the subsystem.

10.3.2.3 User Acceptance

The acceptability of the display workstation can be evaluated by surveying users' responses and analyzing data from a subjective image quality questionnaire. Table 10.10 shows a sample item in a user acceptance survey, and Table 10.11 is a typical subjective image quality survey.

10.3.3 Image Quality Evaluation

A major criterion in determining the acceptance of the PACS by users is image quality in soft copy displays, as compared with the quality available from hard copy. In the preceding section, we briefly noted a subjective image quality survey method. In this section, we discuss a more rigorous analysis based on the receiver operating

Table 10.10   Display Workstation User Survey Form

Attribute	Poor (1)	Fair (2)	Good (3)	Excellent (4)	Average Score
Image quality					
Speed of image display					
Convenience of image layout					
Performance of manipulation functions					
Sufficiency of patient information					
Sufficiency of image parameters					
Ease of use					
Overall impression					

Overall average

characteristic (see Section 6.5.5). Although it is tedious, time-consuming, and expensive to perform, ROC has been accepted in the radiology community as the de facto method for objective image quality evaluation. The ROC analysis consists of the following steps: image collection, observer testing, truth determination, and statistical evaluation. Consider a sample comparison of observer performance in detecting various pediatric chest abnormalities—say, pneumothorax, linear atelectasis, air bronchogram, and interstitial disease—on soft copy (a 2K monitor) versus digital laser-printed film from computed radiography. Sections 10.3.3.1–10.3.3.4 provide basic steps of carrying out an ROC analysis.

10.3.3.1 Image Collection

All routine clinical pediatric CR images are sent to the primary 2K workstation and the film printer for initial screening by an independent coordinator, who selects

Table 10.11   Subjective Image Quality Survey Form for Comparing the Film-and-Light Box Versus the Display Workstation

	Ranking Scales (Perception of Confidence)					
	Least					Most
Display systems	1	2	3	4	5	6
Film and light box						
Display workstation						

images of acceptable diagnostic quality, subtle findings, disease categories, and matched normal images. To ensure an unbiased test, half the selected images should be determined from the soft copy and the other from the hard copy. A reasonably large-scale study should consist of about 350 images to achieve a good statistical power.

The selected images should be screened one more time by a truth committee of at least two experts who have access to all information related to a specific patient, including clinical history and images obtained by means of other radiologic techniques. During this second screening, some images will be eliminated for various reasons (e.g., poor image technique, signal too obvious, overlying monitoring or vascular lines clouding the image, overabundance of a particular disease type). The remaining images are then entered into the ROC analysis database both in hard copy and in soft copy forms.

10.3.3.2 Truth Determination

Truth determination is always the most difficult step in any ROC study. The truth committee usually determines the truth of an image by using the clinical history of each patient, the hard copy digital film image, the soft copy image, all image processing tools available, and biopsy results if they are available.

10.3.3.3 Observer Testing and Viewing Environment

The display workstation should be set up in an environment similar to a viewing room, with ambient room light dimmed and no extraneous disruption. Film images should be viewed in a standard clinical viewing environment.

Observers are selected for their expertise in interpreting pediatric chest X-rays. Each observer is given a set of sample images from which to be trained on four steps: (1) learning how to interpret an image with soft copy display, (2) completing an ROC form (see example, Fig. 10.6), (3) viewing the corresponding hard copy film from a light box, and (4) filling out a second ROC form on the hard copy film from a light box.

10.3.3.4 Observer Viewing Sequences

An experimental design is needed to cancel effects due to the order in which images are interpreted. The image sample from the ROC database can be randomized and divided into four subsets (A, B, C, and D), containing approximately equal numbers of images. Identical subsets are present for both the hard copy and the soft copy viewing. Each observer participates in two rounds of interpretation. A round consists of several sessions (depending on the total number of images). To minimize fatigue, each observer interprets about 30 images during a session. During the first round, the observers interpret all images, half from hard copy and the other from

Case Number_____   Board Number_____

Patient Name_____   Procedure Date_____Time_____

Patient I.D._____   Reading Date_____Size_____

Instructions: If abnormality is present, please indicate your level of confidence.

Confidence Scale:
        0 . . . . 1 . . . . 2 . . . . 3 4

    Sure Not Present   50% sure   100% sure
        (default)   It is Present   It is Present

Radiographic Condition	Enter Confidence Ratings					
	Absent	Diffuse	R.U.	R.L.	L.U.	L.L.
1. Pneumothorax						
2. Interstitial Disease						
3. Linear Atelectasis						
4. Air Bronchograms						

Comments:

Figure 10.6 Structured receiver operating characteristic form used in a typical ROC study. For each disease category, a level of confidence response is required. Chest quadrants assessed were right upper (R.U.), right lower (R.L.), left upper (L.U.), and left lower (L.L.).

soft copy. During the second round, which should be 3–5 months later to minimize the learning effect, the observers again interpret all images, but for each image using the viewing technique not used in round 1. The viewing sequence is shown in Table 10.12.

Table 10.12   Order of Interpreting Image
Sets Used in the ROC Study

Observer No.	Order of Interpreting Technique Subsets*	
	Round 1	Round 2
1	A1, B1, C2, D2	A2, B2, C1, D1
2	A2, B2, C1, D1	A1, B1, C2, D2
3	C1, D1, A2, B2	C2, D2, A1, B1
4	C2, D2, A1, B1	C1, D1, A2, B2
5	C1, D1, A2, B2	C2, D2, A1, B1

*   A, B, C, and D are the four image sets, each with equal
number of images. The number 1 and 2 refer to the technique
(soft or hard copy). For example, observer 1 views image sets
A1, B1, C2, D2 during the first round of interpretation and later
(>3 months) reviews the image sets A2, B2, C1, and D1.

10.3.3.5 *Statistical Analysis*

The two ROC forms for each image modality filled in by each observer are entered
in the database. Results are used to perform the statistical analysis. A standard ROC
analysis program—for example, CORROC2 developed by Charles Metz of the
University of Chicago—can be used to calculate the ROC curve area (see Fig. 6.36)
along with its standard deviation for a given observer's results for the hard copy and
soft copy viewing methods. The ROC area overall data can be compared by disease
category with the paired t-test. The results will provide a statistical comparison of
the effectiveness of using soft copy and hard copy on these sets of images in
diagnosing the four disease categories. This statistical analysis forms the basis of an
objective evaluation of image quality of the hard copy and soft copy displays
derived from this image set.

Picture Archive and Communication System (PACS) V: Current Development Trends and Future Research Directions

11.1 Recent Trends in PACS Development

Recent trends in PACS development focus on three areas of application: large-scale PACS, teleradiology, and intensive care units (ICUs).

11.1.1 Large-Scale PACS

PACS has different definitions depending on the user's perspective. It can be as simple as a film digitizer connected to a display workstation with a local database for ICU application, or it can be as complex as a total hospital-integrated PACS. Dr. Roger Bauman, editor in chief of the *Journal of Digital Imaging,* sent out a survey form in 1993 that set forth three conditions a system had to satisfy to qualify as a large-scale PACS:

- It is in daily clinical use.
- It connects to three or more modalities.
- It makes images available inside and outside the radiology department.

Based on this definition, Bauman identified 13 large-scale PACS systems in 1993, and this list had increased to over 20 by 1995. It is clear from these surveys that one PACS developmental trend is toward large-scale systems. Generally speaking, when a new hospital or a new radiology department is being planned, a large-scale PACS is included. Whether the plan is eventually carried to the implementation stage very much depends on financial issues rather than on operational or technical conditions. Almost all these large-scale plans entail hospital-integrated PACS that interface with other hospital information systems. Implementation of a hospital-integrated PACS is expensive and requires a total commitment from the hospital administration. Most plans use the method 2 approach described in Section 10.1.4. Large-scale PACS is a necessary stimulus for the medical community to adopt a digital-based operation.

11.1.2 Teleradiology

Teleradiology can be used to connect peripheral imaging centers to a major radiology consultation center. For example, the Mayo Clinic in Rochester, Minnesota, maintain peripheral imaging centers in Florida and in Arizona. In this application, an imaging center is equipped with various imaging modalities and has on staff technologists to perform examinations but may not employ a general radiologist to do readings. After an examination, routine diagnosis is performed at the imaging center if a radiologist is present; otherwise, all images, especially those requiring the attention of a specialist, are transmitted through teleradiology to the consultation center for interpretation. Such a setup makes possible the delivery of the best possible radiology service to patients. The peripheral imaging centers provide a convenient examination site, relieving many patients of the need to travel extensively for an examination. The remote diagnosis by the specialist provides the necessary expert care.

Teleradiology has a second application as well: to serve remote and rural areas, where radiologists are scarce. Without teleradiology, a radiologist receives contracts to review images from various rural clinics within a radius of a few hundred miles, traveling among these centers to read cases on certain days of the week. It is not uncommon for a patient in the rural area to wait for several days before a radiologist can arrive on site to review the examination.

Teleradiology becomes very useful when it permits rural clinics to transmit images to a specific location for diagnosis by a radiologist or when it offers a way for images to be transmitted to a metropolitan area where a consultation center is located. In both cases, the reading turnaround time is speeded up by full utilization of the capability of teleradiology. A typical example of this application is found on military bases across the United States.

11.1.3 ICU Modules

In the case of ICU applications, the important factor is the timing requirements that must be satisfied in providing radiologic services under critical conditions. Numerous favorable reports on ICUs with teleradiology demonstrate that PACS improves the efficiency as well as the clinical services in the ICUs. There are two possible system designs. The first method is to have only the display component in the ICU; the digital imaging system, including the transmission component, is located in the radiology department. Examinations performed in the unit are brought to the radiology department for processing either in the film or the digital mode. In the former case, a digitizer is necessary to convert the film to a digital image. A radiologist can perform the wet reading, whereupon the digital image along with the digital voice dictation are transmitted to the ICU referring clinician for immediate service. In the second design, the imaging system, the transmission component, and the display component are all in the ICU. A high resolution display system is also placed in the radiology department. In this arrangement, the digital image from the radiologic examination is generated at the ICU. Images are also transmitted to the radiology department to be read. Digital voice dictation is transmitted from the radiology department to the ICU and is appended to the image.

Both architectures have advantages and disadvantages. In the first design, the technologist is still required to bring the exposed film cassette or CR plate to the radiology department for processing, which normally takes 30 minutes. In the second design, the hospital must place a digital imaging system (e.g., a CR) in the ICU as well as a high resolution display system in the radiology department. Obviously these two additional components will increase the cost of the system. Figure 11.1 shows an architectural design of an ICU PACS module based on the first approach.

ICU PACS Module

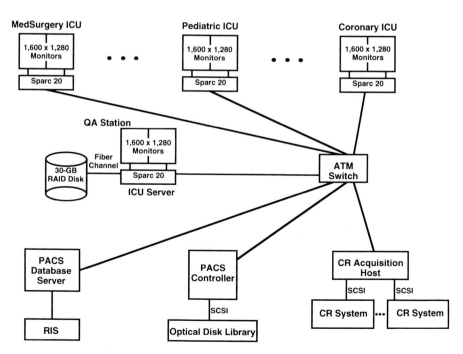

Figure 11.1   Architectural design of an ICU PACS module. In this design, only the display component is in the ICU; digital imaging systems, including the transmission component, are located in the radiology department. QA: quality assurance.

11.1.4 Emergency Room Module

The emergency room (ER) module is used to solve the urgent need for images and their interpretation by ER physicians in an extremely stressful environment, where timely arrival of image-related information means life or death to a critically injured patient. For this reason, it is advantageous to have the required imaging equipment and display system in the ER. The second design of the ICU module described in Section 11.1.3 fits into this application, that is, the imaging system (CR), the transmission component, and the display component are all in the ER. In addition, a high-resolution display system is also placed in the radiology department for immediate interpretation. During an operation, computed radiography images of the critically injured patient are taken at the ER. These images are transmitted immediately to both the ER and radiology reading areas. A radiologist on duty performs a wet reading in the radiology reading area. Voice dictation is transmitted instantaneously to the ER, and is appended to the images by the ER PACS module, ready for the ER physicians to use. A well-organized ER PACS operating system can take less than five minutes to deliver both images and interpretation to the ER reading area after the images are taken. Figure 11.2 depicts the architectural design of an ER PACS module.

11.2 Future Research Directions

PACS originated as an image management system for improving the efficiency of radiology practice. It is evolving into a hospital-integrated system dealing with information media in many different forms, including voice, text, medical records, images, and video recordings. To integrate these various types of information requires the technology of multimedia: hardware platforms, information systems and databases, communication protocols, display technology, and system interfacing and integration. We have discussed most of these topics in earlier chapters. As a PACS grows, so does the content of its database. The richness of information within the PACS provides an opportunity for a complete new approach in medical research and practice via the discipline of medical informatics. This last section in the book touches on some new research frontiers in PACS.

11.2.1 Medical Image Database Management

The PACS environment consists of a vast network of heterogeneous autonomous, and distributed computing resources, including data from HIS, RIS, and PACS. The usefulness of PACS for image content query is seriously limited, however, by the lack of a image database management component in the PACS design. A key challenge in this environment is to create a medical image database server (MIDS) that can provide capabilities for combining this varied collection of databases and information sources into an integrated system, and for allowing uniform and transparent access to multimedia medical data from a single image workstation. When

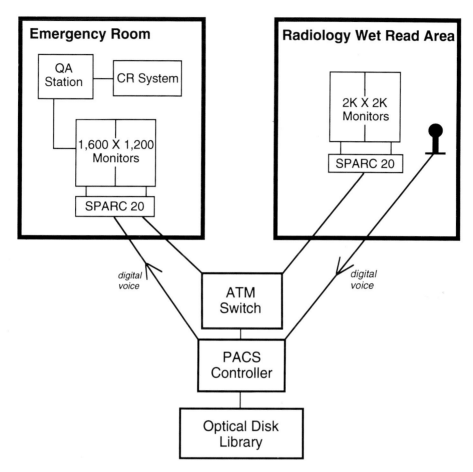

Figure 11.2 Architectural design of an emergency room PACS module. In this design, the imaging system, the transmission component, and the display component are all in the ER. A high resolution workstation is also placed in a radiology reading area for wet reading.

the basic framework is in place, valued-added tools can be developed and incorporated to access integrated information, which in turn will permit the making of better diagnostic or therapeutic decisions. Among these tools of the future will be programs that can reason and extract implicit, previously unknown, but medically relevant information from patient images, demographic records, and related data.

The capabilities of a medical image database server include (1) support for at least one data model, or abstraction, through which the user can view the data, (2) support for certain high level operators or languages that allow the user to define the structure of data, access data from PACS, and manipulate them, and (3) transaction management, or the capability to provide correct, concurrent access to the database through artificial and image content indexing by many users at once.

A MIDS differs from a file system, which does not provide fast access to arbitrary portions of the data. For example, current methods in a database query to a PACS involve a series of complex, time-consuming operations to retrieve *all* related *entire* image files and patient records from the optical disk library and the RIS. The user must review these retrieved data to search for the information needed. Such ineffective data management renders the query operation impractical for clinical use. The concept of MIDS is to provide effective tools for manipulating medical images and free text information, paralleling the handling of records and tables by a relational database system. The physician's desktop retrieval system described in Section 9.6 is the current method available to access PACS data through an artificial indexing, namely, the patient's name or ID. Although not very efficient, this physician's desktop retrieval system does provide a first step toward the concept of MIDS because it can access *all* PACS-related data.

11.2.2 Architecture of the Medical Image Database Server (MIDS)

The core of the MIDS architecture is a distributed object manager program, located between remote client workstations and local medical databases. This architecture extends the object data management system and distributed object management technologies to model and manage multimedia medical data. It is an effective means of satisfying the interconnectivity and interoperability requirements of the hospital-integrated PACS. It has the advantages of both tightly coupled federated systems [e.g., top-down control and a common object (data) model] and loosely coupled federated systems (e.g., modularity and customized queries). At the same time, it avoids many disadvantages such as the difficulty of scaling up database applications and adding new functions (tightly coupled systems), as well as problems in coordinating activities and ensuring timely response (loosely coupled systems). Figure 11.3 shows MIDS architecture.

The MIDS architecture includes at least the following:

- *Distributed object manager* (*DOM*) that contains a collection of objects [i.e., entities having both state (textual or nontextual) data] and a set of functions they can perform, and defines a set of operators to manipulate them. As they model heterogeneous information and computing resources in a hospital-integrated PACS environment, DOM objects are distributed as interacting objects of various levels of granularity (images and textual data, library routines, computing tools, end-user applications, etc.).
- *Client interfaces* that enable clients to request multimedia data objects or the DOM to perform operations, provide the arguments to the operations, retrieve results, and present them in a user-friendly, workstation-based window environment.
- *Communication facilities* that connect the component systems to exchange data and messages reliably and forward client requests to the objects to which they are directed.

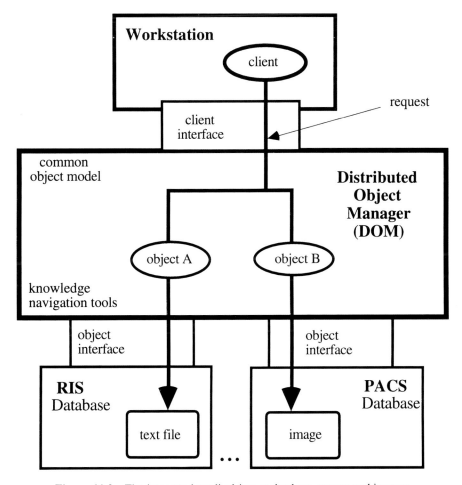

Figure 11.3   The integrated medical image database system architecture.

- *Object interfaces* that allow the DOM to invoke the operations and implementations of objects in support of client requests.
- *Distributed heterogeneous medical databases and systems,* such as PACS, RIS, HIS, digital voice reporting system, and electronic mail and file services, that provide the environment in which the system components run.
- *Image workstation* for multimedia display and 3-D rendering.

The distributed object manager identifies the request from a client workstation as two object data types (i.e., text and image) and routes the queries to the corresponding databases. The DOM will also combine and send the retrieved information to the client in an appropriate form through the same object and client interfaces. This architecture is similar to that of loosely coupled, federated database systems in that it provides a DOM that routes requests among component databases and uses attached components to perform the actual requested operations. In addition, it defines an object data model to provide a common set of abstractions and operations for the user to access and query patient data scattered in component databases. This feature is similar to the motivation for a global data schema in tightly coupled systems. The DOM, however, uses more flexible object modeling to describe the diverse operations implemented by the objects in the system and provides a primitive set of operators to manipulate them. Clients or end-user applications can tailor their query languages for individual scenarios using the defined set of operators.

Clients may be user interface programs, or data objects, running in a medical workstation. Client interfaces can be provided via a library of subroutine calls. To deal with heterogeneous objects, both client and object interfaces must support translation of operation requests, arguments, and results between different image and data representations. Although this may be done in pairwise fashion between each client and object implementation, the use of the common DOM object model reduces the amount of type mapping among components. MIDS serves both *real-time* clients and *regular* clients. "Real-time clients" are in movable and portable workstations for use in operating rooms, wards, and other places where it is critical that information be displayed on demand within a specific time limit. "Regular clients," on the other hand, are those used by individual groups for more complex and time-consuming tasks.

This system architecture describes system components and functionalities of MIDS that are independent of applications. The key idea is to implement the distributed object manager with which all clients and resources may communicate seamlessly. The results are better task coordination, system control, and database administration for health care delivery. The DOM will support multithread, multi-user activities. For a medical application, the user will have to use the common object model provided to define problem details and workup procedures. The physician desktop retrieval system (Section 9.6) provides only file retrieval capabilities; it contains no clinical knowledge to aid decision making. In contrast, MIDS will provide powerful object database management capabilities and will incorporate clinical cases and rules to aid diagnosis. Methodologies in developing the MIDS will be an important research direction in PACS.

11.2.3 Computation and Three-Dimensional Rendering Node

PACS is designed as a data management system; it lacks the computational power for image content analysis at the image workstation or at the PACS controller. To facilitate the effectiveness of the medical image database server, it will be necessary to append a computation and 3-D rendering node as a special facility in the PACS network, to perform high power computations requested by image workstations. Upon the completion of a given computation, the results are distributed with visualization capability to other image workstations through the high speed PACS network. The architecture of a computation and 3-D rendering node in a PACS environment at UCSF is shown in Figure 11.4: the PACS integrated database is at the

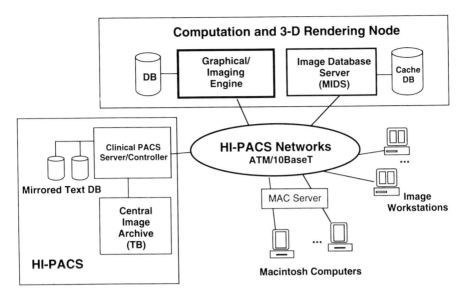

Figure 11.4 Simplified scheme for a HI-PACS (hospital-integrated PACS) network with a computation and 3-D Rendering Node.

left; the computation and 3-D rendering node is on top, connected to the HI-PACS networks, with ATM and with 10 BaseT as the backup. The MAC server (see Section 9.6, Fig. 9.23) provides a connection of the PACS with the Macintosh users, and the image workstations are for clinical use. Let us consider two scenarios.

Scenario 1: Volumetric Visualization of Clinical Images. Suppose that the user wishes to view fusion volumetric images from different imaging modalities (e.g., MRI and PET) in the PACS database, either from the image workstation or from a Macintosh computer through the MAC server. Current PACS controller and image workstation design does not support such a capability. Figure 11.5 shows the steps that would be needed to accomplish this task through the computation node. (1) From the image workstation, the request is sent to the PACS database to retrieve the volumetric image sets; then (2) the image set is sent to the computation node, where (3) computation and 3-D image fusion and volume rendering are performed. When the task is complete, (4) results are sent back to the image workstation for viewing. In step 4, the user can also communicate with the computation node directly for further instructions. In this scenario, we assume that the image workstation has the capability to view 3-D image and graphics.

Scenario 2: Video/Image Conferencing with Image Database Query Support. Now suppose that the referring physician at an image workstation requests a video conference on a patient image case with a radiologist located elsewhere. Figure 11.6 shows the data flow. In this case, we demonstrate how to utilize the medical image database server and the computation node to accomplish the task.

The data flow starts with (1), establishment of a video conference between two

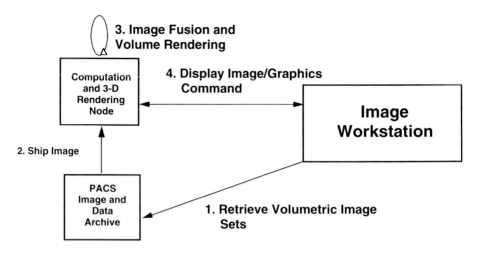

Figure 11.5 Application scenario 1: volumetric visualization of clinical images.

image workstations; then from an image workstation (2), the referring physician requests the case from the PACS database and sends necessary queries to the medical image database server (MIDS). The PACS database transmits data (3), and the MIDS sends synthesized query instructions to the computation node. The computation node performs necessary computation and 3-D rendering and sends results back almost in real time to both image workstations (4), and the results (5) allow a real-time video conference with the 3-D high resolution image set and related data at

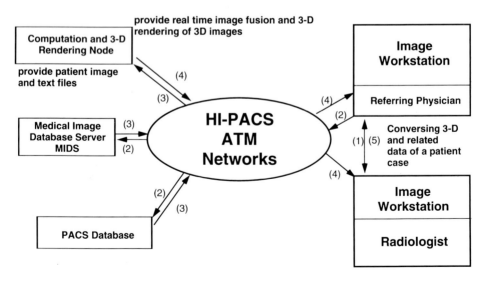

'1.6 Application scenario 2: image conferencing with image database query sup-

both workstations. Note that to accomplish this scenario, three components are necessary in addition to the PACS database: the MIDS, the computation node, and the high speed ATM network.

11.2.4 Image Content Indexing

Current image retrieval is through artificial indexing using a patient's name, ID, age group, disease category, and so on. With the combination of the MIDS and the computation node, it is possible to explore image content indexing. In one-dimensional data, indexing can be through key words, which is a fairly simple procedure. On the other hand, indexing through image content is complicated because the computation node and the MIDS first must understand the image content, which can include abstract terms (e.g., objects of interest), derived quantitative data (e.g., area and volume of the object of interest), and texture information (e.g., interstitial disease). Figure 11.7 shows some preliminary results using indexing via image

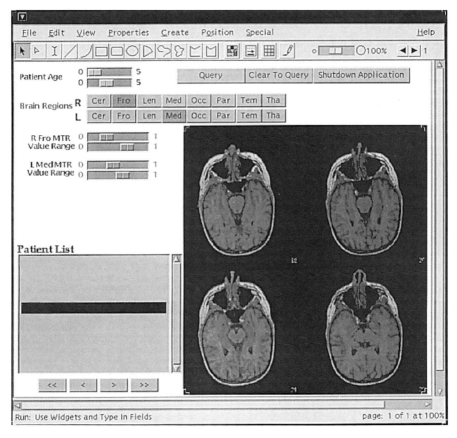

Figure 11.7   Image query by content and features in brain myelination disorders: R (L) FRO MTR, right (left) front magnetization transfer ratio.

Source: Courtesy of Steven Wong.

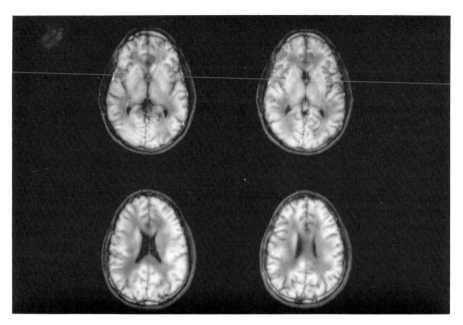

Figure 11.8 Mapping of brain function to anatomy. The four gray level images are from the MR, the color images are from PET of the same patient: red shows high metabolic rates; registration of these two images required sophisticated mathematics and computer programming. (See color plates.)

Source: Courtesy of D. Valentino, 1991.

content in brain myelination disorder research. Indexing via image content is a frontier research topic in image processing, and the PACS-rich database will allow the validation of new theories and algorithms. Figure 11.8 (see color plate) shows the mapping of the brain function (PET, color) to anatomy (MRI, black and white).

11.2.5 Concept of Distributed Computing

The basic idea of distributed computing is that if several computers are networked together, the workload can be divided into smaller pieces for each computer to work on. In principle, when n computers are networked together, the total processing time can be reduced to $1/n$ of single-computer processing time. It should be noted that this theoretical limit is unlikely to be achieved because of the unavoidability of various overheads, most likely due to data communication latency.

Two important factors affect the design of a distributed computing algorithm. Processor speed variations in different computers make it important to implement the mechanism to balance the workload in distributed computing in a way that allows faster computers to be given more work to do. Otherwise, the speed of the processing is essentially dictated by the capabilities of the slowest computers in the network. Data communication speed is another factor to consider. If workstations are connected by conventional Ethernet, with a maximum data transfer rate of 10 Mbit/s, the slow data transfer rate will limit the application of the distributed computing to CPU-intensive problems and areas where data communication is sparse. Increased implementation of the asynchronous transfer mode (ATM) technology will widen the parameter regime in which distributed computing is applicable.

The minimum requirement for distributed computing is a networked computer system with software that can coordinate the computers in the system to work coherently to solve a problem. There are several software implementations available for distributed computing; an example is the parallel virtual machine (PVM) system developed jointly by Oak Ridge National Laboratory, the University of Tennessee, and Emory University. It supports a variety of computer systems, including workstations by Sun Microsystems, Silicon Graphics, Hewlett-Packard, DEC/Microvax, and IBM-compatible personal computers running on a linux operating system.

After the PVM system has been installed in all computer systems, one can start the PVM task from any computer. Other computers can be added to or deleted from the PVM task interactively or by a software call to reconfigure the virtual machine. For computers under the same PVM task, any computer can start new PVM processes in others. Intercomputer communication is realized by passing messages back and forth, thus allowing exchange data among the computers in the virtual machine.

The parameter regimes for applicability of distributed computing are both problem and computer dependent. For distributed computing to be profitable, t_1, the time interval required to send a given amount of data between two computers across the network, should be much shorter than t_2, the time needed to process them in a host computer. In other words, the network data communication rate (proportional to $1/t_1$) should be much higher than the data processing rate (proportional to $1/t_2$). The smaller the ratio of t_1 to t_2 or the higher the ratio of the two rates, the more advantages for distributed computing. If the ratio of the two rates is equal to or less than 1, there is no reason to use distributed computing, since too much time would be spent waiting for the results to be sent across the network back to the host computer. Thus for $t_1 \leq t_2$, it is faster to use a single computer to do the calculation.

While the data communication rate can be estimated based on the network type and the communication protocol, the data processing rate depends both on the computer and on the nature of the problem. For a given workstation, more complex calculations lower the data processing rate. Since the computer system and the network are usually fixed within a given environment, the data processing rate depends more on the nature of the problem. Therefore, whenever a problem is given, one can estimate the ratio of the two rates and determine whether distributed computing is worthwhile. Figure 11.9 depicts the concept of distributed computing based on the data communication rate and processing rate. The graphics were obtained using the Sun SPARC LX computers and the Ethernet communication protocol. Distributed computing is applicable only when the communication rate is above the computation rate. Immediate applications using distributed computing are image compression, unsharp masking, enhancement as well as computer-aided diagnosis, as discussed in Chapter 6 and Section 9.3.

Comm. Rate vs Proc. Rate

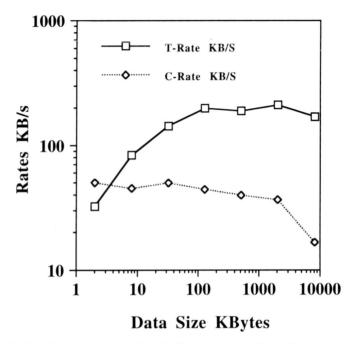

Data Size KBytes

Figure 11.9 Distributed computing in a PACS environment. The solid curve represents the computer-to-computer transmission rate (T-rate) under PVM and TCP/IP Ethernet connection, as a function of data size. The dotted curve represents the data processing rate (C-rate) required to perform a 2-D FFT in a SUN SPARC-LX computer. The squares and diamonds represent the measured data points. Distributed computing is applicable only when the solid curve exceeds the dotted curve.

Source: Courtesy of Xiaoming Zhu.

11.2.6 Distributed Computing in a PACS Environment

Each image workstation in a PACS, when it is not in active use, consumes only a minimum of its capacity for running the background processes. As the number of image workstations grows, this excessive computational power can be exploited to perform value-added image processing functions for PACS images. Image processing is used extensively in the preprocessing stage, as in unsharp masking in CR, but it has not been popular in postprocessing (see Sections 7.6 and 9.3). One reason is that preprocessing can be done quickly through the manufacturer's imaging modality hardware, which is application specific. On the other hand, postprocessing depends on the image workstation which, in general, does not provide hardware image processing functions beyond such simple functions as lookup table and zoom and scroll. For this reason, at the image workstation, the user very seldom uses time-consuming image processing functions even though some, like unsharp masking, are effective. The multi-image workstation PACS environment allows the investigation of distributed computing for image processing by taking advantage of the excessive computational power available from the workstations. Conceptually, distributed computing will allow the acceleration of time-consuming image processing functions, with the result that the user will demand postimage processing tools that can improve medical service by providing near-real-time performance at the image workstation.

In distributed computing, several networked image workstations can be used for computationally intensive image processing functions by distributing the workload to these stations. Thus, image processing time can be reduced at a rate inversely proportional to the number of workstations used. Distributed computing requires several workstations linked together with a high speed network, but these conditions are within the realm of a PACS in its number of workstations and the ATM technology. Figure 11.10 depicts the concept of distributed computing in a PACS network environment using a three-dimensional data set as an example.

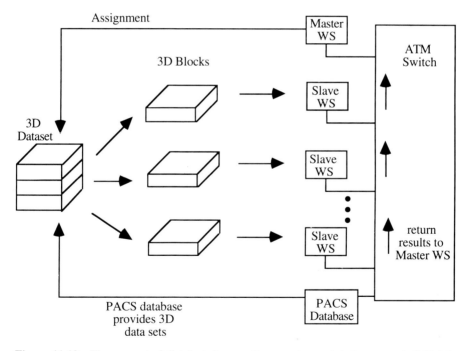

Figure 11.10   The concept of distributed computing: master workstation requests 3-D data from the PACS database and assigns 3-D blocks to each slave workstation (WS) for the computation task. Each slave WS returns results to the master workstation, which compiles all results.

Source: Courtesy of Jun Wang.

11.2.7 Authenticity for PACS Images and Records

11.2.7.1 Background

A digital radiology environment supported by picture archiving and communication systems (PACS) raises a new issue: How to establish trust in multimedia medical data that exist only in the easily altered memory of the computer. Trust is characterized in terms of the integrity and privacy of digital data. Two major self-enforcing techniques can be used to assure the authenticity of electronic images and text—key-based cryptography and digital time stamping.

Key-based cryptography associates the content of an image with the originator, using one or two distinct keys, and prevents alteration of the document by anyone other than the originator (Schneier, 1993). It can be further classified into three general types of algorithms. First, in secret-key algorithms, the encryption key and the decryption key are the same. Second, in public-key algorithms, the public encryption key is different from the private decryption key. Third, in digital signatures, image data are encrypted with the private key and decrypted with the public key. On the other hand, a digital time stamping algorithm does not involve keys. It generates a characteristic "digital fingerprint" for an image when it is first generated, using a mathematical hash function, and checks that it has not been modified since then by anyone. The digital notary concept involving a third party further refines the time-stamping method by blending several sequential time stamp requests into a chain or tree structure (Cipra, 1993).

11.2.7.2 Key-Based Cryptographic Algorithms

There are three general forms of key-based cryptographic algorithms, classified according to the nature of the encryption and decryption keys. This section reviews their principles briefly and provides an example. Secret or private-key algorithms use the encryption key which can be calculated from the decryption key and vice versa. In many such cryptosystems, the encryption and the decryption key are the same. These algorithms require the sender and the receiver to agree on a key before they pass messages back and forth. This key must be kept secret, and therefore the security of such symmetric algorithms rests in the key.

Figure 11.11 illustrates an example of software implementation of a secret key cipher on an eight bit magnetic resonance image where the left hand side is the original, and the right hand side is the encrypted image. The cipher used is the IDEA (International Data Encryption Algorithm) implementation from Phil Zimmermann's PGP (Pretty Good Privacy) package (Davies and Price, 1980). The secret key length is 128 bits and it would require 2^{128} (or 10^{38}) encryptions to recover the key. Figure 11.12 is the corresponding histogram of the encrypted image. Note that the gray level frequencies are very evenly distributed over all gray levels. The main drawback to the private key algorithm is that anyone with the key can both encode and decode messages and images. If the key is intercepted, any message can be compromised. Also, the management of keys involved in a cryptographic protocol

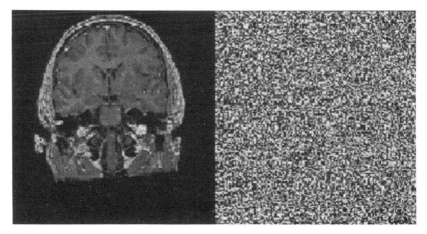

Figure 11.11   An MR image (L) and its encrypted image (R) using the IDEA PGP package.
Source: Courtesy of Steven Wong.

creates a problem, since the total number of keys increases rapidly as the number of users increases.

The key management problem of secret-key ciphers can be alleviated by public-key cryptography. In this case, two different keys are used: one public and one private. Information is encoded by the sender with the recipient's public key but can only be decoded by the recipient who possesses the private key. Moreover, the public key contains no hint as to the nature of the public key. Anyone with the

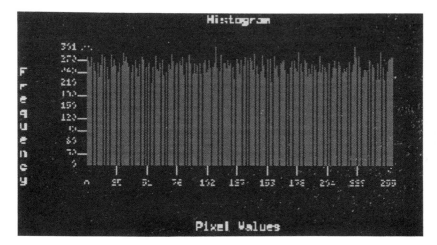

Figure 11.12   The histogram distribution of the encrypted image shown in Figure 11.11 (R).
Source: Courtesy of Steven Wong.

Table 11.1 Three General Types of Key-Based Cryptography

Secret Key Cryptography	Encryption key (e) = Decryption key (d)	e & d are private
Public-key Cryptography	e ≠ d	e public, d private
Digital Signature	e ≠ d	e private, d public

public key (which, presumably, is made public by the owner) can encrypt a message but not decrypt it. Only the person with the private key can decrypt the message. The disadvantage of the public-key encryption algorithm is that it is much slower than conventional single-key encryption, and therefore is impractical for implementation.

Digital signatures can be accomplished in some public-key algorithms by enciphering images with the sender's private key and deciphering them with the sender's public key. Encrypting a medical image using the physician's private key generates a secure digital signature. Often, digital signatures include time stamps. The date and time of the signature are attached to the image and signed along with the rest of the images. The PACS can store this time stamp in its image archive, which can be used for future reference. In practical implementation, public-key algorithms are often too inefficient to encrypt large documents such as medical images. Table 11.1 summarizes the three general types of key based cryptography.

Key-based encryption techniques, along with digital time stamp methods, form the foundation for investigating the authenticity of PACS images. However, as of today, no dedicated research is being carried out in this area. Image authenticity will become a major social issue as more PACS are gradually integrated into daily clinical practice. Concentrated effort by the medical imaging community is needed to resolve this important issue.

References

Aberle, D.R., Hansell, D., and Huang, H.K. Current Status of Digital Projection Radiography of the Chest. *J. Thorac. Imaging,* Vol. 5, 1990, pp. 10–20.

Aberle, D., Gleeson, F.V., Sayre, J.W., Brown, P., Batra, P., Young, D., Stewart, B.K., Ho, B.K.T., and Huang, H.K. The Effect of Irreversible Image Compression on Diagnostic Accuracy in Thoracic Imaging. *Invest. Radiol.,* Vol. 28, 1993, pp. 398–403.

Advanced Archival Products, Inc. AMASS: Storage Management Systems (Version 4.0). Greenwood Village, CO: Advanced Archival Products, 1993.

Allen, P.S. Nuclear Magnetic Resonance Imaging. In *Imaging with Non-ionizing Radiations,* D.F. Jackson, Ed. Glasgow: Surrey University Press, 1983.

Alvarez, R.E., and Macovski, A. Energy-Selective Reconstructions in X-Ray Computerized Tomography. *Phys. Med. Biol.,* Vol. 21, No. 5, 1976, pp. 733–744.

Andriole, K.P., Gooding, C.A., Gould, R.G., and Huang, H.K. Analysis of a High-Resolution Computed Radiography Imaging Plate Versus Conventional Screen–Film Radiography for Neonatal Intensive Care Unit Applications. *Proc. SPIE,* Vol. 2163, 1994, pp. 89–97.

Arenson, R. L., Seshadri, S., Kundel, H.L., et al. Clinical Evaluation of a Medical Image Management System for Chest Images. *Am. J. Roentgenol.,* Vol. 150, 1988, pp. 55–59.

Arenson, R.L., Chakraborty, D.P., Seshadri, S.B., and Kundel, H.L. The Digital Imaging Workstation. *Radiology,* Vol. 176, 1990, pp. 303–315.

Arenson, R.L., Avrin, D.E., Wong, A., Gould, R.G., and Huang, H.K. *Second Generation Folder Manager for PACS.* In *Comp. Appl. Assist. Radiology,* Boehme, J.M., Rowberg, A.H., Wolfman, N.T., Ed. Symposia Foundation, Carlsbad, CA, 1994, pp. 601–605.

Barnes, G.T. Radiographic Mottle: A Comprehensive Theory. *Med. Phys.,* Vol. 9, 1982, pp. 656–667.

Barnes, G.T. Noise Analysis of Radiographic Imaging. In *Recent Developments in Digital Imaging,* D. Doi, L. Lanzi, and P.P. Lin, Eds. New York: American Institute of Physics, 1985, pp. 16–38.

465

Barnes, G.T., et al. Digital Chest Radiography: Performance Evaluation of a Prototype Unit. *Radiology,* Vol. 154, 1985, pp. 801–806.

Barnes, G.T. Digital X-Ray Image Capture with Image Intensifier and Storage Phosphor Plates: Imaging Principles, Performance and Limitations. In *Specifications, Acceptance, Testing, and Quality Control of Diagnostic X-ray Imaging Equipment, Proceedings of The AAPM Summer School,* Vol. II, J.A. Seibert, G.T. Barnes, and R.G. Gould, Eds. College Park, MD: American Association of Physicists in Medicine, 1991.

Barnes, G.T., Morin, R.L., and Staab, E.V. Teleradiology: Fundamental Considerations and Clinical Applications. In *Syllabus: A Special Course in Computers for Clinical Practice and Education in Radiology, 1992,* Radiological Society of North America. Oak Brook, IL: RSNA, 1992, pp. 139–146.

Barrett, H.H., and Swindell, W. *Radiological Imaging: The Theory of Image Formation, Detection, and Processing.* New York: Academic Press, 1981.

Barrett, H.H., and Swindell, W. *Radiological Imaging,* Vols. 1 and 2. New York: Academic Press, 1981.

Bauman, R.A. Large Picture Archiving and Communication Systems (PACS). *Proceedings of Computer Assisted Radiology 95,* pp. 537–541.

Bertram, S. On the Derivation of the Fast Fourier Transform. *IEEE Trans. Audio Electroacoust.,* Vol. AU-18, March 1970, pp. 55–58.

Bidgood, W.D., and Horii, S.C. Introduction to the ACR-NEMA DICOM Standard. In *Syllabus: A Special Course in Computers for Clinical Practice and Education in Radiology, 1992.* Radiological Society of North America. Oak Brook, IL: RSNA, 1992, pp. 37–45.

Bjorkholm, P.J., et al. Digital Radiography. *Soc. Photo-Opti. Instrum. Eng.* Vol. 233, 1980, pp. 137–144.

Blume, H., Roehrig, H., Browne, M., and Ji, T.-L. Comparison of the Physical Performance of High Resolution CRT Displays and Films Recorded by Laser Image Printers and Displayed on Light Boxes and the Need for a Display Standard. *Proc. SPIE,* Vol. 1232, 1990, pp. 97–114.

Boag, J.W. Xeroradiography. *Phys. Med. Biol.,* Vol. 18, 1973, pp. 3–37.

Boyd, D., Herrmannsfeldt, W.B., Quinn, J.R., and Sparks, R.A. X-Ray Transmission Scanning System and Method and Electron Beam X-Ray Scan Tube for Use Therewith. U.S. Patent 4,352,021, September 28, 1982.

Bracewell, R.N. Strip Integration in Radio Astronomy. *Aust. J. Phys.,* Vol. 9, 1956, 198–217.

Bracewell, R. *The Fourier Transform and Its Applications.* New York: McGraw-Hill, 1965.

Bramble, J.M., Huang, H.K., and Murphy, M.D. Image Data Compression. Investigative Radiology. *Invest. Radiol.,* Vol. 23, 1988, pp. 707–712.

Breant, C.M., Taira, R.K., and Huang, H.K. Integration of a Voice Processor Machine in a PACS. *J. Comput. Med. Imaging Graphics,* Vol. 17, 1993, pp. 13–19.

Breant, C.M., Taira, R.K., and Huang, H.K. Interfacing Aspects Between the PACS, RIS, and HIS. *J. Digital Imaging,* Vol. 6, 1993, pp. 88–94.

Brigham, E.O. *The Fast Fourier Transform.* Englewood Cliffs, NJ: Prentice-Hall, 1974, pp. 148–183.

Brody, W.R. *Digital Radiography.* New York: Raven Press, 1984.

Brooks, R.A., and Chiro, G.D. Principles of Computer Assisted Tomography (CAT) in Radiographic and Radioisotopic Imaging. *Phys. Med. Biol.,* Vol. 21, No. 5, 1976, pp. 689–732.

Budinger, T.F., et al. Emission Computer Assisted Tomography with Single-Photon and Positron Annihilation Photon Emitters, *J. Comput. Assist. Tomogra.,* Vol. 1, No. 1, 1977, pp. 131–145.

Budinger, T.F. Physical Attributes of Single-Photon Tomography. *J. Nuclear Med.,* Vol. 21, No. 6, 1980, pp. 579–592.

Carlson, C.R., Cohen, R.W., and Gorog, I. Visual Processing of Simple Two-Dimensional Sinewave Luminance Grating. *Vision Res.,* Vol. 17, 1977, pp. 351–358.

Castleman, K.R. *Digital Image Processing.* Englewood Cliffs, NJ: Prentice-Hall, 1979.

Chan, K.K., Lou, S. L., and Huang, H.K. Full-Frame Transform Compression of CT and MR Image. *Radiology,* Vol. 171, 1989, pp. 847–851.

Chan, K.K., Lou, S.L., and Huang, H.K. Radiological Image Compression Using Full-Frame Cosine Transform with Adaptive Bit-Allocation. *Comput. Med. Imaging Graphics,* Vol. 13, No. 2, 1989, pp. 153–159.

Chang, L.T. A Method for Attenuation Correction in Radionuclide, Computed Tomography. *IEEE Trans. Nuclear Sci.,* Vol. NS-25, No. 1, 1978, pp. 638–643.

Cho, P.S., Huang, H.K., Tillisch, J., and Kangarloo, H. Clinical Evaluation of a Radiologic Picture Archiving and Communication System for a Coronary Care Unit. *Am. J. Roentgenol.,* Vol. 151, 1988, pp. 823–827.

Choplin, R.H., Boehme, J.M., and Maynard, C.D. Picture Archiving and Communication Systems: An Overview. In *Syllabus: A Special Course in Computers for Clinical Practice and Education in Radiology, 1992,* Radiological Society of North America. Oak Brook, IL: RSNA, 1992, pp. 33–35.

Chotas, H.G., Dobbins, J.T., Floyd, C.E., and Ravin, C.E. Single-Exposure Conventional and Computed Radiography Image Acquisition. *Invest. Radiol.,* Vol. 26, 1991, pp. 428–445.

Cipra, B. Electronic time-stamping: The notary public goes digital, *Science,* Vol. 261, 9 1993, 162–3.

Cochran, W.T., et al. What Is the Fast Fourier Transform? *IEEE Trans. Audio Electroacoust.,* Vol. AU-15, June 1967, pp. 45–55.

Cohen, M.D., Katz, B.P., Kalasinski, L.A., White, S.J., Smith, J.A., and Long, B. Digital Imaging with a Photostimulable Phosphor in the Chest of Newborns. *Radiology,* Vol. 181, 1991, pp. 829–832.

Cowart, R.W. Realtime Radiation Exposure Monitor and Control Apparatus. U.S. Patent 4,268,750, May 19, 1981.

Creasy, J.L., Thompson, B.G., Johnston, R.E., and Parrish, D. PACS Development at UNC: Evaluation of the Neuroradiology Service Concept. *Proc. SPIE,* Vol. 767, 1987, pp. 808–811.

Curry, T.S., et al. *Cristensen's Introduction to the Physics of Diagnostic Radiology,* 3rd ed. Philadelphia: Lea & Febiger, 1984.

Curtis, D.J., et al. Teleradiology: Results of a Field Trial. *Radiology,* Vol. 149, 1983, pp. 415–418.

Cushman, W.H. Illumination. In: Salvendy G., Ed. *Handbook of Human Factors.* New York: Wiley, 1987, 670–695.

Dainty, J.C., and Shaw, R. *Image Science.* New York: Academic Press, 1974, Chap. 5.

Das, M., and Burgett, S. Lossless Compression of Medical Images Using Two-Dimensional Multiplicative Autoregressive Models. *IEEE Trans. Med. Imaging,* Vol. 12, No. 4, 1993, pp. 721–726.

Daubechies, I. Orthonormal Bases of Compactly Supported Wavelets. *Commun. Pure Appl. Math.,* Vol. 41, 1988, pp. 909–996.

Davies, D.W., and Price, W.L. The application of digital signatures based on public-key cryptosystems. *Proc. Fifth International Computer Communication Conference,* Oct 1980, pp. 525–530.

de Groot, P.M. Image Intensifier Design and Specifications. In *Specification, Acceptance Testing and Quality Control of Diagnostic X-Ray Imaging Equipment, Proceedings of the AAPM Summer School,* Vol. I, J.A. Seibert, G.T. Barnes, and R.G. Gould, Eds. College Park, MD: American Association of Physicists in Medicine, 1991, pp. 477–510.

De Valk, J.P.J. *Integrated Diagnostic Imaging–Digital PACS in Medicine,* 1992 ed. Amsterdam: Elsevier.

Dick, C.E., and Motz, J.W. Image Information Transfer Properties X-Ray Fluorescent Screens. *Med. Phys.* Vol. 8, 1981, pp. 337–346.

Donovan, J.L. X-Ray Sensitivity of Selenium, *J. Appl. Phys.,* Vol. 50, 1979, pp. 6500–6504.

Duerinckx, A., Ed. Picture Archiving and Communications Systems (PACS) for Medical Applications. *First International Conference and Workshop, Proceedings of SPIE—International Society for Optical Engineering,* Vol. 318, 1982.

Dunn, J.F. Cathode Ray Tube (CRT) Film Recording of Video Based Medical Images. *Society of Photo-Optical Instrumentation Engineers, Picture Archiving and Communication Systems for Medical Applications,* Vol. 318, 1982.

Dwyer, S.J., III, Ed. Picture Archiving and Communication Systems (PACS) for Medical Applications. Second International Conference Workshop for Picture Archiving and Communication Systems (PACS) for Medical Applications. *Proceedings of SPIE—International Society for Optical Engineering,* Vol. 418, 1983.

Dwyer, III, S.J., Stewart, B.K., Sayre, J.W., Aberle, D.R., Boechat, M.I., Honeyman, J.C., Boehme, J.M., Roehrig, H., Ji, T.-L., and Blaine, G.J. Performance Characteristics and Image Fidelity of Gray-Scale Monitors. In *Syllabus: A Special Course in Computers for Clinical Practice and Education in Radiology, 1992,* Radiological Society of North America. Oak Brook, IL: RSNA, 1992, pp. 107–124.

Dwyer III, S.J., Stewart, B.K., Sayre, J.W., and Honeyman, J.C. Wide-Area Network Strategies for Teleradiology Systems. In *Syllabus: A Special Course in Computers for Clinical Practice and Education in Radiology, 1992,* Radiological Society of North America. Oak Brook, IL: RSNA, 1992, pp. 107–115.

Emmel, P.M. System Design Considerations for Laser Scanning. *Laser Scanning and Recording for Advanced Image and Data Handling, SPIE,* Vol. 222, 1980.

Fairchild, CCD Device Catalog, Winston-Salem, NC, 1983–1984.

Frost, M.M., Honeyman, J.C., and Staab, E.V. Image Archival Technologies. In *Syllabus: A Special Course in Computers for Clinical Practice and Education in Radiology, 1992,* Radiological Society of North America. Oak Brook, IL: RSNA, 1992, pp. 69–72.

Fujita, H., Doi, K., Giger, M.L., and Chan, H.P. Investigation of Basic Imaging Properties in Digital Radiography. V. Characteristic Curves of II-TV Digital Systems. *Med. Phys.,* Vol. 13, 1986, pp. 13–18.

Fukushima, E., and Roeder, S.B.W. *Experimental Pulse NMR: A Nuts and Bolts Approach.* Reading, MA: Addison-Wesley, 1981.

Fullerton, G.D., et al. Electronic Imaging in Medicine, *Medical Physics Monogram No. 11.* New York: American Institute of Physics, 1984.

Georinger, F. Medical Diagnostic Imaging Support Systems for Military Medicine in Picture Archiving and Communication Systems (PACS). In *Picture Archiving and Communications Systems, NATO ASI Series F,* Vol. 74, H.K. Huang et al., Eds. Berlin: Springer-Verlag, 1991, pp. 213–230.

Giger, M., and Doi, K. Investigation of Basic Imaging Properties in Digital Radiography. I. Modulation Transfer Function. *Med Phys.,* Vol. 11, 1984, pp. 287–295.

Giger, M., Doi, K., and Metz, C.E. Investigation of Basic Imaging Properties in Digital Radiography. II. Noise Weiner Spectrum, *Med. Phys.*, Vol. 11, 1984, 797–805.

Glass, H.I., and Slark, N.A. PACS and Related Research in the United Kingdom in Picture Archiving and Communication Systems (PACS). In *Picture Archiving and Communications Systems, NATO ASI Series F*, Vol. 74, H.K. Huang et al., Eds. Berlin: Springer-Verlag, 1991, p. 319–324.

Golomb, S.W. Run Length Encodings. *IEEE Trans. Inf. Theory*, Vol. IT-12, 1966, pp. 399–401.

Gonzalez, R.C., and Wintz, P. *Digital Image Processing.* Reading, MA: Addison-Wesley, 1982, pp. 36–88.

Gonzalez, R.C., and Wood, R.E. *Digital Image Processing.* Reading, MA: Addison-Wesley, 1992.

Goodman, J.W. *Introduction to Fourier Optics.* New York: McGraw-Hill, 1968, pp. 21–25.

Graham, L.S. Clinical Applicable Modifications of Anger Camera Technology. In *Nuclear Medicine Annual*, L.M. Freeman and H.S.S. Weissman, Eds. New York: Raven Press, 1983.

Gullberg, G.T. The Attenuated Radon Transform: Theory and Application in Medicine and Biology. Ph.D. Thesis, University of California, Berkeley, 1979, Lawrence Berkeley Laboratory, LBL-7486.

Gur, D. Requirements for PACS: Users' Perspective. In *Syllabus: A Special Course in Computers for Clinical Practice and Education in Radiology, 1992,* Radiological Society of North America. Oak Brook, IL: RSNA, 1992, pp. 65–68.

Hayrapetian, A., Aberle, D.R., Huang, H.K., Morioka, C.R., Valentino, D., and Boechat, M.I. Comparison of 2048 Matrix Digital Display Formats: An ROC Study. *Am. J. Roentgenol.*, Vol. 152, 1989, pp. 1113–1118.

Health Level Seven, Inc. Health Level Seven: An Application Protocol for Electronic Data Exchange in Healthcare Environments (Version 2.1). Ann Arbor, MI: Health Level Seven, 1991.

van der Heiden, G.H., Brauninger, U., Grandjean, E. Ergonomic studies on computer-aided design. In: Grandjean E., Ed. *Ergonomics and Health in Modern Offices.* London: Taylor and Francis, 1984, 119–128.

Heiken, J.P., Brink, J.A., and Vannier, M.W. Spiral (Helical) CT. *Radiology*, Vol. 189, 1993, pp. 647–656.

Hendee, W.R., et al. *Radiologic Physics, Equipment and Quality Control.* Chicago: Year Book Medical Publishers, 1977.

Hillen, W., Schiebel, U., and Zaengel, T. Imaging Performance of a Digital Storage Phosphor System. *Med. Phys.*, Vol. 14, 1987, pp. 744–751.

Hisatoyo, K. Photostimulable Phosphor Radiography Design Considerations. In *Specification, Acceptance Testing and Quality Control of Digital X-ray Imaging Equipment, Proceedings of the AAPM Summer School*, Vol. II, J.A. Seibert, G.T. Barnes, and R.G. Gould, Eds. College Park, MD: American Association of Physicists in Medicine, 1991.

Ho, B.K.T. Automatic Acquisition Interfaces for Computed Radiography, CT, MR, US, and Laser Scanner. *Comput. Med. Imaging Graphics*, Vol. 15, 1991, pp. 135–145.

Ho, B.K.T., and Huang, H.K. Specialized Module for Full-Frame Radiological Image Compression, *Opt. Eng.*, Vol. 30, 1991.

Ho, B.K.T., Chao, J., Wu, C.S., and Huang, H.K. Full-Frame Cosine Transform Image Compression for Medical and Industrial Application. *Machine Vision Appl.*, Vol. 3, 1991, pp. 89–96.

Ho, B.K.T., Chao, J., Zhu, P., and Huang, H.K. Design and Implementation of Full-Frame Bit-Allocation Image-Compression Hardware Module, *Radiology*, Vol. 179, 1991, 563–567.

Hoffman, E.J., et al. ECAT III—Basic Design Considerations. *IEEE Trans. Nuclear Sci.* Vol. NS-30, No. 1, 1983, pp. 729–733.

Hoffman, J.G. Reliability Requirements in a Digital Imaging Environment. *Proc. SPIE,* Vol. 767, 1987, pp. 834–838.

Honeyman, J.C., Messinger, J.M., Frost, M.M., and Staab, E.V. Evaluation of Requirements and Planning for Picture Archiving and Communication Systems. In *Syllabus: A Special Course in Computers for Clinical Practice and Education in Radiology, 1992,* Radiological Society of North America. Oak Brook, IL: RSNA, 1992, pp. 55–64.

Horii, S.C. Electronic Imaging Workstations: Ergonomic Issues and the User Interface. *Syllabus: A Special Course in Computers for Clinical Practice and Education in Radiology, 1992,* Radiological Society of North America. Oak Brook, IL: RSNA, 1992, pp. 125–134.

Horii, S.C., and Bidgood, Jr., W.D. Network and ACR-NEMA Protocols. In *Syllabus: A Special Course in Computers for Clinical Practice and Education in Radiology, 1992,* Radiological Society of North America. Oak Brook, IL: RSNA, 1992, pp. 97–106.

Hounsfield, G.N. A Method and Apparatus for Examination of a Body by Radiation Such as X- or Gamma Radiation. British Patent No. 1,283,915, 1972.

Huang, H.K., et al. Selected Computerized Tommographic Scan Data Format. *Proceedings of the IEEE Computer Society Conference on Pattern Recognition and Image Processing,* Ch 1318-5, 1978, pp. 438–443.

Huang, H.K., and Ledley, R.S. Scanning Methods and Reconstruction Algorithms for Computerized Tomography. In *Medical Imaging Techniques,* K. Preston et al., Eds. New York: Plenum Press, 1979, pp. 313–327.

Huang, H.K., and Wong, C.K. Dual-Potential Imaging in Digital Radiography. *IEEE Proceedings of an International Workshop on Physics of Medical Images,* 1982, pp. 122–129.

Huang, H.K. Recent Development in Medical Digital Radiography. *Trans. Am. Nuclear Soc.,* Vol. 45, October–November, 1983, pp. 249–251.

Huang, H.K., Bassett, L.W., Mankovich, N.J., Cho, P., Kangarloo, H., and Seeger, L. Instruction in Image Processing for Residents in Diagnostic Radiology. *Am. J. Roentgenol.,* Vol. 149, 1987, pp. 435–437.

Huang, H.K., Lo, S.-C., Ho, B.K., and Lou, S.-L., Radiological Image Compression Using Error-Free and Irreversible Two-Dimensional Direct-Cosine-Transform Coding Techniques. *J. Opt. Soc. Am. A,* Vol. 4, 1987, pp. 984–992.

Huang, H.K., *Elements of Digital Radiology.* Englewood Cliffs, NJ: Prentice-Hall, 1987, Chap. 3.

Huang, H.K., Mankovich, N.J., Taira, R.K., Cho, P., Stewart, B., Ho, B., Cho, K., and Ishimitsu, Y. PACS for Radiological Images: State of the Art. *CRC Crit. Rev. Diagn. Imaging,* Vol. 28, 1988, pp. 383–427.

Huang, H.K., Cho, P.S., Ratib, O., et al., Personal Digital Image Filming System. *Radiology,* Vol. 173, 1989, pp. 292.

Huang, H.K., et al. Picture Archiving and Communication Systems in Japan: 3 Years Later. *Am. J. Roentgenol.,* Vol. 154, 1990, pp. 415–417.

Huang, H.K., Aberle, D., Lufkin, R., Grant, E., and Hanafee, W. Advances in Medical Imaging. UCLA Conference. *Ann. Intern. Med.,* Vol. 112, 1990, pp. 157–240.

Huang, H.K., Kangarloo, H., Cho, P.S., et al. Planning a Totally Digital Radiology Department. *Am. J. Roentgenol.,* Vol. 154, 1990, pp. 635–639.

Huang, H.K., Lou, S.L., Cho, P.S., et al. Radiologic Image Communication Methods. *Am. J. Roentgenol.*, Vol. 155, 1990, pp. 183–186.

Huang, H.K., Ratib, O., Bakker, A., and Witte, G., Eds. *Picture Archiving and Communication Systems. NATO ASI Series F*, Vol. 74. Berlin: Springer-Verlag, 1991.

Huang, H.K. Image Storage, Transmission, and Manipulation, *J. Minimally Invasive Ther.*, Vol. 1, 1991, pp. 85–92.

Huang, H.K. PACS—A Review and Perspective. In *Integrated Diagnostic Imaging: Digital PACS in Medicine*. J. de Valk, Ed. Amsterdam: Elsevier, 1992, pp. 39–58.

Huang, H.K. Three Methods of PACS Research, Development, and Implementation. *Radiographics*, Vol. 12, 1992, pp. 131–139.

Huang, H.K., and Taira, R.K. Infrastructure Design of a Picture Archiving and Communication System. *Am. J. Roentgenol.*, Vol. 158, 1992, pp. 743–749.

Huang, H.K., Tecotsky, R.H., and Bazzill, T.A. Fiber-Optic Broadband CT/MR Video Communication System. *J. Digital Imaging*, Vol. 5, 1992, pp. 22–25.

Huang, H.K., Wong, A.W.K., Lou, S.L., and Stewart, B.K. Architecture of a Comprehensive Radiologic Imaging Network. *IEEE J. S.A. Commun.*, Vol. 10, 1992, pp. 1118–1196.

Huang, H.K. Medical Imaging. In *Encyclopedia of Computer Science and Engineering*, 3rd ed., A. Ralston and E.D. Reilly, Eds. New York: Van Nostrand Reinhold, 1993, pp. 842–847.

Huang, H.K., Ultrasonic Picture Archiving and Communication Systems. In *Advances in Ultrasound Technologies and Instrumentation*, P.N.T. Wells, Ed. New York: Churchill Livingstone, 1993, pp. 141–150.

Huang, H.K., and Cho, P.S. Architecture and Ergonomics of Imaging Workstations. In *The Perception of Visual Information*, W.H. Hendee and P.N.T. Wells, Eds. Berlin: Springer-Verlag, 1993, pp. 316–334.

Huang, H.K., Arenson, R.L., Lou, S.L., et al. Second Generation PACS (abstr.). *Radiology*, Vol. 198, 1993, p. 410.

Huang, H.K., Taira, R.K., Lou, S.L., Wong, A.W.K., et al. Implementation of a Large Scale Picture Archiving and Communication System. *J. Comput. Med. Imaging Graphics*, Vol. 17, 1993, pp. 1–11.

Huang, H.K., Arenson, R.L., Lou, S.L., et al. Multimedia in the Radiology Environment: Current Concept. *Comput. Med. Imaging Graphics*, Vol. 18, 1994, pp. 1–10.

Huang, H.K., Arenson, R.L., Dillon, W.P., Lou, A.S.L., Bazzill, T., Wong, A.W.K. Asynchronous Transfer Mode (ATM) Technology for Radiologic Communication. *Am. J. Roentgenol.*, Vol. 164, 1995, pp. 1533–1536.

Huffman, D.A. A Method for the Construction of Minimum-Redundancy Codes. *Proc. IRE V*, Vol. 40, 1952, pp. 1098–1101.

Irie, G. Clinical Experience—16 Months of HI-PACS in Picture Archiving and Communication Systems (PACS). In *Picture Archiving and Communications Systems, NATO ASI Series F*, Vol. 74, H.K. Huang et al., Eds. Berlin: Springer-Verlag, 1991, pp. 183–188.

Ishida, M., Kato, H., Doi, K., and Frank, P.H. Development of a New Digital Radiographic Image Processing System. *SPIE*, Vol. 347, 1982, pp. 42–48.

Ishida, M., Frank, P.H., Doi, K., and Lehr, J.L. High Quality Digital Radiographic Images: Improved Detection of Low-Contrast Objects and Preliminary Clinical Studies. *Radiographics*, Vol. 3, 1983, pp. 325–338.

Ishida, M., et al. Digital Image Processing: Effect on Detectability of Simulated Low-Contrast Radiographic Patterns. *Radiology,* Vol. 150, 1984, pp. 569–575.

Ishimitsu, Y., Arai, K., Taira, R.K., and Huang, H.K. Radiological Laser Film Scanner Sampling Artifact. *Comput. Med. Imaging and Graphics,* Vol. 14, 1990, pp. 25–33.

Jain, A.K. Image Data Compression: A Review. *Proc. IEEE,* Vol. 69, March 1981, pp. 349–389.

Ji, T.-L., Roehrig, H., Blume, H., Seeley, G., and Browne, M. Physical and Psychological Evaluation of CRT Noise Performance. *Proc. SPIE,* Vol. 1444, 1991, pp. 136–150.

Johns, H.E., and Cunningham, J.R. *The Physics of Radiology,* 4th ed. Springfield, IL: Charles C. Thomas, 1983.

Kalender, W.A., Sissler, W., Klotz, E., and Vock, P. Spiral Volumetric CT with Single-Breath-Hold Technique, Continuous Transport, and Continuous Scanner Rotation. *Radiology,* Vol. 176, 1993, pp. 181–183.

Kangarloo, H., Boechat, M.I., Barbaric, Z., Taira, R.K., Cho, P.S., Mankovich, N.J., Ho, B.K.T., Eldredge, S.L., and Huang, H.K. Two-Year Clinical Experience with a Computed Radiography System. *Am. J. Roentgenol.,* Vol. 151, 1988, pp. 605–608.

Kato, H. Photostimulable Phosphor Radiography Design Considerations. In *Specification, Acceptance Testing and Quality Control of Diagnostic X-Ray Imaging Equipment, Proceedings of the AAPM Summer School,* Vol. II, J.A. Seibert, G.T. Barnes, and R.G. Gould, Eds. College Park, MD: American Association of Physicists in Medicine, 1991, pp. 860–898.

Kaufman, L., et al. *Nuclear Magnetic Imaging in Medicine.* New York: Igaku-Shoin, 1982.

Keller, P.A. Cathode-Ray Tube Displays for Medical Imaging. *J. Digital Imaging,* Vol. 3, 1990, pp. 15–25.

Koo, J.I., Lee, H.S., and Kim, Y. Applications of 2-D and 3-D Compression Algorithms to Ultrasound Images. *SPIE Image Capture, Formatting, Display,* Vol. 1653, 1992, pp. 434–439.

Korn, D.M., et al. A Method of Electronic Readout Electrophotographic and Electroradiographic Images. *J. Appl. Photogr. Eng.,* Vol. 4, 1978, pp. 178–182.

Kotsas, P., Piraino, D.W., Recht, M.P., and Richmond, B.J. Comparison of Adaptive Wavelet-Based and Discrete Cosine Transform Algorithms in Image Compression. *Radiology,* Vol. 93(P), 1994, Suppl., pp. 331ff.

Krestel, E. *Imaging Systems for Medical Diagnostics.* Berlin: Siemens Aktiengesellschaft, 1990, p. 334.

Krongauz, V.G., and Parfianovich, I.A. Photostimulated Luminescence of Phosphors. *J. Lumin.,* Vol. 9, 1974, pp. 61–70.

Kruger, R.A., Mistretta, C.A., Houk, T.L., et al. Computerized Fluoroscopy in Real Time for Noninvasive Visualization of the Cardio-Vascular System. Preliminary Studies. *Radiology,* Vol. 130, 1979, pp. 49–57.

Kuhl, D.E., and Edwards, R.Q. Image Separation Radioisotope Scanning. *Radiology,* Vol. 80, No. 4, 1963, pp. 653–661.

Kundel, H.L. Visual Perception and Image Display Terminals. *Radiol. Clin. North Am.* Vol. 24, 1986, pp. 69–78.

Lee, H., Kim, Y., Rowberg, A.H., and Riskin, E.A. Statistical Distributions of DCT Coefficients and Their Application to an Interframe Compression Algorithm for 3D Medical Images. *IEEE Trans. Med. Imaging,* Vol. 12, No. 3, 1993, pp. 478–485.

Leverenz, H.W. *An Introduction to Luminescence of Solids.* New York: Dover, 1962, p. 150.

Lo, S.-C. Radiological Image Compression. Ph.D. Thesis, University of California, Los Angeles, December 1985.

Lo, S.-C., and Huang, H.K. Error-Free and Irreversible Radiographic Image Compression. *Society of Photo-Optical Instrumentation Engineers 536: Picture Archiving and Communication Systems (PACS III) for Medical Applications.* Newport Beach, CA, February 1985, pp. 170–177.

Lo, S.-C., and Huang, H.K. Radiological Image Compression: Full-Frame Bit-Allocation Technique. *Radiology,* Vol. 155, No. 3, 1985, pp. 811–817.

Lo, S.-C., and Huang, H.K. Compression of Radiological Images with 512, 1024, and 2048 Matrices. *Radiology,* Vol. 161, No. 2, 1986, pp. 519–525.

Lo, S.-C., Taira, R.K., Mankovich, N.J., Huang, H.K., and Takeuchi, H. Performance Characteristics of a Laser Scanner and Laser Printer System for Radiological Imaging. *Comput. Radiol.,* Vol. 10, 1986, pp. 227–237.

Lo, S.-C.B., Mun, S.K., and Chen, J. A Method for Splitting Digital Value in Radiological Image Compression. *Med. Phys.,* Vol. 18, No. 5, 1991, pp. 939–946.

Lou, S.L., Huang, H.K., Mankovich, N.J., et al. A CT/MR/US Picture Archiving and Communication System. *Proc. SPIE,* Vol. 1093, 1989, pp. 31–36.

Lou, S.L., Lufkin, R.B., Valentino, D.J., et al. A Neuroradiology Viewing Station. *Proc. SPIE,* Vol. 1232, 1990, pp. 238–245.

Lou, S.L. The Design and Implementation of a CT/MR Picture Archiving and Communication System Applied to Neuroradiology. Dissertation, University of California, Los Angeles, 1991.

Lou, S.L., Loloyan, M., Weinberg, W., et al. Image Delivery Performance of a CT/MR PACS Module Applied in Neuroradiology. *Proc. SPIE,* Vol. 1446, 1991, pp. 302–311.

Lou, S.L., and Huang, H.K. Assessment of a Neuroradiology PACS in the Clinical Environment. *Am. J. Roentgenol.,* Vol. 159, 1992, pp. 1321–1327.

Lou, S.L., Wang, J., Moskowitz, M., Bazzill, T., and Huang, H.K. Methods of Automatically Acquiring Images from Digital Medical Systems. *J. Comput. Med. Imaging Graphics,* 19:4, 369–376, 1995.

Lubinsky, A.R., Owen, J.F., and Korn, D.M. Storage Phosphor System for Computed Radiography: Screen Optics. *SPIE,* Vol. 626, 1986, pp. 120–132.

Lubinsky, A.R., Whiting, B.R., and Owen, J.F. Storage Phosphor System for Computed Radiography: Optical Effects and Detective Quantum Efficiency (DQE). *SPIE,* Vol. 767, 1987, pp. 167–177.

Mallat, S.G. A Theory for Multiresolution Signal Decomposition: The Wavelet Representation. *IEEE Trans. Pattern Anal. Mach. Intellig.,* Vol. 11, No. 7, 1989, pp. 674–693.

Mankovich, N.J., Taira, R.K., Cho, P.S., and Huang, H.K. An Operational Radiological Image Archive and Digital Optical Disks. *Radiology,* Vol. 167, 1988, pp. 139–142.

Mansfield, P., and Morris, P.G. *NMR Imaging in Biomedicine.* New York: Academic Press, 1982.

Masahiro, I., Ed. *Nuclear Medicine in Japan. Instrumentation in Nuclear Medicine.* Tokyo: Takeshi A. Iinuma, International Medical Foundation of Japan, 1975.

Masser, H., Mandl, A., Urban, M., et al., The Vienna Project SMZO in Picture Archiving and Communication Systems (PACS). In *Picture Archiving and Communication Systems, NATO ASI Series F,* Vol. 74, H.K. Huang et al., Eds. Berlin: Springer-Verlag, 1991, pp. 247–250.

McNitt-Gray, M.F., Pietka, E., and Huang, H.K. Image Preprocessing for PACS. *Invest. Radiol.,* Vol. 27, 1992, pp. 529–535.

Medical Imaging Technology. *The Fifth MIT and the Third PACS/PHD Symposia,* Vol. 4, No. 2. Tokyo, 1986.

Mengers, P. Low Contrast Imaging. *Electro-Opt. Syst. Design,* October 1978, pp. 1–5.

Merritt, C.R.B., et al. Clinical Application of Digital Radiography. *Radiographics,* Vol. 5, No. 3, May 1985.

Merritt, C.R.B., Matthews, C.C., Scheinhorn, D., and Balter, S. Digital Imaging of the Chest. *J. Thorac. Imaging,* Vol. 1, 1985, pp. 1–13.

Miller, E.R., McCury, E.M., and Hruska, B.B. Immediate Hospital Wide Access to X-Ray Film Image. *Radiology,* Vol. 192, 1969, pp. 13–16.

MITRE Corporation. Installation Site for Digital Network and Picture Archiving and Communication Systems (DIN/PACS). *RFP B52-1545,* Washington, D.C., 1985.

Miyahara, J., and Kato, H. Computed Radiography. *Oyo Buturi* (in Japanese), Vol. 53, 1984, pp. 884–890.

Murphey, M.D., Huang, H.K., Siegel, E.L., and Hillman, B.J. Clinical Experience in the Use of Photostimulable Phosphor Radiographic Systems. *Invest. Radiol.,* Vol. 26, 1991, pp. 590–597.

Nakazawa, M., et al. Effect of Protective Layer on Resolution Properties of Photostimulable Phosphor Detector for Digital Radiographic System. *SPIE,* Vol. 1231, 1990, pp. 350–363.

Nelson, M. The *Data Compression Book.* M&T Books, San Mateo, CA, 1992.

Oishi, I., *Frequency Characteristics of the Mosaic Type Display System.* Tokyo Television Society of Japan, 1970 (in Japanese).

Olendorf, W.H. Isolated Flying Spot Detection of Radiodensity Discontinuities—Displaying the Internal Structure Pattern of a Complex Object. *IEEE Trans. Biomed. Electron.,* Vol. BME-8, No. 1, 1961, pp. 68–72.

Ophir, J., and Maklad, N. Digital Scan Converters in Diagnostic Ultrasound Imaging. *Proc. IEEE,* Vol. 67, No. 4, April 1979.

Oppenheim, A.V., and Schafer, R.W. Effect of Finite Register Length in Digital Signal Processing. *Digital Signal Processing,* Englewood Cliffs, NJ: Prentice-Hall, Inc., 1975, p. 453.

Osteaux, M. *A Second Generation PACS Concept.* Berlin: Springer-Verlag, 1992.

Papin, P.J. A Prototype Amorphous Selenium Imaging Plate System for Digital Radiography. Ph.D. Dissertation, University of California, Los Angeles, 1985.

Papin, P.J., et al. Sensitivity Characteristics of a Prototype Selenium Detection System for Digital Radiographic Imaging. *Soc. Photo-Opt. Instrum. Eng.,* Vol. 535, 1985, pp. 222–227.

Partain, C.C.L., et al. *Nuclear Magnetic Resonance Imaging.* Philadelphia: Saunders, 1983.

Pietka, E., and Huang, H.K. Orientation Correction for Chest Images. *J. Digital Imaging,* Vol. 5, No. 3, 1992, pp. 185–189.

Queisser, H.J. Luminescence, Review and Survey. *J. Lumin.,* Vol. 24/25, 1981, pp. 3–10.

Ramachandran, G.N., and Lakshminarayanan, A.V. Three-Dimension Reconstruction from Radiographs and Electron Micrographs: Applications of Convolutions Instead of Fourier Transforms. *Proc. Nat. Acad. Sci.,* Vol. 68, No. 9, 1971, pp. 2236–2240.

Ramaswamy, M.R., Wong, A.W.K., Lee, J.K., and Huang, H.K. Accessing a PACS's Text and Image Information Through Personal Computers. *Am. J. Roentgenol.,* Vol. 163, 1994, pp. 1239–1243.

Razavi, M., Sayre, J.W., Taira, R.K., et al. A ROC Study of Pediatric Chest Radiographs Comparing Digital Hardcopy Film and 2K × 2K Softcopy Images. *Am. J. Roentgenol.,* Vol. 158, 1992, pp. 443–448.

Reeve, III, H.C., and Lim, J.S. Reduction of Blocking Effects in Image Coding. *Opt. Eng.,* Vol. 23, No. 1, 1984, pp. 34–37.

Richardson, M.L., and Gillespy, T. An Inexpensive Computer-Based Digital Imaging Teaching File. *Am. J. Roentgenol.,* Vol. 160, 1993, pp. 1299–1301.

Riederer, S.J. The Application of Matched Filtering to X-ray Exposure Reduction in Digital Subtraction Angiography: Clinical Results. *Radiology,* Vol. 146, 1983, pp. 349–354.

Riederer, S.J., and Kruger, R.A. Intravenous Digital Subtraction: A Summary of Recent Development in Radiology. *Radiology,* Vol. 147, 1983, pp. 633–638.

Riskin, E.A., Lookabaugh, T., Chou, P.A., and Gray, R.M. Variable Rate Vector Quantization for Medical Image Compression. *IEEE Trans. Med. Imaging,* Vol. MI-9, 1990, pp. 290–298.

Roehrig, H., Blume, H., Ji, T.-L., and Browne, M. Performance Tests and Quality Control of Cathode Ray Tube Displays. *J. Digital Imaging,* Vol. 3, 1990, pp. 134–145.

Roos, P., and Viergever, M.A. Reversible Interframe Compression of Medical Images: A Comparison of Decorrelation Methods. *IEEE Trans. Med. Imaging,* Vol. MI-10, No. 4, 1991, pp. 538–547.

Roos, P., and Viergever, M.A. Reversible 3-D Decorrelation of Medical Images. *IEEE Trans. Med. Imaging,* Vol. MI-12, No. 3, 1993, pp. 413–420.

Rosenfeld, A., and Kak, A.C. *Digital Picture Processing.* New York: Academic Press, 1976.

Rossman, K. Image Quality. *Radiol. Clin. North Am.,* Vol. VII, No. 3, 1969.

Roth, K. *NMR—Tomography and Spectroscopy in Medicine.* Berlin: Springer-Verlag, 1984.

Rowlands, J.A., and Taylor, K.W. Absorption and Noise in Cesium Iodide X-ray Image Intensifiers. *Med. Phys.,* Vol. 10, 1983, pp. 786–795.

Rowlands, J.A., and Taylor, K.W. Detective Quantum Efficiency of X-Ray Image Intensifiers: Comparison of Scintillation Spectrum and Rms Methods. *Med. Phys.,* Vol. 11, 1984, pp. 597–601.

Sanada, S., Doi, K., Su, X.W., Yin, F.F., Giger, M.L., and MacMahon, H. Comparison of Imaging Properties of a Computed Radiography System and Screen–Film Systems. *Med. Phys.,* Vol. 18, 1991, pp. 414–420.

Sanders, J.N., Cattell, C.L., Bender, N.E., and Tesic, M.M. Design Consideration of a Laser Based Multiformat Camera for Medical Imaging. *Appl. Opt. Instrum. Med. XII, SPIE,* Vol. 454, 1984.

Sayre, J.W., Ho, B.K.T., Boechat, M.I., Hall, T.R., and Huang, H.K. The Effect of Full-Frame Image Compression on Diagnostic Accuracy in Hand Radiographs with Subperiosteal Resorption. *Radiology,* Vol. 185, 1992, pp. 559–603.

Schaetzing, R., Whiting, B.R., Lubinksy, A.R., et al. Digital Radiography Using Storage Phosphors. In *Digital Imaging in Diagnostic Radiology,* J.D. Newell, Jr., and C.A. Kelsey, Eds. New York: Churchill Livingstone, 1990, pp. 107–138.

Schaffert, R.M. The Nature and Behavior of Electrostatic Images. *Photogr. Sci. Eng.,* Vol. 6, 1962, pp. 197–215.

Scheffer, P.A., and Stone, A.H. A Case Study of SREM. *Computer,* Vol. 18, 1985, pp. 47–54.

Schneider, R.H., Dwyer, S.J., III, and Jost, R.G., Eds. Medical Imaging III. *Proc. SPIE,* Vols. 1090, 1091, 1092, and 1093, 1989.

Schneier, B., *Applied Cryptography: Protocols, Algorithms, and Source Code in C*. New York: John Wiley & Sons, 1993.

Seshadri, S.B. Software Suite for Image Archiving and Retrieval. *Syllabus: A Special Course in Computers for Clinical Practice and Education in Radiology, 1992*, Radiological Society of North America. Oak Brook, IL: RSNA, 1992, pp. 73–78.

Shade, O.H. *Image Quality: A Comparison of Photographic and Television Systems*. Princeton, NJ: RCA, 1975, p. 2.

Sheep, L.A., and Logan, B.F. The Fourier Reconstruction of a Head Section. *IEEE Trans. Nuclear Sci.*, Vol. NS-21, No. 3, 1974, pp. 21–43.

Sinha, S., Sinha, U., Kangarloo, H., and Huang, H.K. A PACS-Interactive Teaching Module for Radiological Sciences. *Am. J. Roentgenol.*, Vol 159, 1992, pp. 199–205.

Sones, R.A., and Barnes, G.T. A Method to Measure the MTF of Digital X-Ray Systems. *Med. Phys.*, Vol. 11, 1984, pp. 166–171.

Sonoda, M., et al. Computed Radiography Utilizing Scanning Laser Stimulated Luminescence. *Radiology*, September 1983, pp. 833–838.

Sorenson, J.A., and Phelps, M.E. *Physics in Nuclear Medicine*, 2nd ed. Philadelphia: Grune & Stratton, 1986.

Sprawls, P. *The Physics and Instrumentation of Nuclear Medicine*. Baltimore: University Park Press, 1981.

Stevels, A.L.N., and Pingault, F. $BaCl:Eu^{2+}$: A New Phosphor for X-Ray Intensifying Screen. *Philips Res. Report*, Vol. 30, 1975, pp. 277–290.

Stewart, B.K., and Huang, H.K. Single-Exposure Dual-Energy Computed Radiography. *Med. Phys.*, Vol. 17, 1990, pp. 866–875.

Stewart, B.K. Three-Tiered Network Architecture for PACS Cluster in Picture Archiving and Communication Systems (PACS). In *Picture Archiving and Communications Systems, NATO ASI Series F*, Vol. 74, H.K. Huang et al., Eds. Berlin: Springer-Verlag, 1991, pp. 113–118.

Stewart, B.K., Lou, S.L., Wong, A.W.K., and Huang, H.K. An Ultra-Fast Network for Radiologic Image Communication. *Am. J. Roentgenol.*, Vol. 156, 1991, p. 835–839.

Stewart, B.K. Local Area Network Topologies, Media, and Routing. In *Syllabus: A Special Course in Computers for Clinical Practice and Education in Radiology, 1992*. Radiological Society of North America. Oak Brook, IL: RSNA, 1992, pp. 79–95.

Swank, R.K. Absorption and Noise in X-Ray Phosphors. *J. Appl. Phys.*, Vol. 44, 1973, pp. 4199–4203.

Swank, R.K., et al. The Development of a Self-Contained Instant-Display Erasable Electrophoretic X-Ray Imager. *J. Appl. Phys.*, Vol. 50, 1979, p. 6534.

Sun, H.F., Goldberg, M. Radiographic Image Sequence Coding Using Two-Stage Adaptive Vector Quantization. *IEEE Transactions on Medical Imaging*, Vol. 7, No. 2, June 1988, pp. 118–126.

Swets, J.A., Picket, R.M. *Evaluation of Diagnostic Systems: Methods from Signal Detection Theory*. New York: Academic Press, 1982.

Taira, R.K., Mankovich, N.J., Boechat, M.I., Kangarloo, H., and Huang, H.K. Design and Implementation of a Picture Archiving and Communication System (PACS) for Pediatric Radiology. *Am. J. Roentgenol.*, Vol. 150, 1988, pp. 1117–1121.

Taira, R.K., and Huang, H.K. A Picture and Communication System Module for Radiology. *Comput. Methods Programs Biomed.*, Vol. 30, 1989, pp. 229–237.

Takahashi, K., et al. Mechanism of Photostimulated Luminescence in BaFX:Eu^{2+} (X = Cl, Br) Phosphors. *J. Lumin.,* Vol. 31/32, 1984, pp. 266–268.

Takeuchi, H. et al. Preliminary Experience with a Laser Scanner and Printer System for Radiological Imaging. *Society of Photo-Optical Instrumentation Engineers 536: Picture Archiving and Communications Systems (PACS III) for Medical Applications.* Newport Beach, CA, February 1985, pp. 65–71.

Tasto, M., and Wintz, P.A. Image Coding by Adaptive Block Quantization. *IEEE Trans. Commun. Technol.,* Vol. *COM-19,* 1971, pp. 957–971.

Tsai, M., Ho, B.K., Villasenor, J., and Saipetch, P. Full-Frame Wavelet Video Comparison with Incorporation of Block Classification. *Radiology,* Vol. 93(P), suppl. 1994, p. 140.

U.S. Department of Health and Human Services. Multiple Viewing Station for Diagnostic Radiology: RO1 CA 39063, National Cancer Institute, 1985.

U.S. Food and Drug Administration, *Guidance for the content and review of 510(k) notifications for picture archiving and communication systems and related products.* Center for Devices and Radiological Health, the US Food and Drug Administration, Washington, D.C., Aug. 1993.

Valentino, D.J., Mazziotta, J.C., and Huang, H.K. Volume Rendering of Mulit-Modal Images. *IEEE Trans. Med. Imaging,* Vol. MI-10, 1991, pp. 554–562.

Verhoeven, L. Design Considerations of Digital Fluoroscopy/Fluorography Equipment. In *Specification, Acceptance Testing and Quality Control of Diagnostic X-ray Imaging Equipment, Proceedings of the 1991 AAPM Summer School,* Vol. II, J.A. Seibert, G.T. Barnes, and R.G. Gould, Eds. College Park, MD: American Association of Physicists in Medicine, 1991, pp. 734–789.

Vetterli, M., and Herley, C. Wavelets and Filter Banks: Theory and Design. *IEEE Trans. Signal Process.,* Vol. SP-40, 1992, pp. 2207–2232.

Villasenor, J.D., Belzer, B., and Liao, J. Wavelet Filter Evaluation for Image Compression. *IEEE Trans. Image Process.,* 1995. Vol. 4, N8: 1053–1060.

Wang, J., and Huang, H.K. Film Digitization Aliasing Artifacts Caused by Grid Line Patterns. *IEEE Trans. Med. Imaging,* Vol. MI-13, 1994, pp. 375–385.

Wang, J., Huang, H.K., Three-Dimensional Medical Image Compression Using a Wavelet Transform with Parallel Computing, *Proc. SPIE,* Vol. 2431, 1995, pp. 162–172.

Weinberg, W.S., Loloyan, M., and Chan, K.K. On-line acquisition of CT and MRI studies from multiple scanners. *Proc. SPIE,* Vol. 1446, 1991, pp. 430–435.

Wells, P.N.T. *Biomedical Ultrasonics.* London: Academic Press, 1977.

Wells, P.N.T., *Advances in Imaging Techniques in Advances in Ultrasound Techniques and Instrumentation.* Wells, P.N.T., Ed. Churchill Livingstone, 1993, pp. 47–53.

Wilson, A.J., and West, O.C. Single-Exposure Conventional and Computed Radiography: The Hybrid Cassette Revisited. *Invest. Radiol.,* Vol. 28, 1993, pp. 409–412.

Wintz, P.A. Transform Picture Coding. *Proc. IEEE,* 1972, pp. 809–820.

Wong, C.K., and Huang, H.K. Calibration Procedure in Dual-Energy Scanning Using the Basis Function Technique, *Med. Phys.,* Vol. 10, No. 5, September–October 1983.

Wong, S., Zaremba, L., Gooden, D., and Huang, H.K. Radiologic Image Compression—A Review. *Proc. IEEE,* Vol. 83, 1995, pp. 194–219.

Wong, S., Abundo, M., and Huang, H.K. Authenticity Techniques for PACS Images and Records. *Proc. SPIE,* Vol. 2435, 1995, pp. 68–79.

Wong, A.W.K., Stewart, B.K., Lou, S.L., et al. Multiple Communication Networks for a Radiology PACS. *Proc. SPIE,* Vol. 1446, 1991, pp. 73–80.

Wong, A.W.K., Taira, R.K., and Huang, H.K. Digital Archive Center: Implementation for a Radiology Department. *Am. J. Roentgenol.,* Vol. 159, 1992, pp. 1101–1105.

Wong, A.W.K., and Huang, H.K. Subsystem Throughputs of a Clinical Picture Archiving and Communications System. *J. Digital Imaging,* Vol. 5, 1993, pp. 252–261.

Wong, A.W.K., Huang, H.K., Arenson, R.L., and Lee, J.K. Multimedia Archive System for Radiologic Images. *Radiographics,* Vol. 14, 1994, pp. 1119–1126.

Yin, L., Ramaswamy, M.R., Wong, A.W.K., et al. Access of Medical Information and Radiological Images through a Local Area Network. *Proc. SPIE,* Vol. 2165, 1994, pp. 21–26.

Yuste, M., Taurel, L., Rahmani, M., and Lemoye, D. Optical Absorption and ESR Study of F Centers in BaFCl and SrCIF Crystals. *J. Phys. Chem. Solids,* Vol. 37, 1976, pp. 961–966.

Zeman, R.K., Fox, S.H., Silverman, P.M., et al. Helical (Spiral) CT of the Abdomen. *Am. J. Roentgenol.,* Vol. 160, 1993, pp. 719–725.

Zhang, Y.-Q., Loew, H., and Pickholtz, R.L. A Combined-Transform Coding (CTC) Scheme for Medical Images. *IEEE Trans. Med. Imaging,* Vol. MI-11, No. 2, June 1992, pp. 196–202.

Index